The Clinician's Guide to Liver Disease

K. Rajender Reddy, MD
University of Pennsylvania
Philadelphia, Pennsylvania

Thomas Faust, MD
University of Pennsylvania
Philadelphia, Pennsylvania

SLACK
INCORPORATED
An innovative information, education, and management company
6900 Grove Road • Thorofare, NJ 08086

ISBN 10: 1-55642-6755
ISBN 13: 9-781556-42675-9

The procedures and practices described in this book should be implemented in a manner consistent with the professional standards set for the circumstances that apply in each specific situation. Every effort has been made to confirm the accuracy of the information presented and to correctly relate generally accepted practices. The authors, editor, and publisher cannot accept responsibility for errors or exclusions or for the outcome of the material presented herein. There is no expressed or implied warranty of this book or information imparted by it.

Care has been taken to ensure that drug selection and dosages are in accordance with currently accepted/recommended practice. Due to continuing research, changes in government policy and regulations, and various effects of drug reactions and interactions, it is recommended that the reader carefully review all materials and literature provided for each drug, especially those that are new or not frequently used.

Any review or mention of specific companies or products is not intended as an endorsement by the author or publisher.

The work SLACK Incorporated publishes is peer reviewed. Prior to publication, recognized leaders in the field, educators, and clinicians provide important feedback on the concepts and content that we publish. We welcome feedback on this work.

Printed in the United States of America.

The clinician's guide to liver disease / [edited by] K. Rajender Reddy,
Thomas Faust.
p. ; cm.
Includes bibliographical references and index.
ISBN-13: 978-1-55642-675-5 (soft cover)
ISBN-10: 1-55642-675-9 (soft cover)
1. Liver--Diseases. I. Reddy, K. Rajender. II. Faust, Thomas.
[DNLM: 1. Liver Diseases. WI 700 C64115 2006]
RC845.C565 2006
616.3'62--dc22

2005020660

Published by: SLACK Incorporated
6900 Grove Road
Thorofare, NJ 08086 USA
Telephone: 856-848-1000
Fax: 856-853-5991
www.slackbooks.com

Contact SLACK Incorporated for more information about other books in this field or about the availability of our books from distributors outside the United States.

Last digit is print number: 10 9 8 7 6 5 4 3 2 1

THE CLINICIAN'S GUIDE TO
Liver Disease

CONTENTS

Acknowledgments

I would like to acknowledge my wife Vanaja and my children Pranay and Smita for their unconditional support of my career. My mentors Eugene Schiff and the late Leon Schiff and Dame Sheila Sherlock have been instrumental in shaping my career as a Hepatologist and to whom I am greatly indebted.

Additionally, I would like to thank the contributing authors and the SLACK Incorporated staff, particularly Carrie Kotlar, for their hard work on this book.

–KRR

I would like to acknowledge my wife Margaret and my children, T.J. and Millis, for their unconditional support of my career. My mentor, Mike Sorrell, has been instrumental in shaping my career as a Hepatologist and to whom I am greatly indebted. I would also like to thank Anil Rustgi and Raj Reddy for giving me the opportunity to work in a world class gastroenterology and hepatology section at the University of Pennsylvania.

–TF

About the Editors

K. Rajender Reddy, MD is Professor of Medicine and Surgery in the Division of Gastroenterology at the University of Pennsylvania in Philadelphia, Pennsylvania. He is also the Director of Hepatology and the Medical Director of Liver Transplantation at the University of Pennsylvania School of Medicine.

Dr. Reddy received his medical education from Osmania Medical College in Hyderabad, India. He then completed a residency in internal medicine at New York Medical College Hospitals, a fellowship in Gastroenterology at East Tennessee State University College of Medicine, and a fellowship in Hepatology at the University of Miami School of Medicine. Subsequently he joined the faculty at the University of Miami in the Division of Hepatology and moved up the ranks to become a Professor of Medicine. In October 2001, Dr. Reddy moved to the University of Pennsylvania to the current position.

A fellow of the American College of Physicians and the American College of Gastroenterology, Dr. Reddy is also a member of the American Association for the Study of Liver Diseases, the American Gastroenterological Association, and the American Society of Gastrointestinal Endoscopy. He has held several visiting professorships at medical schools throughout the world.

Dr. Reddy has authored or coauthored over 200 peer-reviewed papers on a spectrum of hepatobiliary topics that include liver transplantation, chronic C viral hepatitis, HIV and the liver, and hepatocellular carcinoma. In addition, he has contributed to several textbooks and has participated in numerous scientific presentations at national and international meetings. He serves on the editorial boards of prestigious journals such as *Liver Transplantation* and is an ad-hoc reviewer for several journals, including the *New England Journal of Medicine.*

Dr. Reddy also has participated in a number of clinical trials that have advanced the understanding of the therapy of chronic viral hepatitis. He has been the recipient of both federal and nonfederal funding for clinical research. His current research interests include areas of liver transplantation, viral hepatitis, and hepatocellular carcinoma.

Thomas Faust, MD is Assistant Professor of Medicine in the Division of Gastroenterology at the University of Pennsylvania in Philadelphia, Pennsylvania.

Dr. Faust received his medical education from the University of Tennessee College of Medicine, Memphis, Tennessee. He then completed an internship and residency in internal medicine at Yale-New Haven Hosptial, a fellowship in gastroenterology at the University of Texas Southwestern Medical Center at Dallas, and a fellowship in hepatology and transplant hepatology at the University of Nebraska. Dr. Faust has served as a faculty member both at the University of Chicago and the University of Pennsylvania.

A fellow of the American College of Physicians and the American College of Gastroenterology, Dr. Faust is also a member of the American Association for the Study of Liver Diseases, the American Gastroenterological Association, the American Society of Transplantation, the International Liver Transplant Society, and the American Society of Gastrointestinal Endoscopy.

In additition to authoring many articles on liver transplantation, autoimmune liver diseases, and vascular diseases of the liver, Dr. Faust has contributed to several textbooks and has participated in a variety of scientific presentations at national meetings.

Dr. Faust has participated in a number of clinical trials that have advanced the understanding of the therapy of chronic viral hepatitis. His current research interests include medical and bioethical issues pertaining to hepatology and liver transplantation. Dr. Faust has also received numerous teaching awards while at the University of Chicago and the University of Pennsylvania, and also directs the pathophysiology course in gastroenterology for first-year medical students at Penn.

Contributing Authors

Raúl J. Andrade, MD
Professor of Medicine
Liver Unit
Gastroenterology Service
Virgen de la Victoria University Hospital and School of Medicine
Málaga, Spain

Anne Burke, MD
Assistant Professor
University of Pennsylvania Health System
Philadelphia, Pennsylvania

Rena Desai Callahan, MD
Resident in Internal Medicine
UCLA School of Medicine
Los Angeles, California

Mical S. Campbell, MD
Gastroenterology Division
University of Pennsylvania Health System
Philadelphia, Pennsylvania

Jayanta Choudhury, MD
Instructor in Internal Medicine
Division of Gastroenterology
Virginia Commonwealth University Medical Center
Richmond, Virginia

Stanley Martin Cohen, MD
Associate Director
Section of Hepatology
Rush University
Chicago, Illinois

Lawrence S. Friedman, MD
Professor of Medicine
Harvard Medical School
Assistant Chief of Medicine
Massachusetts General Hospital
Boston, Massachussetts
Chair, Department of Medicine
Newton-Wellesley Hospital
Newton, Massachussetts

Richard K. Gilroy, MBBS, FRACP
Section of Gastroenterology and Hepatology
University of Nebraska Medical Center
Omaha, Nebraska

Wolfram Goessling, MD, PhD
Instructor in Medicine
Harvard Medical School
Fellow, Gastrointestinal Unit
Massachusetts General Hospital
Fellow in Hematology/Oncology
Dana-Farber Cancer Institute
Brigham and Women's Hospital
Boston, Massachussetts

Steven-Huy B. Han, MD
Associate Clinical Professor of Medicine and Surgery
David Geffen School of Medicine at UCLA
Los Angeles, California

Josh Levitsky, MD
Assistant Professor of Medicine
Northwestern University
Feinberg School of Medicine
Chicago, Illinois

M. Isabel Lucena, MD
Professor of Pharmacology
Clinical Pharmacology Service
Virgen de la Victoria University Hospital and School of Medicine
Málaga, Spain

Paul Martin, MD
Professor of Medicine
Associate Director
Division of Liver Diseases
Mt. Sinai Medical Center
New York, New York

Timothy McCashland, MD
Associate Professor of Medicine
University of Nebraska Medical Center
Omaha, Nebraska

Barbara A. Piasecki, MD, MSCE
Gastroenterology Division
Kaiser Permanente Medical Center
Denver, Colorado

Arie Regev, MD
Associate Professor of Medicine
Division of Hepatology, Center for Liver Diseases
University of Miami School of Medicine
Miami, Florida

Javier Salmerón, MD
Professor of Medicine.
Liver Section, Gastroenterology Service
San Cecilio University Hospital and School of Medicine
Granada, Spain

Arun J. Sanyal, MD
Professor of Medicine
Chief, Division of Gastroenterology
Medical College of Virginia
Richmond, Virginia

Kirti Shetty, MD
Division of Transplantation
Georgetown University Hospital
Washington, DC

Michael F. Sorrell, MD
Robert L. Grossom Professor of Medicine
Department of Internal Medicine
University of Nebraska Medical Center
Omaha, Nebraska

John C. Sun, MD
University of Pennsylvania Health System
Philadelphia, Pennsylvania

Tram T. Tran, MD
Assistant Professor of Medicine, UCLA
Cedars Sinai Medical Center
Los Angeles, California

Preface

The field of hepatobiliary diseases has evolved considerably in the past decade. The discovery of hepatitis C virus has helped in the diagnosis of a large number of chronic infections caused by this virus and also has lead to a better understanding of the natural history. Advances in liver transplantation has been instrumental in providing a life saving opportunity for some of our patients. Yet challenges remain in the area of hepatocellular carcinoma, particularly with regard to early diagnosis and effective treatments for the majority of patients with this deadly malignancy that has been on the rise. Nonalcoholic fatty liver disease presents another challenge and we are only seeing the "tip of the iceberg" of this condition.

The challenges are daunting and the researchers and clinicians continue to work hard to improve the understanding of the diseases,provide better patient care,make therapeutic advances and thus overall have an impact on the lives of our patients. It is intended that this book will serve as a resource for trainees and clinicians in the medical and surgical fields: those that frequently diagnose and take care of patients with a spectrum of hepatobiliary diseases. To this end we have sought the help of nationally and internationally recognized authors to provide the reader with a concise and current understanding about liver diseases.

chapter 1

Evaluation of the Liver Patient

Wolfram Goessling, MD, PhD and Lawrence S. Friedman, MD

The evaluation of the patient with liver disease has become more complex and advanced in recent years. Whereas liver disease is often suspected after careful history-taking and physical examination, an increasing array of biochemical and serologic tests allows us to diagnose disease earlier, assess prognosis more accurately, and improve outcomes for certain diseases.

HISTORY

Liver disease is often detected incidentally on a routine screening blood examination before a patient receives medical attention for symptoms. Early symptoms of acute and chronic liver disease are nonspecific, and the value of the patient's history in the initial diagnosis of liver disease has been underemphasized. In fact, chapters on history-taking and physical examination have been eliminated from recent editions of leading hepatology textbooks. There are, however, symptoms that should alert the clinician to the possibility of underlying liver disease, thereby leading to an earlier diagnosis and improved outcome.

FATIGUE AND MALAISE

Fatigue is common in patients with liver disease. It is a nonspecific symptom that can occur with many other diseases. Tiredness and easy fatigability may be present for years in a patient with undiagnosed chronic liver disease. Typically, these symptoms worsen during the day, whereas fatigue that is most prominent in the early morning is typical of depression. The absence of associated cardiac or respiratory symptoms makes a cardiovascular or pulmonary cause of fatigue unlikely.

Malaise, the generalized feeling of lack of well-being, is present in about one-third of patients with acute and chronic liver disease. In patients with acute liver disease, malaise may persist long after biochemical and serologic recovery.

Nausea and Vomiting

Nausea is a frequent complaint in patients with liver disease. It can occur in both acute and chronic liver disease. In patients with cholestasis, nausea may precede the onset of jaundice. Vomiting is common in patients with biliary obstruction.

Anorexia

Anorexia is common in patients with acute viral hepatitis and in those with neoplasms of the liver, biliary tree, pancreas, or colon.

Weight Loss and Weight Gain

Weight loss in patients with acute and chronic liver disease may result from anorexia in patients with acute viral hepatitis and signifies the loss of muscle mass in patients with advanced liver disease. Unintentional weight loss of 10 pounds or more should always raise the suspicion of malignancy.

Weight gain in patients with advanced liver disease is typically caused by ascites and edema and may precede other symptoms of liver disease.

Abdominal Pain

Abdominal pain is a common complaint in patients with liver disease and is typically located in the right upper quadrant of the abdomen below the right rib cage. Both the character and timing of the pain may provide clues to the diagnosis of liver disease. The pain tends to be constant and worse with motion as a result of the stretching of the liver capsule.

By contrast, in patients with symptomatic gallstones, right upper quadrant or epigastric pain (biliary "colic") is typically acute in onset and steady in nature; attacks often begin after a meal or in the early hours of the morning and last 30 to 90 minutes. Similarly, acute cholecystitis may present with steady right upper quadrant pain that may radiate to the right shoulder and is often exacerbated by respiration because of diaphragmatic irritation.

A rapidly enlarging liver resulting from tumor growth, inflammation, or congestion may cause the onset of right upper quadrant pain over several weeks. Splenomegaly, as a result of portal hypertension, can provoke left upper quadrant discomfort. Ascites can cause generalized abdominal discomfort.

Focal pain over the liver, with associated point tenderness on examination, can occur with liver abscesses and tumors.

Pain that is localized in the lower half of the abdomen is rarely related to liver disease.

Increased Abdominal Girth and Edema

Ascites is a common complication of acute and chronic liver disease and increasing abdominal girth may be the presenting symptom of liver disease. Leg edema is also common. Rapidly increasing abdominal fullness over several weeks in a patient with known cirrhosis should raise the suspicion of a neoplasm.

Table 1-1

CAUSES OF DARK URINE

Color	*Causes*
Red	Blood
	Beets
	Cranberries
	Drugs
Orange	Bilirubin
	Rhubarb
Black	Alkaptonuria
	Tyrosinosis
	Myoglobin
Purple	Porphyrins
	Phenolphthalein laxatives

ICTERUS AND JAUNDICE

Jaundice is a characteristic presentation of liver disease and refers to the yellow coloration of the patient's skin caused by the deposition of bilirubin glucuronides in the tissue. Icterus is the term used to denote yellow sclerae resulting from hyperbilirubinemia. Family or friends may note the jaundice before the patient does. A history of jaundice may suggest prior episodes of acute hepatitis.

DARK URINE

Like jaundice, darkening of the urine resulting from urinary excretion of bilirubin can be observed in patients with liver disease. The differential diagnosis of dark urine is shown in Table 1-1.

ABNORMAL STOOL

A mild increase in the frequency or decrease in the consistency of bowel movements is often seen in patients with liver disease; constipation is infrequent. Diarrhea may result from a decrease in the concentration of intestinal bile salts, leading to an increase in fecal fat.

In patients with cholestasis or acute hepatitis, the stool is typically pale or "clay-colored" as a result of decreased bilirubin excretion into the intestinal lumen. It is important to question patients with chronic liver disease about melenic (dark, tarry) stool, which indicates upper gastrointestinal bleeding.

Pruritus

Pruritus, or itching, is a common symptom in patients with cholestatic liver disease. The pathophysiology of pruritus is poorly understood. The itching typically affects the extremities more than the trunk and face and is usually worse at night. The scratching associated with pruritus may cause fleeting skin excoriations.

Easy Bruisability

Spontaneous bruising and mucosal bleeding may indicate impaired hepatic synthesis of coagulation factors in patients with chronic liver disease.

Sleep Disturbance

In patients with known or suspected end-stage liver disease, a disruption of the normal sleep pattern may be the earliest symptom of hepatic encephalopathy. Patients may have trouble falling asleep, interrupted sleep at night, or daytime somnolence. The sleep disturbance is thought to result in part from changes in melatonin secretion in cirrhotic patients.

Change in Mental Status

Patients with worsening hepatic encephalopathy may experience mental impairment, ranging from lethargy and confusion to stupor and coma. Encephalopathy can be associated with personality changes, depression, irritability, and inappropriate and disinhibited behavior. These symptoms are typically not noted by the patient but reported by friends and family.

Leg Cramps

Patients with end-stage liver disease have a high frequency of muscle cramps, typically in the legs and mostly at night.

Physical Examination

Liver disease may be suspected initially on the basis of a careful physical examination. Certain findings can also provide clues about the nature and severity of the liver disease.

Jaundice

Jaundice must be distinguished from yellow discoloration of the skin caused by other yellow pigments, as that which occurs with excessive ingestion of carrots. Bilirubin levels below 2 to 3 mg/dL generally cannot be detected on physical examination. Although scleral icterus is the most commonly described manifestation of hyperbilirubinemia, detection of yellow discoloration of the palate and tympanic membranes is an even more sensitive indicator of hyperbilirubinemia.

Skin Findings

Spider angiomata and palmar erythema are frequent in patients with severe or advanced liver disease, especially patients with alcoholic cirrhosis. The underlying pathophysiology of these changes is not fully explained but relates in part to increased circulating estrogen levels. Spontaneous bruising may be observed in patients with hepatic synthetic dysfunction and impaired coagulation. Petechiae may result from thrombocytopenia in patients with hypersplenism or bone marrow suppression.

Other skin abnormalities can provide clues to the nature of the underlying liver disease. Xanthomas and xanthelasma, as well as hyperpigmentation, are typical of primary biliary cirrhosis. Palpable purpura and livedo reticularis raise the possibility of polyarteritis nodosa, which can be seen in patients with hepatitis B infection; palpable purpura caused by leukocytoclastic vasculitis can be seen in patients with cryoglobulinemia associated with hepatitis C infection.[1] Skin fragility with the formation of blisters and hyperpigmentation in sun-exposed areas is indicative of porphyria cutanea tarda, which is also associated with hepatitis C infection. Palmar erythema, typically localized to the thenar and hypothenar regions of the hand, is commonly found in patients with cirrhosis and results from vasodilatation.

Gynecomastia

In male patients with liver disease, enlargement of breast tissue—palpable underneath the areola—may be detected and should not be confused with generalized breast enlargement associated with obesity. Spironolactone to treat ascites may exacerbate gynecomastia. Like gynecomastia, Dupuytren's contractures (characterized by thickening of the flexor tendons of the hand) and parotid gland enlargement are common in patients with advanced alcoholic liver disease. Gynecomastia can occur physiologically during the neonatal period and puberty and is also associated with hormone-producing neoplasms, renal disease, and hyperthyroidism.[2]

Lymphadenopathy

Enlarged lymph nodes are not typical in patients with liver disease. If found in a patient with liver disease, lymphadenopathy suggests the possibility of underlying Epstein-Barr virus infection or lymphoma.

Abdominal Examination

Inspection

Inspection of the abdomen may reveal enlarged veins in the abdominal wall. The term caput medusae refers to the appearance of enlarged veins radiating from the umbilicus in patients with portal hypertension. High portal venous pressures may open up the umbilical vein, which normally ends in the left portion of the portal vein during fetal development. The blood follows the ligamentum teres and eventually reaches the abdominal wall veins through the umbilicus. These veins are seen better if the skin is stretched and are thus most prominent in patients with ascites. By contrast, enlarged veins that run longitudinally along the side of the abdomen are suggestive of obstruction of the inferior vena cava. In this case, the veins are fed by lower abdominal or leg veins.

Bulging flanks may be the earliest indicator of ascites. With larger amounts of ascites, the abdomen becomes grossly distended, often with splaying of the lower ribs.

Palpation

The liver can be palpated by placing the examiner's hand below the right costal margin, applying soft pressure, and asking the patient to take a deep inspiration. As the liver moves down with the diaphragm, the lower edge can be felt with the edge or tips of the fingers. Alternatively, the curved fingers of the palpating hand can slide down over the costal margin from above, and the liver can be palpated on inspiration; this technique is also known as the Middleton method. The normal liver edge should be sharp and smooth, but not hard. The left lobe is typically not palpable. A palpable liver edge does not necessarily mean an enlarged liver, and assessment of true liver volume on physical examination is generally not accurate.[3] In patients with emphysema, the entire liver may be pushed down by the diaphragm.

The liver may be tender in acute hepatitis. Focal tenderness over the liver may be present in patients with a liver abscess or hepatic neoplasm. Rebound tenderness indicates inflammation of the peritoneum.[4] A pulsatile liver can be found in severe tricuspid regurgitation and constrictive pericardial disease.

A normal gallbladder generally cannot be palpated. An enlarged gallbladder can often be palpated between the lateral border of the right rectus abdominis muscle and the right costal margin. This finding typically indicates obstruction of the common bile duct below the level of the cystic duct, by gallstone impaction, tumor in the head of the pancreas, or cholangiocarcinoma.

Splenomegaly can be found in patients with cirrhosis and portal hypertension and in those with acute hepatitis, especially when caused by Epstein-Barr virus infection. Subtle enlargement of the spleen may be difficult to detect and commonly requires ultrasonographic confirmation.

Percussion

Percussion of the liver complements palpation in detecting the lower edge of the liver in patients who are obese or have well-exercised abdominal muscles. Percussion may also suggest a small liver size. The liver is generally percussed in the midclavicular line or in the midline of the abdomen. The measured liver span by percussion of both the upper and lower liver edges varies by percussion technique and position. Light percussion typically yields a bigger liver span than does hard percussion, thereby accounting for the great interobserver variability noted in several studies.[5]

Auscultation

Auscultation of the abdomen can reveal bruits, which are systolic sounds due to turbulent blood flow. Common causes of abdominal bruits are atherosclerosis of the aorta and compression of the celiac axis. Bruits of hepatic origin occur as a result of alcoholic hepatitis, hepatocellular carcinoma, hepatic artery aneurysm, traumatic hepatic arteriovenous fistula, and portosystemic shunts.

"Scratch" auscultation refers to the technique of listening over the right quadrant with the stethoscope while scratching over the skin. Transmission of the sound is supposedly less muted over the area where the liver is next to the abdominal wall; however, the method is unreliable for detecting the span of the liver below the costal margin.[6]

Detection of Ascites

A large volume of ascites is generally apparent on inspection. Ascites can also be detected by eliciting a fluid wave or shifting dullness on percussion.[7] To detect a fluid wave, the examiner taps the flank of the recumbent patient with one hand, while the other hand feels for an impulse on the opposite flank. A second examiner or, when possible, the patient places the ulnar border of his or her hand along the midline of the abdomen to block transmission of the impulse through abdominal wall fat. To detect shifting dullness, the examiner percusses the recumbent patient's abdomen, moving from the umbilicus towards one side until there is dullness to percussion. The patient is then rolled toward the opposite side, and, after 15 to 20 seconds to allow for fluid redistribution, the examiner percusses for dullness again. The fluid will have shifted and the previously dull area will now sound resonant.

Laboratory Evaluation

The liver performs a multitude of functions, and no single test can adequately assess liver function in any clinical scenario. A broad spectrum of different biochemical tests is used to evaluate injury to and function of the liver. Use of the term "liver function tests" (LFTs) has been criticized because many of these blood tests are used to detect liver injury rather than the synthetic, metabolic, or excretory function of the liver. However, the term LFTs is still commonly used and rarely misunderstood.

LFTs are often used as screening tests in asymptomatic patients to detect asymptomatic liver disease. The pattern of abnormalities can suggest different diagnostic possibilities and guide further diagnostic testing. In patients with known liver disease, LFTs can give information about the severity and progression of the disease. However, these tests vary in sensitivity and specificity throughout the course of the patient's disease. A patient with cirrhosis caused by chronic hepatitis, for example, may have normal serum aminotransferase levels. Moreover, the test results are nonspecific; the measured enzymes can derive from tissues other than the liver, either as isoenzymes (eg, alkaline phosphatase from bone, kidney, intestine, placenta) or as the same enzyme (eg, aspartate aminotransferase from muscle).

The localization of the various liver enzymes in the hepatocyte is shown in Figure 1-1. The different tests can be categorized in groups reflecting 1) hepatocellular or bile duct injury, 2) transport capacity of the liver for organic anions and bile salts, and 3) metabolic function or synthetic capacity. Other specific tests may be used to confirm a suspected diagnosis; these include serologic and molecular tests to detect viral hepatitis, serologic markers for autoimmune liver disease, and genetic tests for hemochromatosis and α-1 antitrypsin deficiency.

Tests that Reflect Hepatic and Biliary Injury

Aminotransferases

Elevated levels of alanine aminotransferase (ALT, previously called serum glutamic pyruvic transaminase, SGPT) and aspartate aminotransferase (AST, previously called serum glutamic oxaloacetic transaminase, SGOT) indicate hepatocyte injury and necrosis. The enzymes catalyze the transfer of α-amino groups of alanine and aspartate to ketoglutaric acid, thereby forming pyruvic and oxaloacetic acid. Whereas ALT is a cytosolic enzyme that is found in highest concentrations in the liver,[8] AST is located

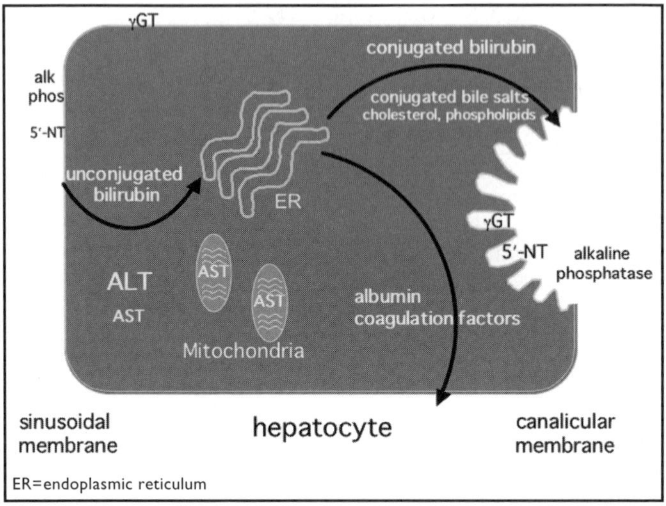

Figure 1-1. Localization in the hepatocyte of commonly measured serum markers of liver disease.

predominantly in the mitochondria (80%) and also in the cytosol (20%) of liver, heart, skeletal muscle, kidney, brain, pancreas, lungs, leukocytes, and erythrocytes (see Figure 1-1). In addition to liver disease, AST levels are typically elevated in muscle and cardiac disease and were used in the past for the diagnosis of myocardial infarction.

The aminotransferases are routinely measured photometrically by coupling the enzymatic reduction of oxaloacetate and pyruvate with the oxidation of the reduced form of nicotinamide adenine dinucleotide (NADH) to NAD.

Serum aminotransferase levels are elevated in almost all forms of liver disease. Their absolute level in serum does not correlate with the extent of hepatocellular injury and is not specific for the etiology of liver disease or predictive of outcome. Very high enzyme elevations of more than 15-fold the upper normal limit are typically limited to acute viral hepatitis, toxin- or drug-induced liver damage, ischemic injury (shock liver), hepatic artery ligation, Budd-Chiari syndrome, and fulminant Wilson's disease. Moderate elevations can be seen in many forms of acute and chronic liver disease, including viral and autoimmune hepatitis, alcoholic hepatitis, and hepatic injury caused by metabolic diseases such as hemochromatosis or Wilson's disease. Mildly elevated (up to 5-fold) aminotransferase levels can be seen in patients with nonalcoholic fatty liver and nonalcoholic steatohepatitis, chronic hepatitis B or C, celiac disease, and many other disorders (Table 1-2).[9]

The ratio of AST to ALT may provide an important clue as to the etiology of hepatic injury. An AST:ALT ratio of greater than 2.0 is typically seen in patients with alcoholic liver disease, in which ALT levels are often normal or only mildly elevated. This is thought to be the result of two mechanisms: 1) patients with alcohol dependence are often deficient in pyridoxal 5'-phosphate, which is a cofactor for both ALT and AST and deficiency of pyridoxal 5'-phosphate decreases ALT activity to a greater extent than AST activity; and 2) alcohol-induced liver injury leads to increased release of mitochondrial AST, thereby further increasing the AST:ALT ratio.[10]

Table 1-2

CAUSES OF MILD ALT OR AST ELEVATIONS

Hepatic: Predominantly ALT
Chronic hepatitis C
Chronic hepatitis B
Acute viral hepatitis (A to E, EBV, CMV)
Steatosis/steatohepatitis
Hemochromatosis
Medications/toxins
Autoimmune hepatitis
α1-antitrypsin deficiency
Wilson's disease
Celiac disease
Hepatic: Predominantly AST
Alcohol-related liver injury
Steatosis/steatohepatitis
Cirrhosis
Nonhepatic
Hemolysis
Myopathy
Thyroid disease
Strenuous exercise
Macro-AST

Adapted from Green R, Flamm S. AGA technical review on the evaluation of liver chemistry tests. *Gastroenterology.* 2002; 123:1367-1384.

Low serum aminotransferase levels are typically seen in patients on chronic hemodialysis.[11]

Alkaline Phosphatase

Alkaline phosphatases catalyze the hydrolysis of phosphate esters at an alkaline pH. This family of enzymes comprises several isoenzymes that are all zinc-dependent. In humans, alkaline phosphatase is found in liver, osteoblasts, intestinal enterocytes, placenta, kidney, and leukocytes and can be detected in serum, urine, bile, and lymph. In the liver, two isoforms of the enzyme can be detected; their exact role is unknown. Alkaline phosphatase is associated with the sinusoidal and canalicular membranes of the hepatocyte and with the biliary epithelium. Elevations in serum enzyme levels after biliary injury result from induction and *de novo* synthesis of the protein, rather than release of stored enzyme or impaired clearance. Therefore, a rise in serum alkaline phosphatase levels may not be detected immediately after biliary injury and may be preceded by an elevation in serum aminotransferase levels.

Alkaline phosphatase is measured photometrically and fluorimetrically by various methods, and depending on the assay, the activities of the different isoenzymes are weighed differently. Elevated serum levels of alkaline phosphatase typically have a liver origin but may be caused by bone disease or derive from the placenta in pregnant women. Traditionally, the bone and hepatic isoforms of the enzyme have been distinguished by their heat stability. Whereas heat inactivates virtually all bone alkaline phosphatase, 30% to 50% of hepatic alkaline phosphatase activity remains after heating. This method of distinguishing hepatic from bone alkaline phosphatase has been replaced by more specific markers of cholestatic injury, such as the 5'-nucleotidase.[12]

Serum levels of alkaline phosphatase of hepatic origin are highest in patients with acute or chronic cholestatic liver disease, including primary biliary cirrhosis or primary sclerosing cholangitis and cholestatic drug reactions, and are often associated with elevated serum bilirubin levels. It is not possible to distinguish intrahepatic from extrahepatic cholestasis based on the serum level of alkaline phosphatase. Isolated elevation of the alkaline phosphatase in serum may be found in patients with hepatocellular carcinoma, lymphoma, and metastatic disease in liver or bone. In addition to malignant tumors, other infiltrative diseases such as granulomatous disease, sarcoidosis, tuberculosis, fungal infections, hepatic abscesses, and amyloidosis can cause an isolated elevation of the serum alkaline phosphatase level.[9]

Alkaline phosphatase levels may be elevated in conjunction with bilirubin levels in patients with sepsis or after extensive trauma or surgery.

Low levels of alkaline phosphatase can result from zinc deficiency, hypothyroidism, and pernicious anemia. Low levels of alkaline phosphatase in patients presenting with fulminant Wilson's disease are attributed to displacement of zinc, a co-factor for alkaline phosphatase activity, by copper.

5'-Nucleotidase

5'-nucleotidase catalyzes the hydrolysis of nucleotides by releasing inorganic phosphate from the 5'-position of the pentose ring. It is present in the liver, intestine, brain, heart, blood vessels, and endocrine pancreas. In the liver, 5'-nucleotidase is located at the basolateral and canalicular plasma membranes; its function is not known. Elevated levels are generally of hepatobiliary origin, as it is believed that only the hepatic enzyme can be released into the serum.

The enzyme activity of 5'-nucleotidase is assessed by measuring the released inorganic phosphate or the remaining adenosine moiety.

Serum levels of 5'-nucleotidase are measured to confirm the hepatic origin of an isolated alkaline phosphatase elevation. This is particularly useful in adolescent and pregnant patients in whom alkaline phosphatase levels are elevated physiologically but 5'-nucleotidase levels are unaffected. One study, however, has suggested that an elevated 5'-nucleotidase level is not sensitive enough to detect all patients with a hepatic source of an elevated alkaline phosphatase level.[13]

γ-Glutamyl Transpeptidase

γ-glutamyl transpeptidase catalyzes the transfer of γ-glutamyl groups to other amino acids. γ-glutamyl transpeptidase is found in the cell membranes of many tissues, including liver, kidney, seminal vesicles, pancreas, spleen, heart, and brain. In the liver, γ-glutamyl transpeptidase is localized to hepatocytes and the common bile duct. The enzyme is measured spectroscopically in a reaction with γ-L-glutamyl-p-nitroanilide that releases p-nitroaniline.

Serum γ-glutamyl transpeptidase levels are elevated in many forms of hepatobiliary disease as well as in chronic alcohol abuse, pancreatic disease, cardiac disease, renal failure, diabetes, chronic obstructive pulmonary disease, and chronic inflammatory disorders. In liver disease, an elevated serum γ-glutamyl transpeptidase level is a sensitive marker of hepatobiliary disease and closely correlated with serum alkaline phosphatase levels. It is, however, not specific for liver disease and is therefore not suitable for screening or diagnosis of liver disease. The enzyme is induced by alcohol, phenytoin, and rifampin and has been used as a marker of surreptitious alcohol use. Traditionally, measurement of γ-glutamyl transpeptidase in serum has been used to establish the hepatic origin of elevated alkaline phosphatase levels; however, elevated 5'-nucleotidase levels are more specific for this purpose.

Tests That Measure the Capacity for Organic Anion Transport

The metabolic function of the liver was first studied by the rate of removal of bromosulfophthalein (BSP) from the circulation. Because of side effects of BSP and the inability of such testing to distinguish hepatocellular from obstructive jaundice, the BSP test was ultimately replaced by the measurement of endogenous compounds, specifically bilirubin and bile acids.

Bilirubin

Bilirubin is the primary breakdown product of hemoglobin metabolism. It is transported to the liver bound to albumin and lipoproteins and conjugated by uridine diphosphoglucuronate (UDP)-glucuronosyltransferase in the endoplasmic reticulum to bilirubin monoglucuronide and bilirubin diglucuronide. Although unconjugated bilirubin cannot be excreted by the kidneys, conjugated bilirubin is found in the urine of patients with conjugated hyperbilirubinemia. However, in prolonged cases of conjugated hyperbilirubinemia, bilirubin binds covalently to albumin and assumes the plasma half-life of albumin, accounting for the slow decline in bilirubin levels even after resolution of acute liver injury.

Bilirubin is measured photometrically in the van den Bergh reaction, which separates the more hydrophilic conjugates that can be measured directly after addition of a diazo reagent from the hydrophobic unconjugated bilirubin that is measured indirectly, by first determining the total bilirubin concentration in the presence of an accelerator such as caffeine-benzoate and then calculating the difference between total and direct bilirubin. The van den Bergh reaction is not entirely accurate, as it overestimates the conjugated bilirubin at low serum levels when compared to high performance liquid chromatography and may cause misinterpretation of the results in cases of low unconjugated hyperbilirubinemia.

Table 1-3 lists the various causes of hyperbilirubinemia. Excessive bilirubin production from hemolysis, impaired uptake into hepatocytes, and reduced conjugation can result in unconjugated hyperbilirubinemia. Conjugated hyperbilirubinemia results from impaired hepatic secretion caused by drugs or enzyme defects, intrahepatic cholestasis, and extrahepatic obstruction.

Urinary Bilirubin and Urobilinogen

Bilirubin in the urine is always conjugated and therefore associated with causes of conjugated hyperbilirubinemia. The detection of bilirubinuria is only helpful when found in patients with a low serum bilirubin level, as it indicates liver disease. In patients with marked hyperbilirubinemia, however, bilirubinuria does not provide additional information. Urinary urobilinogen can result from increased production of bilirubin, as in hemolysis, and hepatocellular dysfunction. This test is no longer used.

Serum Bile Acids

Bile acids are synthesized from cholesterol in the liver, conjugated with glycine and taurine, and excreted into bile. Elevated levels of serum bile acids indicate impaired biliary excretion and are more sensitive than elevated bilirubin levels in detecting mild hepatic dysfunction.

Bile acids can be measured by various methods. Gas chromatography is widely used, and radioimmunoassays have been developed to measure levels of individual bile acids, although measurement of serum bile acids is not routinely done in clinical practice. The ratio of cholic acid to chenodeoxycholic acid can suggest the cause of liver disease. The ratio is typically 0.1 to 0.5 in cirrhotic patients, 0.5 to 1.0 in normal persons, and 0.96 to 3.6 in patients with extrahepatic obstruction. Clearance of bile acids after intravenous loading, postprandial bile acids, and bile acid levels after administration of cholecystokinin are additional methods of assessing liver function. These tests are rarely used in routine practice.

Quantitative Liver Tests to Measure the Metabolic Capacity of the Liver

Tests of Synthetic Function

The liver produces and secretes a large number of proteins. Among these, albumin, coagulation factors, and lipoproteins can be routinely measured and reflect the synthetic capacity of the liver.

Albumin

Albumin is the most abundant protein produced by the liver; 12 to 15 grams of albumin are synthesized daily. The plasma half-life of albumin is 14 to 20 days, and therefore, levels are rarely affected in the early phases of acute liver disease. Albumin levels reflect not only hepatic synthetic capacity, but also nutritional and catabolic status and osmotic pressure. Nephrotic syndrome, protein-losing enteropathy, and extensive burns may also cause low plasma albumin levels. In cirrhotic patients, plasma albumin levels correlate with prognosis.

Prothrombin Time and Coagulation Factor Levels

The liver plays a central role in the maintenance of normal hemostasis. It synthesizes the coagulation factors I, II, V, VII, IX, and X, which are involved in the extrinsic coagulation pathway and can be assessed by measurement of the prothrombin time by the method of Quick. Factors II, VII, IX, and X are dependent on vitamin K for γ-carboxylation. Vitamin K deficiency, vitamin K antagonists, congenital coagula-

Table 1-3

CAUSES OF HYPERBILIRUBINEMIA

Unconjugated Hyperbilirubinemia

Hemolysis

Wilson's Disease

Hemolytic anemias

- Blood transfusion
- Ineffective erythropoiesis

Abnormal conjugation

- Gilbert's syndrome
- Crigler-Najjar syndrome, type I
- Crigler-Najjar syndrome, type II

Immature enzyme system

- Impaired bilirubin uptake
- Maternal milk jaundice
- Maternal serum jaundice (Lucey-Driscoll syndrome)

Increased intestinal absorption

Conjugated Hyperbilirubinemia

Hapatocellular disease

Intrahepatic cholestasis

Biliary obstruction

Total parenteral nutrition

Impaired organic anion transport

- Inherited
    - *Rotor's syndrome*
    - *Dubin-Johnson syndrome*
    - *Progressive familial intrahepatic cholestasis*
- Acquired
    - *Cholestastis of sepsis*
    - *Drugs*
- Anatomical anomalies
    - *Alagille syndrome*

Adapted from Adams PC, Arthur MJ, Boyer TD, et al. Screening in liver disease: report of an AASLD clinical workshop. *Hepatology.* 2004;39:1204-1212.

tion factor deficiencies, and acquired coagulation factor abnormalities can affect the prothrombin time. Factor V is not dependent on vitamin K, and serum levels of factor V correlate with the severity of liver disease even in the presence of vitamin K deficiency. The half-life of all coagulation factors is relatively short (eg, 12 to 15 hours for factor V) and prolongation of the prothrombin time can occur soon after acute liver failure. Prolongation of the prothrombin time has been found to be more predictive of prognosis in patients with chronic liver disease than are serum aminotransferase, bilirubin, and albumin levels. Prolongation of the prothrombin time is also a predictor of outcome in patients with acute liver failure caused by acetaminophen and acute alcoholic hepatitis.

Plasma Lipids and Lipoproteins

The liver has a central role in the production and metabolism of plasma lipoproteins. The liver is the major source of all lipoproteins, except chylomicrons, and the hepatic enzymes lecithin-cholesterol acyltransferase (LCAT) and hepatic lipase play major roles in modifying the composition of lipoproteins.

Increased plasma levels of triglycerides and decreased levels of cholesterol esters are found in acute hepatocellular injury. In addition, low-density lipoprotein triglyceride levels are often increased, and the electrophoretic pattern of lipoproteins is changed, presumably because of loss of LCAT activity, with a wide β band and absent α and pre-β bands. Lipoprotein abnormalities in patients with chronic liver disease are similar but may be less pronounced.

Patients with intrahepatic or extrahepatic cholestasis often have highly elevated plasma cholesterol and phospholipid levels.

Screening Tests for Specific Liver Diseases

There are an ever increasing number of laboratory tests to screen asymptomatic patients for the presence of specific liver diseases. Screening is typically indicated when early diagnosis and treatment will lead to an improved outcome.[14] The diseases for which screening is often undertaken are listed, with the corresponding screening strategies, in Table 1-4, and the most established screening approaches are discussed in the following section.

Hemochromatosis

Hemochromatosis is the most common autosomal recessive disease among Whites and is readily treatable when detected early. Standard screening tests for hemochromatosis are the transferrin saturation and serum ferritin level. With the discovery of disease-specific mutations in the *HFE* gene, genetic testing for hemochromatosis has become available. Homozygosity for the most common mutation, *C282Y,* is responsible for 85% to 90% of cases of hemochromatosis, and genetic testing can be used to screen relatives of affected patients. However, because many patients with *C282Y* homozygosity never develop clinical disease, the advisability of population-wide screening has been questioned.

Hepatitis C

Screening for hepatitis C virus (HCV) infection is recommended for high-risk persons. Early detection of HCV infection permits initiation of treatment and possible containment of the disease. All blood donors have been screened for HCV in the United States since the availability of anti-HCV antibody assays in 1992. Table 1-5 lists the persons for whom screening has been recommended by the American Association for the Study of Liver Diseases.[14]

Table 1-4

SCREENING FOR LIVER DISEASE

Screening Target	*Available Screening Options*	*Characteristics*
Hemochromatosis	Transferrin saturation, ferritin *HFE* genotype for *C282Y*	Transferrin saturation and ferritin detect iron overload; *HFE* genotype detects predisposition to iron overload
Hepatitis B	HBsAg for active infection Anti-HBs for immunity status and need for vaccination	Asymptomatic carriers may be subjected to unnecessary tests
Hepatitis C	Anti-HCV	Testing for high-risk groups
Hepatotoxicity	Serial measurements of ALT, alkaline phosphatase	Stop drug if ALT >3 times the upper normal limit; toxicity of drugs that cause cholestasis may be slow to reverse
Cirrhosis	Different test combinations/algorithms under study	Many currently used tests are nonspecific
Portal hypertension	Endoscopy for esophageal varices	Risk of bleeding must be weighed against side effects of treatment
Hepatocellular carcinoma	Serial imaging (US, CT) α-fetoprotein	Efficacy of screening uncertain

Adapted from Adams PC, Arthur MJ, Boyer TD, et al. Screening in liver disease: report of an AASLD clinical workshop. *Hepatology.* 2004;39:1204-1212.

Hepatitis B

As for hepatitis C, persons at high risk of hepatitis B viral (HBV) infection should be screened. Persons for whom screening is recommended include pregnant women, health care workers, hemodialysis patients, recipients of clotting factor concentrates, household contacts of patients with chronic HBV, injection drug users, institutionalized persons, men who have sex with men, and patients with HCV or human immu-

Table 1-5

INDICATIONS FOR SCREENING FOR HEPATITIS C VIRUS INFECTION

Persons with a history of intravenous drug use

Persons with the potential for exposure to HCV because of other medical problems:

- Patients undergoing hemodialysis
- Patients who received clotting factor concentrations before 1997

Persons with persistently elevated serum aminotransferase levels

Recipients of transfusions or organ transplants:

- Blood transfusion before July 1992
- Recipients of known HCV-infected blood transfusion
- Patients who received an organ transplant before July 1992

Health care workers with needlestick injury

Children born to HCV-positive mothers

Patients from an area of high HCV prevalence

Adapted from Adams PC, Arthur MJ, Boyer TD, et al. Screening in liver disease: report of an AASLD clinical workshop. *Hepatology.* 2004;39:1204-1212

nodeficiency virus (HIV) infection. In the United States, all newborns should be vaccinated against HBV.

HEPATIC IMAGING

The importance of hepatic imaging and the number of imaging modalities available have increased considerably over the past several decades. Hepatic imaging often complements the findings of the patient's history and physical examination, laboratory evaluation, and histologic assessment. Liver imaging is particularly useful in the evaluation of focal liver lesions, diffuse liver disease, and biliary diseases. Based on the clinical presentation of the patient, different imaging strategies are employed. Table 1-6 summarizes the imaging modalities used in several clinical situations. Imaging is generally indicated in the evaluation of the patient with jaundice or abnormal LFTs and in the patient with suspected or established mass lesions of the liver. In addition, imaging may allow the assessment of cirrhosis and portal hypertension. Cirrhosis is suggested by the presence of caudate lobe hypertrophy and atrophy of the right lobe of the liver. In addition, an enlarged gallbladder fossa, splenomegaly, and portocaval collateral vessels may be detected.

PLAIN ABDOMINAL AND CHEST X-RAYS

Plain abdominal x-rays are typically not helpful in the evaluation of liver disease. Incidental calcifications may suggest gallstone disease or echinococcal infection. An

Table 1-6

Clinical Presentation and Use of Liver Imaging Studies

Clinical Presentation	*Initial Imaging Study*	*Additional Imaging Modalities*
Jaundice	US or CT to detect biliary obstruction, liver masses, or obvious hepatic parenchymal disease	CT to detect obstructing lesion, mass in the pancreas, or enlarged porta hepatis lymph nodes. MRCP or ERCP to determine site and exact cause of dilated bile ducts. Endoscopic ultrasound can be helpful to guide biopsy and stage disease
Hepatic parenchymal disease	US MRI	US with Doppler or MRI with flow-weighted images if a vascular abnormality is suspected
Screening for liver mass	US CT	MRI
Detection of liver metastases	CT	MRI US- or CT-guided biopsy
Characterization of known liver mass		
- Suspicion of malignancy	US- or CT-guided biopsy	MRI
- Suspicion of benign lesion	MRI	US- or CT-guided biopsy if uncertainty remains Radionuclide scan (Tc-^{99}m red cell scan for suspected hemangioma)
- Suspicion of abscess	US or CT Image-guided aspiration if indicated	Radionuclide imaging (gallium or In-111 white blood cell scan)

continued

Table 1-6 (continued)

Clinical Presentation and Use of Liver Imaging Studies

Clinical Presentation	*Initial Imaging Study*	*Additional Imaging Modalities*
Detection of biliary duct abnormalities	US to detect bile duct dilatation, stones, or mass MRCP or ERCP to assess ductal anatomy	CT or endoscopic ultrasound to detect stones or cause of extrinsinc compression

Adapted from Friedman LS, Martin P, Munoz SJ. Laboratory evaluation of the patient with liver disease. In: Zakim D, Boyer TD, eds. *Hepatology: a textbook of liver disease. Vol. I*. Philadelphia: Saunders; 2003:661-708.

elevated right hemidiaphragm can result from a pyogenic liver abscess or advanced hepatocellular carcinoma. A right-sided pleural effusion in a patient with ascites suggests hepatic hydrothorax.

Ultrasound

Ultrasound is noninvasive, readily available, fairly inexpensive, and the most common initial imaging modality for liver disease. Ultrasound is indicated in patients with jaundice to characterize the nature of biliary disease, specifically bile duct obstruction, gallstones, and gallbladder inflammation. The sensitivity of ultrasound for the evaluation of biliary obstruction is 85%, and the specificity is 90%; these rates are lower than those for abdominal computed tomography (CT) (90% and 90%, respectively) and for ERCP, the gold standard (95% and 99%, respectively). However, gallstones in the gallbladder are more accurately identified on ultrasound than on CT scan. Ultrasound can also detect parenchymal liver disease, hepatic mass lesions, and, with Doppler imaging, vascular occlusion or compromise. Ultrasound is often superior to other imaging techniques in characterizing hepatic cysts.

The introduction of harmonic imaging, enhanced Doppler ultrasonography, and liver-specific contrast agents has broadened the scope of ultrasound examinations, but limitations remain. For example, ultrasound cannot penetrate bone or air, and unenhanced B-mode ultrasonography cannot sensitively detect subcentimeter hepatic lesions, although the introduction of contrast-enhanced phase-inversion ultrasound imaging, using microbubble contrast agents, has markedly improved the ability to detect small lesions. Ultrasound cannot generally differentiate benign from malignant liver lesions. Galactose-based intravascular contrast agents can characterize the vascularity of liver lesions.

Moderate to marked steatosis of the liver is often seen on ultrasound as increased echogenicity, with a characteristically bright liver, often with hepatomegaly. With real-time imaging, ultrasound is used to guide biopsies and drain abscesses.

Computed Tomography

CT has become the most frequently used imaging modality in industrialized countries for the evaluation of the liver. CT is commonly used in the evaluation of hepatic mass lesions and in some patients with abnormal LFTs. Oral contrast is required to visualize the intestinal lumen, and intravenous contrast is often administered, especially for imaging hepatic mass lesions and vascular abnormalities in the liver. The choice of intravenous contrast agent remains controversial. Ionic contrast agents have a higher risk of allergic reactions, and nonionic agents are often used in patients with multiple allergies or significant cardiopulmonary disease, when high infusion rates of the contrast agent are required. Characterization of hepatic lesions by CT in a cirrhotic patient can be difficult because the appearance of hepatocellular carcinoma can be heterogeneous, and benign changes such as nodular regenerative hyperplasia can coexist.[15] Lipiodol is an iodinated ethyl ester of the fatty acid of poppy seed oil with 37% iodine content and is preferentially retained in hepatocellular carcinoma cells after arterial injection. Very small hepatic lesions (<5 mm) can be detected on delayed imaging 7 to 28 days after injection.

Technical advances in CT, including helical CT and multidetector CT, have led to increases in the speed and resolution of imaging. Helical CT, also called spiral CT, permits imaging of the entire abdomen in a single breath by using slip-ring technology that lets the Roentgen tube and x-ray detector rotate in a directional spiral, as opposed to multiple single circles on older CT scanners. The advent of helical CT has led to substantial decreases in acquisition time and a great reduction in motion artifact that, in the past, was a result of breathing between the scanning of single slices. Helical CT also permits the imaging of multiple phases in the same study after intravenous contrast administration, for example, the arterial phase after 10 to 30 seconds and the portal venous phase between 50 and 70 seconds, thereby increasing the sensitivity for the detection of hepatic tumors (Figure 1-2) and contrasting them with hepatic metastases (Figure 1-3). These two phases reflect the unique dual blood supply of the liver (75% to 80% of blood flow is supplied by the portal vein and the remaining 20% to 25% by the hepatic artery). Liver tumors generally receive most of their blood supply from the hepatic artery and are best imaged during the arterial phase or with use of an intra-arterial contrast agent like lipiodol.

Helical CT also enables multiplanar and three-dimensional reconstruction of the images. These techniques are of particular importance in preoperative evaluation for surgical hepatic resection.

Noncontrast CT scans are occasionally performed to evaluate diffuse liver disease; the liver density in these scans is compared to that of the spleen. Hemochromatosis can present with an increased liver density on noncontrast CT due to the attenuation of the Roentgen beam by the high liver iron content. However, CT is neither sensitive nor specific for hemochromatosis, and high attenuation of the liver can also result from other conditions associated with an increased liver metal content (Wilson's disease), storage diseases (glycogen storage disease, type 1), drugs (amiodarone or gold), and toxins (arsenic). Diffuse hepatic steatosis often can be identified by decreased attenua-

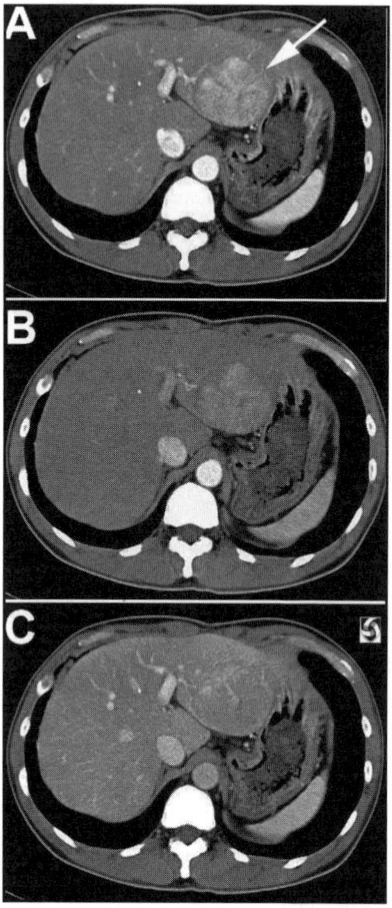

Figure 1-2. Computed tomography of hepatocellular carcinoma. Three contrast-enhanced images from a computed tomography (CT) study are shown. Image A represents the early arterial phase. A heterogeneously enhancing mass (arrow), approximately 4-5 cm in size, is visible in the liver. There is no evidence of calcifications. Image B shows the late-arterial phase image, which demonstrates additional enhancement of the mass. On the portal venous phase image in Image C, the enhancement has decreased. The mass is iso-attenuating with the rest of the liver.

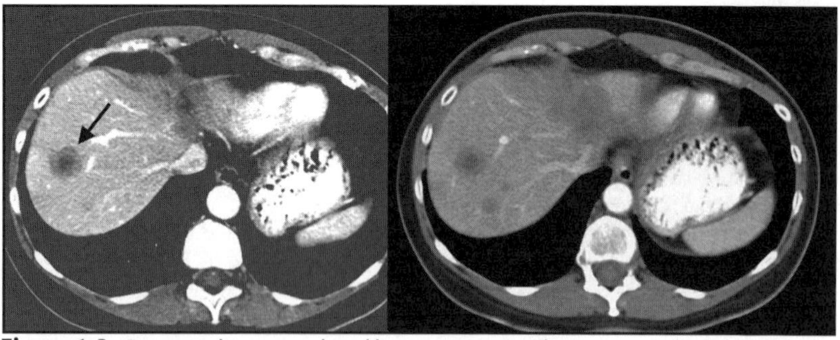

Figure 1-3. Computed tomography of liver metastasis. The image on the left shows the arterial phase, which demonstrates a liver lesion (arrow) in a patient with colon cancer. The lesion is hypointense, reflecting the hypovascularity of the lesion. The image on the right shows the lesion on the venous contrast phase.

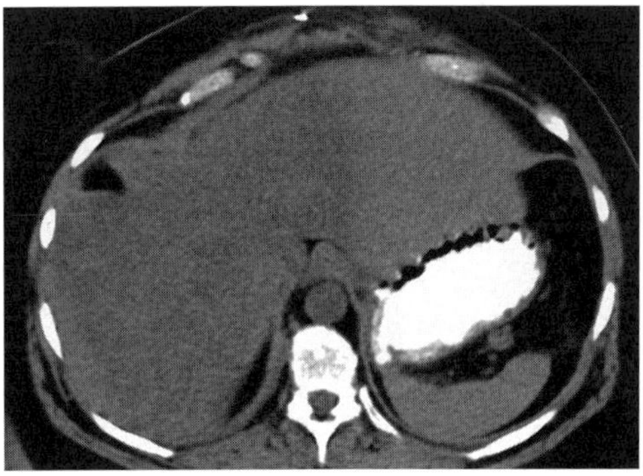

Figure 1-4. Computed tomography of hepatic steatosis. Regional steatosis involving the right lobe of the liver is depicted in this noncontrast CT scan. The steatotic liver parenchyma is hypointense when compared with the spleen and the left liver lobe

tion on a noncontrast CT scan (Figure 1-4). In patients with cirrhosis, areas of confluent fibrosis appear as hypoattenuated lesions on noncontrast CT but as isoattenuated areas on contrast CT, and both modes of image acquisition should be done in these patients to fully characterize the liver disease and exclude a neoplasm.

Magnetic Resonance Imaging

Instead of detecting attenuation of x-rays, as in CT, magnetic resonance imaging (MRI) uses the magnetic properties of protons in hydrogen atoms as signals and does not involve ionizing radiation. Typically, axial T1-weighted and T2-weighted sequences are obtained. Imaging planes can be acquired in axial, longitudinal, and coronal orientation as well as in any oblique direction, an advantage that can be used to image subdiaphragmatic processes. MRI is expensive and not as widely available as CT, especially in less industrialized nations. Patients with metallic devices, such as cardiac pacemakers and certain prostheses, cannot undergo MRI.

MRI is useful in detecting and characterizing focal hepatic parenchymal disease, biliary disease, and vascular abnormalities. Recent developments include faster imaging acquisition and improved imaging sequences, specialized body surface coils, and new contrast agents that allow improved identification of hepatic lesions and definitive diagnosis, in some cases without the need for histologic analysis. The sensitivity and specificity of MRI for hepatic lesions surpass those of dynamic contrast-enhanced CT but have not been compared to those for multidetector CT. Magnetic resonance cholangiopancreatography (MRCP) uses special imaging sequences to visualize the biliary tree and pancreatic duct and is a noninvasive alternative to endoscopic retrograde cholangiopancreatography when the likelihood for an intervention such as sphincterotomy or gallstone extraction is estimated to be low.

Several intravenous contrast agents are used to increase the sensitivity and specificity for the detection of liver lesions on MRI, and their major characteristics are summarized in Table 1-7.[16] Extracellular gadolinium chelates are widely used and essential for standard MRI of the liver. They diffuse freely in the interstitial space and are excreted by the kidneys. MRI with gadolinium is most useful for detecting hepatocellular carcinomas and differentiating them from other hypervascular lesions, such as hemangiomas (Figure 1-5). Ferumoxides, which are taken up specifically by the Kupffer cells in the liver as well as the reticuloendothelial cells in spleen and bone marrow, are most useful

Table 1-7

Characteristics of Hepatic Magnetic Resonance Imaging Contrast Agents

	Extracellular Fluid Agent	*Hepatobiliary Agent*	*Reticuloendothelial Agent*
Effective sequence	TI	TI	T2
Contrast effect	White liver on TI Black lesion on TI	White liver on TI Black lesion on TI	Black liver on T2 White liver on TI
Duration of liver enhancement after injection	2 hours	4 hours	7 days
Possibility of dynamic study	Yes	Yes	No
Uptake by hepato-cellular neoplasm	Probable, but not constant	Probable for well-differentiated lesions	Constant for well-differentiated lesions

Adapted from Ji H, Ros PR. Magnetic resonance imaging. Liver-specific contrast agents. *Clin Liver Dis.* 2002;6:73-90.

in evaluating liver metastases and intrahepatic cholangiocarcinoma. Liver lesions that contain reticuloendothelial cells, such as focal nodular hyperplasia, characteristically have contrast enhancement similar to that of normal liver. Mangafodipir trisodium is a complex of manganese with a chelating agent that is taken up directly by hepatocytes and allows characterization of liver tumors, especially detection of metastases that do not take up this agent. Because mangafodipir is hepatically excreted, it can also be used to evaluate hepatocyte function and the biliary tree. Gadolinium benzyloxypropionictetraacetate and gadolinium ethoxybenzyldiethylenetriminepentaacetic acid are agents that combine characteristics of a perfusional extracellular contrast agent with hepatocyte-selective uptake and are particularly useful in differentiating primary liver tumors from metastases.

Radionuclide Imaging

Radionuclide imaging is used less now to evaluate liver disease than in the past. Technetium-^{99}m (Tc-^{99}m)-HIDA (hepatobiliary iminodiacetic acid) scanning can be used to assess bile flow, hepatocyte function, and biliary excretion and is useful for the diagnosis of acute cholecystitis. Tc-^{99}m sulphur colloid is taken up by the Kupffer cells and can be used to differentiate focal nodular hyperplasia from other hepatocellular and nonhepatocellular focal liver lesions, although MRI is preferred. Gallium-67 can be used to detect hepatocellular carcinoma in cirrhotic livers. Tc-^{99}-labeled erythro-

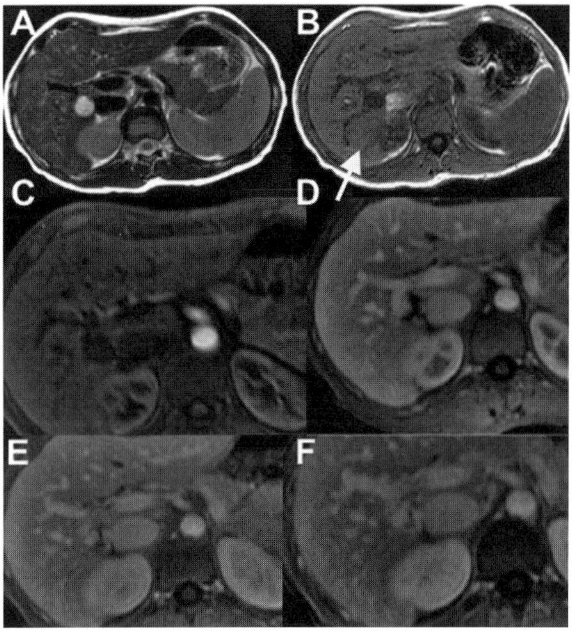

Figure 1-5. Magnetic resonance imaging of a hemangioma. Image A shows a T2-weighted and Image B a T1-weighted image of a hemangioma (arrow). The hemangioma is typically hyperintense on the T2-weighted image and hypointense on the T1-weighted image. Dynamic T1-weighted images following gadolinium administration in Images C to F show the early peripheral and nodular enhancement of the lesion during the arterial phase.

cytes can be used to characterize the blood volume and blood flow in vascular lesions, especially hemangiomas.

Positron Emission Tomography

Positron emission tomography (PET) is technically another radionuclide imaging technique, but it deserves special mention because of its higher resolution than other radionuclide imaging methods due to its use of positron emission radiopharmaceuticals that generate two photons simultaneously. The most commonly used contrast agent is 18-F fluorodeoxyglucose, an analogue of glucose, which is taken up preferentially in metabolically active tissues. Tumor metastases in the liver can be detected with great sensitivity by PET. Because well-differentiated hepatocellular carcinoma takes up little glucose, the use of PET to detect primary hepatocellular carcinoma is limited.

Liver Biopsy

Paul Ehrlich performed the first percutaneous liver biopsy in 1883, but the procedure increased in popularity after 1958, when Menghini described a fast ("1-second") technique for obtaining a liver specimen.

Liver biopsy remains an important tool in the evaluation of patients with suspected liver disease. Often it provides a definitive diagnosis, and serial liver biopsies have provided invaluable information about the characteristic pathological features and natural history of liver disease. Although the specificity of liver imaging techniques continues to increase, in many instances imaging cannot replace liver biopsy for definitive determination of the nature and extent of hepatic damage. However, liver biopsy is an

Table 1-8

Indications for Liver Biopsy

- Evaluation of persistently abnormal liver biochemical tests and hepatomegaly
- Evaluation and staging of chronic hepatitis
- Identification and staging of alcoholic liver disease
- Recognition of systemic inflammatory or granulomatous disorders
- Evaluation of fever of unknown origin
- Evaluation of the type and extent of drug-induced liver injury
- Identification and determination of the nature of intrahepatic masses
- Diagnosis of multisystem infiltrative disorders
- Evaluation and staging of cholestatic liver disease (primary biliary cirrho sis, primary sclerosing cholangitis)
- Screening of relatives of patients with familial diseases
- Obtaining of tissue to culture infectious agents (eg, mycobacteria)
- Evaluation of effectiveness of therapies for liver diseases (eg, Wilson's disease, hemochromatosis, autoimmune hepatitis, chronic viral hepatitis)
- Evaluation of liver test abnormalities following transplantation

invasive procedure, with a risk, albeit small, of potentially life-threatening complications, and controversy persists about specific indications and contraindications and optimal technique.

Indications

The indications for liver biopsy are listed in Table 1-8. In patients with abnormal LFTs that cannot be explained by other findings, liver biopsy can help exclude serious liver disease or disclose the nature and severity of liver disease. However, following exclusion of known causes of liver disease by thorough biochemical and serologic evaluation, liver biopsy leads to a specific diagnosis in only 10% of patients, and treatment is changed by the results in only 12% of patients.

In patients with chronic hepatitis, liver biopsy demonstrates the degree of inflammation, type of inflammatory infiltrate, extent of fibrosis, and in some cases the presence of viral antigens—this information is important for the diagnosis, prognosis, and choice of therapy. Liver biopsy can yield important information in patients with suspected drug-induced hepatic injury and can determine the nature of hepatic masses that are not clearly defined by imaging alone.

Liver biopsy is also indispensable in the care of the patient who has undergone liver transplantation and is especially important in distinguishing graft rejection from recurrence of the disease for which liver transplantation was performed.

Certain indications for liver biopsy remain controversial. The degree of otherwise unexplained serum aminotransferase level elevations that should lead to liver biopsy is uncertain. The need for liver biopsy in suspected nonalcoholic fatty liver disease remains equally controversial. Steatosis can be detected quite sensitively by imaging techniques, but the extent of inflammation and fibrosis can only be assessed reliably by liver biopsy. Liver biopsy in patients with HCV infection prior to antiviral therapy has been standard practice in recent years but is now often deferred in patients infected with HCV genotypes 2 or 3, in whom response rates to treatment are high. The need for liver biopsy in patients with suspected primary biliary cirrhosis and primary sclerosing cholangitis has been questioned; diagnosis can be made by serologic testing in the former and cholangiography in the latter, and scoring systems based on clinical and laboratory findings can be used to estimate prognosis without the need for a liver biopsy.

Requirements

Liver biopsy requires an adequately trained physician and a cooperative patient. Blood transfusion services and a surgeon should be available if needed. In the United States, liver biopsy is routinely performed as an outpatient procedure. Patients should be monitored for 6 hours after the procedure and remain near the hospital for 24 hours.

Contraindications

Coagulopathy is present in many patients with advanced liver disease and is a contraindication to liver biopsy. An elevated prothrombin time of 3 to 4 seconds above the control or thrombocytopenia with a platelet count of less than 60,000/mm^3 generally disqualifies a patient from undergoing liver biopsy. Some hepatologists also measure the bleeding time prior to liver biopsy to determine the clinically relevant risk for bleeding. In patients with a mild prolongation of the prothrombin time, transfusion of fresh frozen plasma may allow the procedure to be performed safely. Aspirin and other nonsteroidal anti-inflammatory drugs (NSAIDs) are generally discontinued at least 1 week before the procedure, although there is no evidence that the risk of bleeding is increased in patients taking these medications.

Tense ascites prohibits liver biopsy because the liver may bounce away from the biopsy needle, thereby reducing the chance that an adequate sample of liver tissue will be obtained. Other contraindications for liver biopsy are extrahepatic bile duct obstruction, biliary infection, and a suspicion of hemangioma.

Technical Aspects

Cutting or suction needles are used for percutaneous liver biopsy. Trucut (Baxter International, Newark, New Jersey) and Vim Silverman needles are examples of cutting needles, which provide larger specimens but probably cause more complications than suction needles, such as Menghini or Klatskin needles. Suction needles are less expensive, remain in the liver for a shorter period of time, and are generally easier to use. Biopsy guns, which have a spring-loaded mechanism that drives a modified Trucut needle, have been used increasingly and are now the instrument of choice in many centers.[17]

The use of ultrasound guidance for liver biopsy is still a subject of controversy. Ultrasound can be used to mark the optimal position for liver biopsy *before* the procedure or for real-time guidance *during* the procedure. Ultrasound decreases the frequency of pain, hypotension, and bleeding, and appears to lead to better samples than do "blind" biopsies. Many centers now use ultrasound to routinely mark the biopsy site, and up to one third of hepatologists in the United States refer patients to a radiologist to perform liver biopsy under real-time ultrasound guidance. In countries where gastroenterologists routinely perform ultrasound examinations themselves, virtually all liver biopsies are done under ultrasound guidance.

A liver biopsy specimen that is adequate for pathologic evaluation is typically 1 to 4 cm long and weighs 10 to 50 mg. The minimal core diameter should be 1.0 mm. Menghini needles yield an average specimen size of 1.8 ± 0.8 cm, often in several fragments; at least 6 (and preferably 11) portal triads are desirable. Too short a specimen typically leads to underestimation of the grade of inflammation and stage of fibrosis. Cirrhosis often leads to a fragmented biopsy specimen and can be missed because of sampling error in up to 20% of cases. Fine-needle aspiration with a 20-gauge or smaller needle should only be used to biopsy focal liver lesions and not diffuse parenchymal disease.

In patients who are at high risk of bleeding because of uncorrectable coagulopathy or have ascites or a small cirrhotic liver, transjugular biopsy is safer than percutaneous biopsy. In this procedure, a catheter is inserted into a hepatic vein via the jugular vein, and a needle is advanced into the liver. The specimen is taken from within the vascular system, thereby minimizing the risk of bleeding; the mortality rate is low (0% to 0.5%). The biopsy specimens are typically smaller than those obtained by percutaneous biopsy. This technique also allows the direct measurement of hepatic venous pressures.

Laparoscopic liver biopsy is indicated for staging abdominal cancer and evaluating patients with peritoneal disease and ascites of unknown origin. Under direct laparoscopic vision, focal hepatic lesions can be targeted. Bacterial peritonitis, intestinal obstruction, cardiopulmonary disease, morbid obesity, coagulopathy, and a large ventral hernia are contraindications to this procedure.

Complications

The most common complication of liver biopsy is pain, which occurs in more than 30% of patients and is moderate to severe in 4.5%. The pain can be in the right upper quadrant or referred to the right shoulder.

Serious complications are most likely to occur within 24 hours of the procedure, and 60% occur within 2 hours; 1% to 3% of patients require hospitalization. The most common serious complication is bleeding, which may not be heralded by pain. Bleeding from a liver laceration can be brisk, resulting in hypotension and shock. The risk of serious hemorrhage is about 0.3% and increases with age, malignancy in the liver, and the number of needle passes used for biopsy. The type of needle may also be important, with cutting needles posing a slightly larger risk than suction needles. Bleeding after liver biopsy is generally detected by ultrasonography or CT. Where required, angiography allows selective embolization of the affected artery. Rarely, surgical ligation is necessary to stop the bleeding.

Puncture of the gallbladder can result in biliary peritonitis and death. Any surrounding organ, such as lung, colon, or kidney can be punctured. As a result, pneumothorax, subcutaneous emphysema, and pleural effusions can occur. There is a small (1% to 3%) risk that biopsy of malignancies may cause seeding of the biopsy track by tumor. Bacteremia can be demonstrated in 5.8% to 13.5% of patients after liver biopsy, and antibiotic prophylaxis is recommended for patients at risk of endocarditis and with biliary sepsis.

Acknowledgment

The authors greatly appreciate the invaluable help of Dr. Mehmet Erturk and Dr. Pablo Ros from the Department of Radiology at Brigham and Women's Hospital and Harvard Medical School, Boston, for providing the radiologic images in this chapter.

References

1. Jones AM, Warken K, Tyring SK. The cutaneous manifestations of viral hepatitis. *Dermatol Clin.* 2002;20:233-47, vi.
2. Braunstein GD. Gynecomastia. *N Engl J Med.* 1993;328:490-495.
3. Zoli M, Magalotti D, Grimaldi M, et al. Physical examination of the liver: is it still worth it? *Am J Gastroenterol.* 1995;90:1428-1432.
4. Naylor CD. The rational clinical examination. Physical examination of the liver. *JAMA.* 1994;271:1859-1865.
5. Gilbert VE. Detection of the liver below the costal margin: comparative value of palpation, light percussion, and auscultatory percussion. *South Med J.* 1994;87:182-186.
6. Tucker WN, Saab S, Rickman LS, Mathews WC. The scratch test is unreliable for detecting the liver edge. *J Clin Gastroenterol.* 1997;25:410-414.
7. Williams JW, Jr., Simel DL. The rational clinical examination. Does this patient have ascites? How to divine fluid in the abdomen. *JAMA.* 1992;267:2645-2648.
8. Kaplan MM. Alanine aminotransferase levels: what's normal? *Ann Intern Med.* 2002;137:49-51.
9. Green R, Flamm S. AGA technical review on the evaluation of liver chemistry tests. *Gastroenterology.* 2002;123:1367-1384.
10. Sorbi D, Boynton J, Lindor KD. The ratio of aspartate aminotransferase to alanine aminotransferase: potential value in differentiating nonalcoholic steatohepatitis from alcoholic liver disease. *Am J Gastroenterol.* 1999;94:1018-1022.
11. Yasuda K, Okuda K, Endo N, et al. Hypoaminotransferasemia in patients undergoing long-term hemodialysis: clinical and biochemical appraisal. *Gastroenterology.* 1995;109:1295-1300.
12. Pratt DS, Kaplan MM. Evaluation of abnormal liver-enzyme results in asymptomatic patients. *N Engl J Med.* 2000;342:1266-1271.
13. Pagani F, Panteghini M. 5'-Nucleotidase in the detection of increased activity of the liver form of alkaline phosphatase in Serum. *Clin Chem.* 2001; 47:2046-2048.
14. Adams PC, Arthur MJ, Boyer TD, et al. Screening in liver disease: report of an AASLD clinical workshop. *Hepatology.* 2004;39:1204-1212.
15. Mortele KJ, McTavish J, Ros PR. Current techniques of computed tomography. Helical CT, multidetector CT, and 3D reconstruction. *Clin Liver Dis.* 2002;6:29-52.
16. Ji H, Ros PR. Magnetic resonance imaging. Liver-specific contrast agents. *Clin Liver Dis.* 2002;6:73-90.
17. Bravo AA, Sheth SG, Chopra S. Liver biopsy. *N Engl J Med.* 2001;344:495-500.

18. Friedman LS, Martin P, Munoz SJ. Laboratory evaluation of the patient with liver disease. In: Zakim D, Boyer TD, eds. *Hepatology: A Textbook of Liver Disease. Vol. 1.* Philadelphia: Saunders; 2003:661-708.

Recommended Reading

McIntyre N. Symptoms and signs of liver disease. In: Bircher J, Benhamou J-P, McIntyre N, Rizzetto M, Rodes J , eds. *Oxford Textbook of Clinical Hepatology.* Oxford, UK: Oxford University Press; 1999:479-499.

Detailed discussion of the symptoms and signs in patients with liver disease, a rare find in current hepatology textbooks.

Friedman LS, Martin P, Muñoz SJ. Laboratory evaluation of the patient with liver disease. In: Zakim D, Boyer TD, eds. *Hepatology: A Textbook of Liver Disease. Vol. 1.* Philadelphia: Saunders; 2003:661-708.

A comprehensive chapter on the laboratory evaluation and imaging of the patient with liver disease.

Green R, Flamm S. AGA technical review on the evaluation of liver chemistry tests. *Gastroenterology.* 2002;123:1367-1384.

Recent comprehensive overview of the common liver biochemical tests.

Adams PC, Arthur MJ, Boyer TD, et al. Screening in liver disease: report of an AASLD clinical workshop. *Hepatology.* 2004;39:1204-1212.

Current summary of an American Association for the Study of Liver Diseases conference on screening tests for liver disease.

Ros PR (guest ed.). Hepatic imaging and intervention. *Clin Liver Dis.* 2004.

An entire issue devoted to hepatic imaging, with detailed discussions of each modality.

Friedman LS. Controversies in liver biopsy: who, where, when, how, why? *Curr Gastroenterol Rep.* 2004;6:30-36.

A detailed overview of indications, contraindications, and controversies regarding liver biopsy.

chapter 2

Cirrhosis and Its Complications

Jayanta Choudhury, MD and Arun J. Sanyal, MD

Introduction

Cirrhosis is the end result of chronic liver injury from a variety of causes. It is defined by marked disruption of hepatic architecture with extensive fibrosis and fibrotic encirclement of regenerative nodules. There are a large number of conditions that can lead to cirrhosis (Table 2-1). The prevalence of cirrhosis is 3.6 per 1000 individuals in North America. It is the seventh leading cause of death in the United States, and is responsible for 25,000 deaths and 10.6 million days of work loss annually. Portal hypertension develops as a consequence of cirrhosis and is present in 60% of subjects at the time of diagnosis. The development of portal hypertension and its complications (Table 2-2) contribute substantially to the morbidity and mortality associated with cirrhosis. Consequently, the prevention and treatment of these complications is one of the cornerstones of the management of the cirrhotic patient. In this chapter we will review the complications of cirrhosis and the current management strategies used to deal with them.

Etiology of Cirrhosis and Its Diagnoses

Over the past decade, chronic hepatitis C (HCV) has replaced alcohol as the leading cause of cirrhosis. Approximately 26% of newly diagnosed cases of cirrhosis are caused by chronic HCV while alcoholic cirrhosis comes a close second with an estimated prevalence of 21%. There is, however, considerable overlap between these groups, and a substantial proportion of subjects with HCV also have a history of alcohol abuse. It is currently felt that regular alcohol consumption, even in modest amounts, may contribute to the progression of other liver diseases towards cirrhosis.

In 10% to 20% of cases of cirrhosis, the cause of the cirrhosis is not apparent despite clinical assessment, serologic and biochemical studies. The cirrhosis in such cases was referred to be cryptogenic in origin. It is now known that up to 70% to 80% of cases of cryptogenic cirrhosis are associated with the metabolic syndrome and

Table 2-1

ETIOLOGY OF CIRRHOSIS

1. Chronic hepatitis C (26%)
2. Alcoholic liver disease (21%)
3. Cryptogenic causes (18%)*
4. Hepatitis B ± hepatitis D (15%)
5. Miscellaneous causes:
    - Nonalcoholic fatty liver disease (NAFLD)
    - Hemochromatosis
    - Wilson's disease
    - α-1 antitrypsin deficiency
    - Autoimmune hepatitis
    - Primary biliary cirrhosis
    - Secondary biliary cirrhosis (extrahepatic biliary obstruction)
    - Primary sclerosing cholangitis
    - Chronic hepatic venous outflow obstruction (Budd-Chiari syndrome)
    - Drug-induced (Methotrexate, Amiodarone)

*May include some cases of NAFLD

development of fatty liver as well as steatohepatitis after liver transplantation. It is also known that as nonalcoholic steatohepatitis (NASH) evolves into cirrhosis, the degree of steatosis decreases and may disappear along with other findings of steatohepatitis such as cytologic ballooning and Mallory's hyaline. Based on these considerations, many cases of cryptogenic cirrhosis are now believed to result from nonalcoholic steatohepatitis (NASH).

The diagnostic evaluation of an individual with suspected cirrhosis involves a three-pronged approach: 1) to establish the presence of cirrhosis, 2) to establish the cause of cirrhosis, and 3) to evaluate the prognosis of the individual patient.

ESTABLISHMENT OF THE DIAGNOSIS OF CIRRHOSIS

The majority of the clinical and the laboratory abnormalities that are detected in cirrhosis are nonspecific and, by themselves, are not diagnostic of the presence of cirrhosis (Table 2-3). However, in a relevant clinical setting they provide useful adjunctive data that helps in confirming the clinical suspicion of cirrhosis. The presence of cirrhosis may be suspected or inferred under the following circumstances:

1. When an individual presents with liver failure and features of portal hypertension.
2. When an individual presents with complications related to cirrhosis eg, hepatocellular cancer or portal hypertension (eg, ascites).

Table 2-2

COMPLICATIONS OF CIRRHOSIS

Portal Hypertension Related	Portal Hypertension Unrelated
Variceal bleeding	Coagulopathy (?-synthesis of factors II, V, VII,IX, X)
Ascites	Hepatocellular carcinoma
Spontaneous bacterial peritonitis	
Hepato-renal syndrome	
Splenomegaly	
Thrombocytopenia	
Hepatic encephalopathy	

Table 2-3

CLINICAL FEATURES AND LAB ABNORMAITIES IN CIRRHOSIS

Clinical Findings	Lab Abnormalities
Spider angioma	Hyperbilirubinemia
Palmer erythema	Elevated aminotransferases
Dupuytren's contracture	Elevated alkaline phosphatases (usually less than 3 times normal except in PBC and PSC)
Muehrcke's and Terry's nails*	Hypoalbuminemia
Gynecomastia	Abnormal coagulation profile
Loss of axillary and pubic hair	Thrombocytopenia
Testicular atrophy	Elevated A-glutamyl transpeptidase
Ascites	Hyperglobinemia
Hepatomegaly or shrunken liver	Hyponatremia
Splenomegaly	
Caput medussae/dilated abdominal veins	
Fetor hepaticus	
Asterexis	
Cruveilhier Baumgarten's sign**	

* Muehrcke's nails: white bands separated by normal appearing nails; Terry's nail: proximal part two third of the nail is white while the distal third is normal color. Both of these are nonspecific and are tought to result from periods of hypoalbuminemia.

** Cruveilhier Baumgarten's sign: venous hum heard best over the epigastrium due to portosystemic collaterals between the portal vein and umbilical vein.

Table 2-4

CLASSIFICATION OF SPONTANEOUS BACTERIAL PERITONITIS

	Cell Count (PMN)	*Culture* (Ascitic fluid)
A. SBP	≥250/mm^3	Monomicrobial
B. SBP variants:		
1. Monomicrobial non-neutrocytic bacterascites	≤250/mm^3	Monomicrobial
2. Culture-negative neutrocytic bacterascites	≥250/mm^3	Negative
3. Polymicrobial bacterascites	≤250/mm^3	Polymicrobial
C. Secondary Bacterial Peritonitis	≥250/mm^3	Polymicrobial

3. When an abnormal liver morphology is detected on imaging studies or during unrelated surgery the liver appearance and consistency is felt to be abnormal.
4. Reversal of AST/ALT ratio to values over 1 and/or development of thrombocytopenia in a patient known to have chronic liver disease. The presence of abnormal liver enzymes suggest the presence of liver disease and do not connote the presence of cirrhosis per se.

The gold standard for the diagnosis of cirrhosis is a liver biopsy. Cirrhosis is often diagnosed when a liver biopsy is performed to stage various chronic liver diseases (eg, hepatitis B [HBV] or HCV) or when a biopsy is performed for diagnostic evaluation (eg, NASH). However, a biopsy is not essential in all cases and a diagnosis of cirrhosis can be made with confidence when liver failure, complications of cirrhosis, and portal hypertension are present.

ESTABLISHMENT OF THE CAUSE OF CIRRHOSIS

As noted above, there are numerous causes of cirrhosis. The diagnosis of the cause of cirrhosis usually involves an adequate clinical assessment and laboratory studies that indicate the presence of the specific cause of cirrhosis. A list of such causes and the appropriate laboratory tests used to diagnose these conditions are shown in (Table 2-4).

ASSESSMENT OF THE PROGNOSIS

The prognosis of a patient with cirrhosis depends on two major variables: 1) the degree of liver failure, and 2) the presence of complications associated with cirrhosis. Several algorithms and scoring systems have been developed to quantify survival probability in patients with cirrhosis using these parameters. Of these, the Child-

Table 2-5

CHILD-PUGH CLASSIFICATION OF SEVERITY OF CIRRHOSIS

Parameter	*1 Point*	*2 Points*	*3 Points*
Ascites	Absent	Slight	Moderate
Bilirubin, mg/dL	≤2	2 to 3	>3
Albumin, g/dL	>3.5	2.8 to 3.5	<2.8
Prothrombin time			
Seconds over control	1 to 3	4 to 6	>6
INR	<1.7	1.8 to 2.3	>2.3
Encephalopathy	None	Grade 1 to 2	Grade 3 to 4

Scores: 5 to 6 Child A (well compensated disease), 7 to 9 Child B (some functional compromise), and 10 to 15 Child C (decompensated disease)

Note: 2-year survival of 85% in Child A, 60% in Child B and 35% in Child C

Pugh-Turcotte (CPT) score (Table 2-5) has been used most. Recently, a model for end-stage liver disease (MELD) scoring system has been developed that includes the serum bilirubin, creatinine, and international normalized ratio (INR).[1] This has the advantage of avoiding the ceiling and floor effects present with the CPT score and is also a continuous scale permitting better separation of subjects with varying prognosis. These considerations were the basis for supplanting the CPT score with the MELD score for organ allocation for liver transplantation.

Liver function is assessed clinically by the serum bilirubin and albumin concentrations and the prothrombin time. Liver failure is characterized by an increase in conjugated bilirubin, decrease in albumin and prolongation of the prothrombin time. It must however be remembered that each of these abnormalities may result from alternate causes and that a diagnosis of liver failure should be made, keeping the clinical picture of the individual patient in perspective.

The key complications of cirrhosis include the development of hepatocellular cancer, variceal hemorrhage, ascites, and encephalopathy. Ascites may be further complicated by spontaneous bacterial peritonitis and hepatorenal syndrome. Of these complications, variceal hemorrhage, ascites, and encephalopathy are directly related to the presence of portal hypertension and porta-systemic collateral circulation. These complications are a major cause of morbidity and mortality associated with cirrhosis. The evaluation and management of these complications is, therefore, a cornerstone of the management of cirrhosis.

MANAGEMENT OF THE CIRRHOTIC PATIENT

The management of the cirrhotic subject requires a clear understanding of the natural history of cirrhosis, the pathophysiology and natural history of its complications, and the utility of specific treatments in the context of the patient's natural history.

General Measures

Nutrition

No dietary interventions are indicated in those with compensated cirrhosis unless they are malnourished for other reasons. Na restriction is required once ascites develops. Protein restriction is not necessary except in those with encephalopathy. Use of branched chain amino acid enriched diets have not been shown to produce significant improvement in quantity or quality of life and are not routinely recommended.

Activity

No significant restrictions are imposed on the well-compensated cirrhotic. Those with large varices may be advised to avoid lifting heavy objects due to the theoretical risks of variceal rupture. Many patients note improvement in their quality of life if they take a short nap in the afternoon.

Immunization

Pneumococcal and influenza vaccines are administered as indicated. Hepatitis A (HAV) and HBV vaccines may be administered to those at risk.

Complications of Cirrhosis

Portal Hypertension

Portal hypertension is an almost inevitable consequence of cirrhosis and is seen at the time of diagnoses in 60% of patients with decompensated cirrhosis and in 40% of patients with compensated cirrhosis. Conversely, cirrhosis is the most common cause of portal hypertension and accounts for 95% of the cases encountered in clinical practice. Normal portal pressure (3 to 5 mmHg) is the difference between the wedged hepatic venous pressure (WHVP) and the free hepatic venous pressure (FHVP). This measurement is referred to as hepatic venous pressure gradient (HVPG) and is a good indirect indicator of the actual portal pressure. Ascites develops when the portal pressure (HVPG) exceeds 8 mmHg while varices appear when the HVPG is greater than 12 mmHg.

The pressure in the portal vein is directly proportional to the amount of venous inflow and the resistance to outflow from the portal venous system. In cirrhosis, portal hypertension is initiated by an increase in outflow resistance at the level of the hepatic sinusoids and is referred to as sinusoidal portal hypertension. This is due to both a relatively static component from fibrotic distortion of the hepatic architecture and a dynamic component from constriction of the hepatic sinusoids. Hepatic sinusoidal constriction results from constriction of myofibroblast-like cells (Stellate cells) that are wrapped around individual sinusoids (Figure 2-1). These cells constrict or relax in response to specific substances (ie, endothelin and nitric oxide [NO]). It has been shown that diminished hepatic sinusoidal NO production contributes to an exaggerated constrictive response by the stellate cells thereby producing sinusoidal constriction. Besides increased resistance to portal blood flow, the pathophysiology of portal hypertension also involves increased portal blood flow secondary to splanchic vasodilatation.

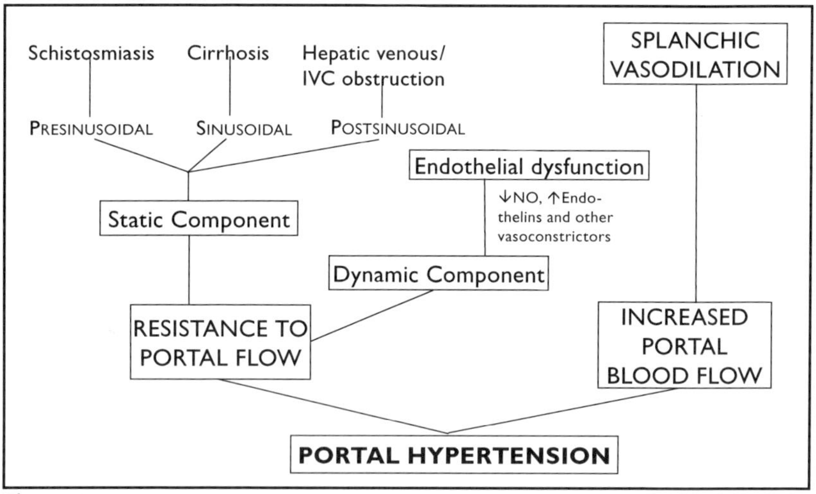

Figure 2-1. Pathophysiology of portal hypertension.

Variceal Bleeding

A major consequence of portal hypertension is the development of a collateral circulation that returns blood to the systemic venous circulation from the portal circulation. A common location of such collaterals is the gastroesophageal junction where these collaterals enlarge and become tortuous esophageal and gastric varices. Varices are classified according to their location as well as their size (Table 2-6). The incidence of varices in a patient with newly diagnosed cirrhosis is about 2% to 5% per year. Factors that are associated with increased risk of variceal bleeding include the variceal size, presence of red wale sign and the severity of liver failure. As dictated by Laplace's law, the larger the variceal diameter, the greater the wall tension. Hence, large varices are at higher risk of rupture. Red wale signs and the presence of hemocystic spots on the variceal surface on the other hand reflect areas of weakness on the variceal wall, and are often indicative of an impending variceal bleed.

The mortality following an episode of acute variceal bleed is approximately 20% at 6 weeks.[2,3] Severe and/or recurrent bleeding, liver failure, and development of complications are risk factors for mortality in this setting. Those with a HVPG greater than 20 mmHg are more likely to continue to bleed or fail first-line therapies for a control of bleeding. Following initial hemostasis, there is a period of high risk of rebleeding that is greatest in the first 48 hours and then subsides to baseline values by 6 weeks. The risk factors for such early rebleeding include age, sepsis, renal failure, spurting varices, and liver failure. In the long-term, over 70% of survivors of an index bleed experience further hemorrhage if left untreated. The risk factors for such late rebleeding include variceal size, liver failure, alcohol abuse, and hepatocellular cancer.

The management strategy that is employed in dealing with variceal hemorrhage can be divided into three broad categories: 1) prevention of variceal hemorrhage (primary prophylaxis, 2) management of acute variceal hemorrhage, and 3) prevention of rebleeding after the index bleed.

Table 2-6

CLASSIFICATION OF VARICES

Esophageal Varices (Based on Variceal Size)

- F1: Small straight varices
- F2: Enlarged tortuous varices occupying less than one third of the lumen
- F3: Enlarged tortuous varices occupying more than one third of the lumen

(To prevent overestimation of variceal size, esophageal insufflation should always be performed prior to measurement)

Gastric Varices

- Gastroesophageal varices (GOV) 1: Direct continuity with lesser curvature of stomach
- Gastroesophageal varices (GOV) 2: Direct continuity with greater curvature of stomach
- Isolated gastric varices (IGV) 1: Isolated fundal varices
- Isolated gastric varices (IGV) 2: Gastric varices in locations other than gastric fundus

Prevention of Variceal Hemorrhage (Primary Prophylaxis)

Primary prophylaxis of varices should be considered in all patients who present with moderate to large varices and in those with stigmata of impending bleed such as red wale signs or hemocystic spots. Preventive measures aimed at reducing the risk of bleeding following detection of varices can be divided in to two broad categories: 1) measures aimed at reducing the portal pressures, and 2) measures aimed directly at the varices themselves (Table 2-7). These interventions assume importance as approximately one-third of all patients who have varices go on to develop variceal hemorrhage, and there is a 30% risk of mortality with each episode of variceal hemorrhage.

Reducing the Portal Pressures

Portal pressures can be reduced by either pharmacologic agents such as nonselective β-blockers and nitrates or by mechanical measures aimed at creating portosystemic shunts such as TIPS or surgical anastomoses.

Nonselective β-blockers such as propranolol and nadolol cause mesenteric vasoconstriction as a result of unopposed alpha adrenergic effects and consequently reduce portal inflow and HVPG. These agents have been shown in several controlled trials to reduce the risk of first episode of variceal hemorrhage by 30% to 50% compared to placebo. Clinically, the therapeutic aim is to reduce the resting heart rate to approximately 55 to 60 beats/minute and the dosage of the β-blocker is titrated until this target is reached or adverse symptoms appear. Adverse effects that may prompt discontinuation of therapy include bronchoconstriction, congestive heart failure and impotence. Although β-blockers are therapeutic agents of choice in primary prophy-

Table 2-7

PRIMARY PROPHYLAXIS FOR VARICES

1. Cirrhotics without varices: No therapy
2. Cirrhotics with small varices (<5mm): No therapy
3. Cirrhotics with moderate to large varices but have never bled: β-blockers (propranolol or nadolol). Those who have contraindications or are intolerant to β-blockers, consider EVL
4. Cirrhotics who have suboptimal response to maximum tolerated dosage of β-blockers should have HVPG measurement (if facilities are available) and if the HVPG is over 12 mmHg, then consider addition of isosorbide mononitrate

laxis, there are no conclusive data demonstrating survival advantage with these agents compared to placebo. The factors that are associated with failure of β-blocker therapy include younger age, larger variceal size, advanced liver failure, and inadequate dosage of β- blockers. Also there is no evidence to suggest that primary prophylaxis with β-blockers in patients with cirrhosis and no varices prevents appearance of varices.

Oral nitrates have also been shown to reduce portal pressures in cirrhotics. However, studies have shown that there is no advantage with nitrate monotherapy in primary prophylaxis compared to β-blockers alone. Moreover, nitrate monotherapy has been associated with increased mortality in patients above the age of 50. Hence, at this time, nitrate monotherapy for primary prophylaxis is not recommended even in those patients who cannot tolerate β-blockers.

Data for combination therapy with β-blockers and nitrates for primary prophylaxis have been inconclusive. Some studies have shown reduced risk of bleeding with the combination compared to β-blockers alone while others have failed to show the same. Hence, given the adverse effect profile of nitrates, combination therapy cannot be recommended as an initial measure for primary prophylaxis for prevention of variceal hemorrhage.

Other measures that may lower portal pressures include TIPS and surgical porto-systemic anastomosis. There are currently no data supporting the use of TIPS for primary prophylaxis of variceal hemorrhage, and, therefore, it is not recommended. Insofar as surgical anastomoses is concerned, available data suggest that although these eradicate the varices and reduce risk of bleeding, there is an overwhelmingly high incidence of crippling encephalopathy. Moreover, some of the studies comparing surgical with medical therapy have shown the advantage of medical therapy over the surgical option. Hence, currently, surgery is not recommended for primary prophylaxis.

Measures Aimed Directly at Varices

Given the high rate of success of both sclerotherapy (EST) and endoscopic variceal band ligation (EVL) in the treatment of variceal hemorrhage, these measures were tested as therapeutic option for primary prophylaxis.

Data for EST suggest that when compared to β-blockers, EST is less effective in preventing variceal hemorrhage with some studies showing excess mortality in the

EST group. Similar results were obtained when EST was combined with β-blockers in comparison to β-blockers alone. Therefore, currently, there is no role for EST in the primary prophylaxis of variceal hemorrhage.

EVL, as a primary prophylactic measure, has been shown in several studies to decrease the incidence of variceal hemorrhage and bleeding related mortality. However, varices tend to recur after initial eradication and continued endoscopic surveillance is necessary to ensure therapeutic effectiveness. Thus given the cost and inconvenience of EVL in comparison to β-blocker therapy, EVL should only be used in patients who have moderate to large varices and are unable to tolerate β-blockers.

Summary of Recommendation for Primary Prophylaxis

Patients with cirrhosis who present for the first time should have a diagnostic upper GI endoscopy to look for varices. Those that have moderate to large (F2 and F3) varices should be started on β-blockers. In facilities where HVPG can be measured, nitrates may be added in those patients who are showing inadequate response to β-blockers. EVL is a therapeutic option inpatients who are unable to tolerate β-blockers and are considered to be at high risk for variceal hemorrhage.

Management of Acute Variceal Hemorrhage

Hemodynamic Support

The extent of hemodynamic compromise can be effectively assessed at the bedside by the measurement of the orthostatic drop in systolic blood pressure by greater than 20 mmHg or the presence of resting tachycardia. The initial aim is to maintain a hematocrit of about 25% to 30%, achieve hemodynamic stability and a normal urine output. Overly aggressive volume resuscitation leads to a loss of protective reflex splanchic vasoconstriction that serves to lower the portal pressures during the bleed and contributes to early rebleeding. When large volumes of blood are required, the platelet counts and ionized calcium levels should be monitored periodically.

General Medical Management

In addition to providing hemodynamic support, it is imperative to provide aggressively supportive medical care. The airway must be protected in those who are unable to do so themselves or are having massive hemorrhage. Alcohol withdrawal should be managed appropriately if present or suspected. Nasogastric aspiration should be done to prepare the patient for endoscopy. It also contributes to the assessment of the severity of bleeding and keeps the GI tract relatively clear of blood that causes reflex splanchnic vasodilation and increase in portal pressures. Urine output and electrolytes should be closely monitored and the cardiopulmonary status maintained in a relatively stable state. Blood cultures should be drawn and a diagnostic paracentesis should be performed in those with ascites. A third-generation cephalosporin should be given intravenously to start with on empirical grounds. The use of prophylactic antibiotics pre or post endoscopic therapy following an acute bleeding episode has been studied in several controlled trials.[4-6] It has been seen that the use of antibiotics in this setting reduces mortality (relative risk 0.75, 95% CI) as well as incidence of bacterial infections (relative risk 0.4, 95% CI), such as spontaneous bacterial peritonitis, urinary tract infection, and septicemia.

Therapies to Achieve Hemostasis and Prevent Further Bleeding

The pharmacologic management of an acute variceal bleeding episode centers on the use of agents that reduce the portal pressure by causing splanchic vasoconstriction.

Somatostatin (250 μg IV bolus followed by 250 μg/hour) and octreotide (50 μg IV bolus followed by 50 μg/hour) causes decreased portal venous flow and portal pressures by inhibiting the actions of vasodilatory hormones. The effect begins immediately after administration of the bolus dosage and persists for the duration of the infusion. However, tachphylaxis has been reported both after repeated bolus injections and after infusion of octreotide. These agents reduce the risk of rebleeding in most studies if continued for up to 5 days after the initial bleed. In several studies, octreotide has been seen to be as effective as sclerotherapy for achieving hemostasis in acute variceal bleed. Adverse effects are usually mild and may include bradycardia, hyperglycemia, diarrhea, and abdominal cramps.

Vasopressin (0.4 U IV bolus followed by 0.4 to 1 U/hour) and its analogue terlipressin act by causing direct vasoconstriction of the mesenteric arterioles lowering the portal pressures and stopping variceal bleeding in 60% to 80% of the cases.[7] However, the use of vasopressin in the management of acute variceal bleeding is limited by its deleterious systemic vasoconstricting effect and the consequent cardiac, bowel, and cerebral ischemia. To counteract some of these unwanted systemic vasoconstrictions, systemic nitroglycerin has been used. Current recommendations advise that when used, vasopressin should always be combined with nitroglycerin (10 to 50 μg/min). Transdermal nitroglycerin is less effective than the intravenous form and the latter should be the preferred route if the management involves the use of vasopressin. Terlipressin has a better adverse effect profile than vasopressin and has also been shown to improve survival in the setting of acute variceal hemorrhage.[8] It is not currently available in the United States.

These medications have been seen in several studies to be more effective in the control of acute bleeding episodes than placebos.[9-11] However, when compared with one another somatostatin is preferred over vasopressin in the control of an acute bleed mainly due to its relative lack of adverse effects. Neither vasopressin nor somatostatin improves overall mortality.

Figure 2-2 presents treatment strategies for acute variceal hemorrhage.

Endoscopic Management

Currently, the definitive treatment of acute variceal hemorrhage involves either endoscopic sclerotherapy (EST) or band ligation (EVL). Both diagnostic as well therapeutic endoscopic procedures can be completed at the bedside with minimal risk of complications within 12 hours of an acute bleeding episode by an experienced endoscopist (Table 2-8).

Several randomized trials have demonstrated that sclerotherapy is superior to vasopressin, placebo and balloon tamponade and is as effective as somatostatin in achieving hemostasis.[12-17] The nature of the sclerosant (Na morrhuate, alcohol, Na teradecyl sulfate) and the type of injection (intra- vs paravariceal) does not influence the outcome of sclerotherapy. The combination of octreotide and EST is superior to EST alone for prevention of early rebleeding and for composite 5-day control of bleeding but does not improve survival. The common adverse effects of EST include ulceration, bleeding, esophageal stricture, dysmotility, esophageal perforation, mediastinitis, as well as sepsis. There is an increased incidence of portal hypertensive gastropathy following successful EST of esophageal varices.

Endoscopic variceal band ligation (EVL) involves the placement of elastic bands around varices in the lower 5 cm of the esophagus. It is more effective than EST in preventing the incidence of rebleeding, and has a lower risk of complications.[18,19]

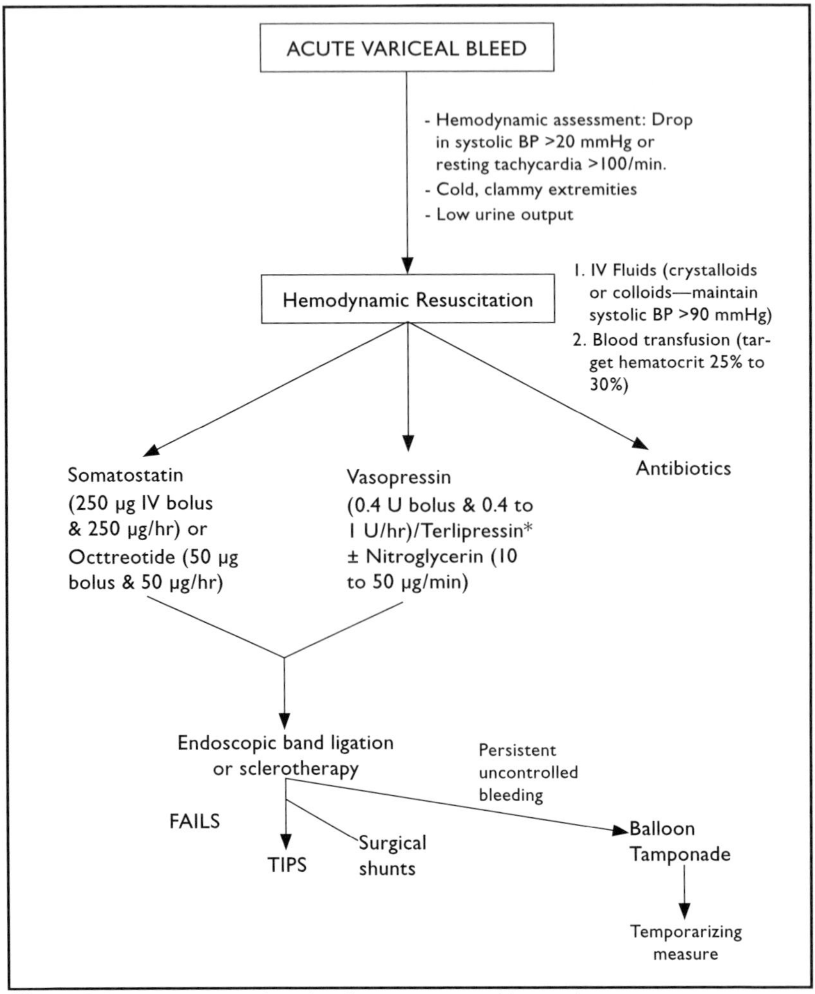

Figure 2-2. Management algorithm for acute variceal hemorrhage.

However, in the setting of acute bleeding, the efficacy of EVL is similar to that of EST. The main disadvantage of EVL during an acute bleeding episode is related to decreased field of vision with EVL. The combination of octreotide with EVL is superior to EVL alone for 5-day control of bleeding. However, the overall long-term mortality was similar in both groups. The current literature suggests that EVL is superior to EST in the long term, but insofar as an acute episode is concerned, either of these modalities are reasonable choices and the final decision depends on the expertise of the endoscopist and the local practices.

Table 2-8

FREQUENCY OF ENDOSCOPY IN CIRRHOTICS

1. Cirrhotics who have never bled: 2 to 3 years.
2. Cirrhotics who have documented varices and have never bled: 1 to 2 years.
3. Cirrhotics with history of variceal bleeding and moderate to large varices at endoscopy: endoscopic variceal ligation (EVL) every 2 to 3 weeks until the varices have been obliterated and then 3 to 6 monthly for 1 year, and if eradication persists, yearly thereafter.

Management of Refractory Variceal Hemorrhage

The incidence of failure of endoscopic therapy can be as high as 10% to 20%, and a second endoscopy with either sclerotherapy or band ligation may be a reasonable therapeutic option at that juncture. However, the recurrence of bleeding after the second procedure should prompt the use of either balloon tamponade or creation of porto-systemic shunts.

Balloon Tamponade

In the event of failure of endoscopic therapy or when endoscopic therapy is not recommended, balloon tamponade may be used as a temporizing measure before definitive measures can be instituted. Initial control of bleeding is achieved in 30% to 90% of patients. Several tubes are currently available. These typically have an esophageal and gastric port for aspiration and vary in the presence and size of the esophageal and gastric balloons. The airway needs to be protected by endotracheal intubation prior to insertion of the balloon to prevent aspiration of oral secretions. The major drawbacks of this procedure include a high incidence of rebleeding following deflation of the balloon and an increased risk of major complications such as esophageal rupture.

Transjugular Intrahepatic Porto-Systemic

Transjugular intrahepatic porto-systemic (TIPS) shunt involves the creation of a portacaval communication in the liver parenchyma that is kept patent by deployment of a metal stent across the tract via a transjugular route under local anesthesia. This procedure is indicated following an acute variceal bleed when there is failure of both pharmacologic and endoscopic therapy. It achieves control of bleeding in more than 90% of patients and survival in high-risk patients (poor surgical risks due to associated co-morbidities and/or advanced liver disease) both after the first week and at 30 days is better than what would have been observed following shunt surgery (63% vs 20%).[20] In patients who are otherwise good surgical candidates, the data are not conclusive, with some studies showing increased incidence of rebleeding and failure of therapy after TIPS compared to conventional surgical shunts.

TIPS also has a role in the prevention of variceal bleeding in those patients who have variceal hemorrhage despite two sessions of endoscopic therapy 2 weeks apart. Although the initial control of bleeding is greater than 90%, the long-term course is complicated by hepatic encephalopathy and inevitable TIPS stenosis. Also, it has no effect on survival and, at best, should be used as a bridge to liver transplantation in those patients that failed to respond to pharmacologic and endoscopic therapy.

The predominant problem with long-term use of TIPS is stenosis of the shunt requiring either angioplasty or replacement of the shunt. Patients with TIPS also have an increased incidence of hepatic encephalopathy following the procedure, requiring closer follow up. In addition, the cost of the procedure (~$26,000) and the need for ultrasound to determine patency during follow up, makes it only applicable in a selected subgroup of patients.

Surgical Shunts

These may be nonselective, selective, or partial and involve surgical decompression of the portal system. In nonselective shunts such as portacaval shunts, the entire portal system is decompressed, while both in the selective (distal spleno-renal) and partial shunts, there is selective decompression of the variceal system, while maintaining some degree of hepatic sinusoidal perfusion. The success rate for achieving hemostasis is very high with these procedures. The principal limitations of surgery include 1) lack of improvement in long-term survival, 2) development of encephalopathy in 30% to 50% of patients, and 3) increasing the technical difficulty of a subsequent liver transplant if surgery involving the hepatic hilum has been performed.

Gastric Varices

The management of bleeding gastric varices is similar in principle to esophageal variceal bleed, but is technically more difficult. The initial therapeutic strategy should include somatostatin or octreotide together with balloon tamponade and endoscopy is only necessary for establishing the initial diagnosis. In case of rebleeding, TIPS should be the first option, although it should be remembered that the presence of spleno-renal collaterals reduces the effectiveness of TIPS in this setting. Although several studies have looked at endoscopic therapeutic options (sclerosants, cyanoacrylate, banding, and intravariceal thrombin injections), they should currently be avoided except in settings of randomized controlled trials.

Prevention of Rebleeding

Pharmacologic agents such as nonselective β-blockers and oral nitrates started after hemodynamic stabilization following an acute variceal hemorrhage have been shown to reduce the risk of rebleeding. Nonselective β-blockers like propranolol or nadolol reduce the risk of rebleeding by approximately 40% while decreasing the risk of death by 20%.[21] A sustained drop in HVPG to values less than 12 mmHg or by 20% from baseline have been associated with a virtually 100% reduction in bleeding risk. Ideally, pharmacologic treatment should be monitored by HVPG measurements. However, this is not practical or feasible in many centers. In general, the dose of β-blockers is titrated to achieve a resting heart rate of approximately 60 beats per minute.

Oral nitrates by themselves are not indicated because they worsen the vasodilated state and have been associated with a higher mortality than β-blockers in those over the age of 50 years. On the other hand, combination therapy with a nonselective β-blocker and a nitrate has been shown to be more effective than sclerotherapy but do not improve survival.

EVL is currently the treatment of choice for the prevention of recurrent esophageal variceal hemorrhage. It is more effective than EST and accomplishes variceal eradication with fewer sessions of endoscopy. It is also associated with a trend toward improved survival in the long-term.

TIPS is generally reserved for those who have experienced recurrent bleeding despite adequate endoscopic variceal hemorrhage. In those with well-preserved liver functions, surgery may also be considered to be an option. For those who may be transplant candidates, a distal splenorenal shunt or mesocaval shunt is generally preferred because they do not involve extensive dissection of the hepatic hilum.

Summary of Recommendations

As a general rule, all survivors of a variceal bleed should be considered as potential candidates for liver transplant. Patients who have well compensated liver disease (Child-Pugh class A) should receive either a pharmacologic agent like a β-blocker with or without nitrates, or EVL. Patients who either fail these measures or are poor candidates of the same should be considered for surgical shunts or TIPS. In patients with advanced liver disease (Child-Pugh class B and C), EVL is the first-line treatment for prevention of recurrent bleeding. If EVL fails, a TIPS is performed ideally as a bridge to liver transplant.

Ascites

Ascites is one of the most common manifestations of cirrhosis with portal hypertension, and its appearance suggests the progression of the underlying liver disease. Ascites is associated with greater than 50% mortality at 2 years. The principal mechanism underlying the development of ascites is systemic arterial vasodilation. This typically is inversely related to the degree of portal hypertension. Systemic vasodilatation results in decreased effective blood volume due to redistribution of fluid in the vascular space. As a consequence, there is compensatory renal retention of sodium and water. Simultaneously, hepatic lymph flow increases based on Starling's forces resulting from sinusoidal hypertension. The excess Na and water ends up in the peritoneum as a result of increased hepatic lymph flow that overwhelms normal mechanisms to return to the circulation and spills into the peritoneal cavity.

In a patient presenting with ascites for the first time, analysis of ascitic fluid should be done to determine the underlying etiology. The tests that may provide useful information in the initial assessment of the patient with ascites includes serum albumin to ascitic fluid albumin gradient (SAAG), cell count, total protein levels, and ascitic fluid culture. Of these tests, SAAG provides the most useful information regarding the etiology of ascites. A value ≥1.1 diagnoses portal hypertension as an etiology in the formation of ascites with a sensitivity and specificity greater than 95%.[22,23] The low albumin level in ascites reflects the deposition of collagen and a basement membrane under the sinusoidal endothelium and ultrastructural changes in the endothelium itself, which decreases the permeability of the sinusoidal wall and decreases protein content of the hepatic lymph.

Therapeutic interventions used in the management of ascites includes both measures to reduce portal hypertension, as well as correction of the neurohormonal abnormalities associated with this sodium and water retention. The various management strategies used in the treatment of ascites include 1) dietary sodium restriction, 2) diuretics, 3) large volume paracentesis, 4) TIPS, and 5) peritoneo-venous shunts.

Sodium Restriction

Sodium restriction forms the cornerstone in the management of ascites as renal sodium and water retention is the initiating pathophysiological trigger. Failure to comply with Na restriction may markedly decrease the efficacy of diuretic therapy. Hence it is recommended that all patients who have ascites be put on a 2 gm/day (88 mmol) Na restricted diet.[23,24] However, sodium restriction alone is rarely successful in achieving control of ascites and should always be used as an adjunct to other therapeutic strategies. When a patient accumulates more ascites despite Na restriction and diuretic therapy, it is often valuable to check urinary Na excretion. When ascites worsens despite an alleged negative Na balance, dietary noncompliance should be suspected.

Diuretics

Diuretics are the initial therapy of choice in the management of mild-to-moderate ascites. The optimal diuretic choice should include a potassium sparing diuretic in combination with a loop diuretic. In cirrhosis due to the presence of hyperaldosteronism and increased sodium delivery to the distal tubules, potassium sparing diuretics such as spironolactone are more effective than normally more potent loop diuretics like furosemide.

The aim of diuretic therapy is to achieve a weight loss of ~1kg/day in patients with both ascites and peripheral edema and 0.5 kg/day if only ascites is present. The initial starting dosage of spironolactone is 50 to 100 mg/day given as a single daily dosage increasing to a maximum of 400 mg/day. The half-life of spironolactone is 3 days and hence multiple daily dosing is not required in achieving therapeutic serum levels. A therapeutic response is seen in more than 75% of patients and the most common adverse effect is gynecomastia.[25,26] In patients with renal impairment, hyperkalemia and metabolic acidosis may complicate therapy and force cessation of treatment. Tamoxifen, used in the dosage of 20 mg/day has been shown in a double-blind study to be useful in the treatment of spironolactone induced gynecomastia.[27] In patients who are unable to tolerate spironolactone or in whom spironolactone is contraindicated, another distally acting diuretic such as amiloride can be used in the dosage of 5 to 20 mg/day. Furosemide is usually started at 40 mg/day and increased to a maximum of 160 mg/day. The major complications that are observed are hyponatremia, hypokalemia and azotemia.

The term refractory ascites is used to describe the failure to lose 1.5 kg/day in weight despite therapy for 1 week with 160 mg/day of furosemide and 400 mg/day of spironolactone or failure of targeted weight loss due to inability to use maximal diuretic dosage as a result of appearance of diuretic associated complications. The options that can be used include large volume paracentesis (LVP), TIPS, and peritoneovenous shunts.

Large Volume Paracentesis

This is currently the therapeutic procedure of choice in dealing with tense or refractory ascites. It involves the removal of >5L of ascitic fluid up to every 2 weeks. The major complications include postparacentesis circulatory dysfunction (PPCD), azotemia and electrolyte abnormalities. PPCD is seen after removal of >5 L of ascitic fluid and is manifested by azotemia, hyponatremia, and elevated renin levels. The risk of PPCD may be decreased by the concurrent administration of 6 to 8 g of albumin intravenously per liter of ascitic fluid removed. Other synthetic plasma volume expanders such as dextran and polygeline have been found to be inferior to albumin. Unless clinically symptomatic and severe coagulopathy exists, LVP can usually be performed safely. In general, it is not necessary to correct coagulopathy before an LVP in most cases.

TIPS

In patients with refractory ascites, TIPS is the recommended primarily as a bridge to liver transplantation in those in whom LVP is unsuccessful in achieving an adequate ascites free interval. Following TIPS, diuresis occurs gradually over the next few weeks and involves decreased proximal tubular Na reabsorption. Once ascites is mobilized, an ascites-free state can often be maintained as long as the shunt is patent and the patient continues to restrict Na intake. When liver failure develops in a person with a functioning TIPS, it often manifests as worsening edema.

Although TIPS corrects some of the neurohormonal abnormalities associated with portal hypertension, it does not affect overall outcome or long-term survival. The mortality following TIPS is particularly high when renal or florid liver failure is present. Thus, TIPS is a poor treatment option for those with a bilirubin >3 mg/dL, an INR >2 and a serum creatinine >2 mg/dL.

Peritoneovenous Shunts

This involves the placement of a silicone tube with a pressure sensitive one way valve between the peritoneal cavity and the thoracic venous system. It has largely been abandoned due to poor patency rate and high-risk of serious complications without any obvious survival benefits. Moreover, it complicates subsequent liver transplantation by causing peritoneal fibrosis in about a third of patients.[28]

Complications of Ascites

Spontaneous Bacterial Peritonitis

Spontaneous bacterial peritonitis (SBP) refers to bacterial infection of the ascitic fluid without the presence of a surgically treatable cause in a patient with advanced cirrhosis. It is associated with development of hepatorenal syndrome and a mortality rate of up to 20%. The predominant mechanism involved in the genesis of SBP involves bacterial translocation across an edematous gut wall to the mesenteric lymph nodes and subsequent peritoneal seeding. A diagnostic paracentesis should be performed in all patients with new onset ascites, hospitalized patients with ascites and those with ascites and clinical deterioration. Based on the results of the ascitic fluid analysis SBP has been classified in to several subgroups (see Table 2-7). The presence of either a positive ascitic fluid culture for a single organism or ascitic fluid polymorphonuclear leukocyte count ≥250 forms the underlying basis for this classification. The routine use of blood culture bottles for ascitic fluid culture increases the rate of positive culture and may help to optimize the appropriate antimicrobial therapy. The presence of a polymicrobial flora in the ascitic fluid indicates secondary bacterial peritonitis due to perforation of gut mucosa during paracentesis or due to a pathologic process. Therapy should be instituted with any third generation cephalosporins in a suspected patient soon after the diagnostic paracentesis and continued for at least 7 to 10 days if the diagnosis of SBP is confirmed. In clinically stable patients, particularly those with incidentally diagnosed SBP, alternate antibiotic choices include oral therapy with quinolones, and amoxicillin-clavulanic acid combination have been used successfully.

If there is a failure of clinical improvement after 48 hours of antibiotic therapy, repeat paracentesis should be considered. About 30% to 40% of patients who get SBP go on to develop renal dysfunction which is a leading cause of morbidity in this group of patients. High doses of albumin (1 g/kg), along with appropriate antibiotic therapy, reduce the incidence of renal dysfunction and improve in hospital as well as 3-month mortality.[29] However, given the high cost of albumin and the large number of patients with ascites and SBP, it remains to be seen whether this will be a cost-effective measure in an unselected group of patients with SBP.

Patients with cirrhosis and upper gastrointestinal bleeding are vulnerable to an SBP and should receive primary prophylaxis with an oral quinolone (eg, norfloxacin [400 mg/day for 10 to 14 days]). In those who survive an episode of SBP, the risk of recurrence is approximately 70%, which provides the rationale for secondary prophylaxis. This is also usually accomplished with an orally-administered quinolone (eg, norfloxacin or ciprofloxacin). Trimethoprim-sulfamethoxazole has been used successfully for secondary prophylaxis of SBP.

Hepato Renal Syndrome

Hepato renal syndrome (HRS) is defined as progressive renal dysfunction in patients with advanced liver disease and portal hypertension with histologically normal appearing kidneys. Intense renal vasoconstriction in response splanchic vasodilatation and low systemic arterial pressure is considered to be the pathophysiologic basis for the appearance of this syndrome. In contrast to acute tubular necrosis, the tubular function is preserved and accounts for the intense sodium and water retention that is observed in this state.

Clinically, two forms of HRS are recognized: Type I HRS is defined by a greater than 100% increase in the serum creatinine levels to a value ≥2.5 mg/dL within a span of less than 2 weeks. This is associated with a greater than 90% mortality unless a liver transplant is performed. Type II HRS includes all those patients with renal impairment but who do not meet the criteria for type I HRS. The progression of renal impairment is much slower in these patients and the predominant problem is progressively increasing refractory ascites. The underlying pathophysiology in Type I HRS and Type II HRS is similar (Figure 2-3).

HRS may be precipitated in any patient with advanced cirrhosis in whom there is an episode of circulatory dysfunction and renal hypoperfusion. However the common precipitating factors include an episode of spontaneous bacterial peritonitis (SBP), an upper gastrointestinal bleed, or PPCD. HRS typically presents with rising serum creatinine levels (≥2.5 mg/dL) and low urinary sodium levels (<10 meq/L). Moreover, as features of prerenal azotemia is very similar to HRS, the patient should be withdrawn from diuretics or other nephrotoxic agents and given an adequate trial of volume expansion before making the diagnoses of HRS.

The prognosis of HRS is dependant on the type of HRS and the stage of liver disease (Child-Pugh score). Patients with type I HRS have an in hospital mortality rate close to 90%, and most die within 2 weeks unless they receive a liver transplant.[30] In addition, patients with advanced liver disease (Childs-Pugh score >13) and HRS have a worse prognosis compared to those with less severe hepatocellular dysfunction. However, patients with HRS have a higher MELD score and, consequently, greater probability of receiving a liver transplant, even though they may have a relatively preserved liver function.

The use of albumin (1.5 g/kg on day 1 and 1 g/kg 48 hours later) along with antibiotics in the management of hospitalized patients with SBP has been shown to reduce the incidence of HRS and improve survival in comparison to antibiotics alone.[29] However, given the high cost of albumin, further evidence is needed from larger studies before this recommendation can be implemented in to the management algorithm.

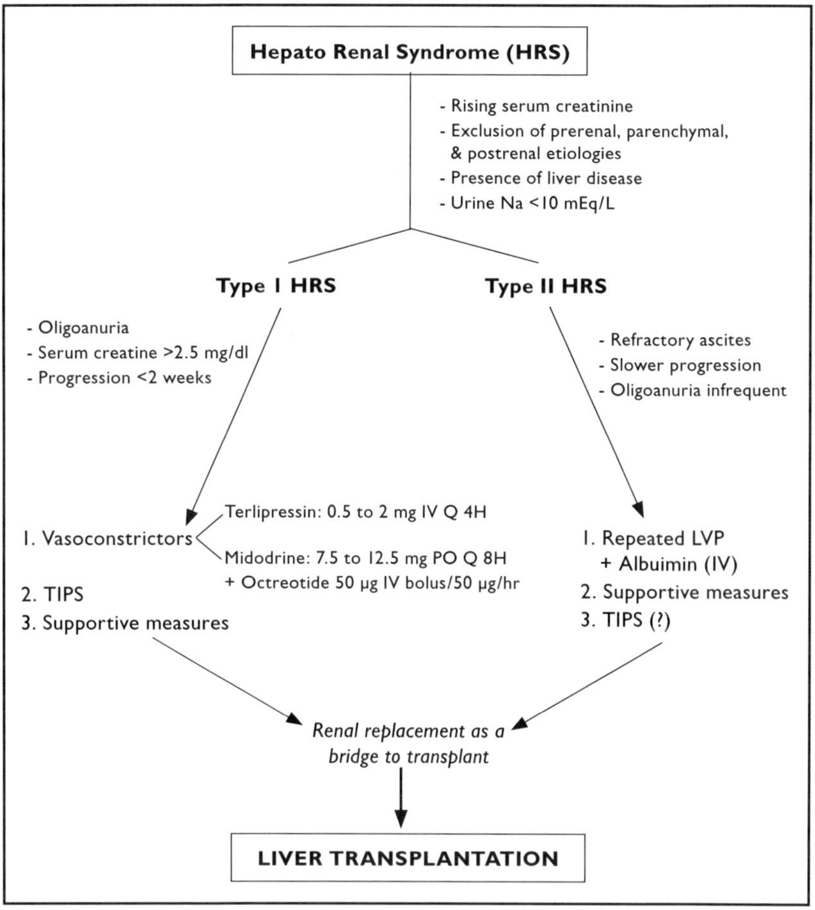

Figure 2-3. Management of hepato renal syndrome.

In patients with alcoholic hepatitis, pentoxyfylline (400 mg tid) has reduced the incidence of HRS when compared to control subjects.[31]

The definitive treatment that reverses the renal impairment in both type I and II HRS is orthotopic liver transplant (OLT). Hence, patients who have no contraindications should be assessed and early referral made to a transplant center. Supportive measures that have been found useful in HRS include fluid and salt restriction, use of vasoconstrictors (eg, terlipressin, norepinephrine, or midodrine) and TIPS. The presence of profound splanchnic vasodilatation and consequent activation of endogenous vasoconstrictor system provides the rationale behind the effectiveness of this form of therapy. In numerous small reports, various systemic vasoconstrictors have been found to produce, at least short-term, improvement in renal function. Of all the agents used, the greatest published experience is with terlipressin. The agent that has been most widely studied in this group of disorders is terlipressin, a synthetic long acting vasopressin analogue. This is used in the dosage range of 0.5 to 2 mg IV every 4 hours and can be continued up to 15 days. In type I HRS, this agent has been shown to bring about improvement in renal function and urine output in 50% to 75% of the patients.[32,33] The incidence of adverse effects is about 5% to 10% and mainly includes bowel and cardiac ischemic complications. Despite the current popularity of octreotide and midodrine for HRS, there are very limited published data to support its use on a large-scale basis. It is also currently unclear if the observed biochemical improvements following any type of vasoconstrictor therapy reflect a short-term reprieve or a true cure for the HRS. In type II HRS, the effectiveness of vasoconstrictors has not been clearly established and its use is currently not recommended on a routine basis.

The value of TIPS in well-established type I HRS remains controversial. Again, the principle mechanism behind the effectiveness of TIPS is lowering of portal pressures and removal of stimulus for endogenous vasoconstriction. Limited data suggest that, in type I HRS, TIPS brings about improvement in renal function in about 60% of patients but there are no data to suggest that this translates into improved survival. Hence, the role of TIPS remains experimental or as a last-ditch effort to save a dying patient.

Supportive measures in the setting of acute onset HRS in patients that do not respond to medical therapy include various forms of renal replacement therapies. Acute hemodialysis in this group of patients is associated with a high mortality due to increased risk of hypotension and circulatory dysfunction, and, therefore, should be avoided as an initial measure in majority. However, continuous veno-venous or arterio-venous hemofiltration may be successfully used in selected patients as a bridge to eventual transplant.

Hepatic Encephalopathy

Hepatic encephalopathy (HE) refers to a heterogenous group of nonspecific abnormalities of central nervous system (CNS) function that are observed in patients with advanced hepatocellular failure. It can present acutely with confusion and coma, or more chronically with cognitive disturbances and abnormalities of higher mental function detectable on neuropsychiatric assessment. Interference with neural transmission in the CNS by nitrogenous substances derived from the gut as a result of either impaired clearance from the liver or porta-systemic shunting forms the pathophysiologic basis for development of HE. In an acute setting, it usually follows a specific precipitating factor such as gastrointestinal bleed, sepsis, SBP, or constipation, but occasionally, specific causal factors may not be apparent. On the other hand, recurrent episodes of HE in the absence of specific precipitating factors should raise the suspicion of a spontaneous splenorenal shunt. HE should be a diagnosis of exclusion as there are no specific clinical or biochemical indicators specific for its diagnosis and other metabolic and structural causes of CNS dysfunction always needs to be excluded.

Elevated arterial levels of ammonia can be used as an initial diagnostic aid, but currently there is no role for serial monitoring of blood ammonia levels in the diagnostic conundrum of HE. This is mainly due to increased permeability of blood-brain barrier in cirrhotics to ammonia and the fact that the some of the neurotoxic effects of ammonia occur after its metabolism in the astrocytes. Both these factors result in poor correlation between the levels of ammonia in the peripheral circulation and the actual central nervous system effects seen in patients with HE.

The principal tenet in the management of HE involves reduction of the nitrogenous load entering the portal circulation from the gut. While protein restriction was widely used in the past to reduce the nitrogenous burden, it has a very limited role in the current management of HE because of the adverse effects related to malnutrition associated with a very low protein diet. Routinely, patients should be advised a protein intake of 1 to 1.5 g/kg of body weight and nutritional advice should be sought for substituting vegetable protein in place of animal protein. The use of branched chain amino acids and zinc supplementation has been seen in small nonrandomized trials to have some beneficial effects in selected patients but recommendations regarding the use of these compounds in the routine management of HE cannot be made at this time.

The mainstay of treatment for HE are nonabsorbable disaccharides such as lactulose that lower the intraluminal pH of the gut (pH ~5), thus favoring the conversion of ammonia (NH3) to nonabsorbable ammonium ion (NH4). This traps the ammonia in the bowel lowering the ammonia levels in the portal circulation. In addition, lactulose also acts as an osmotic laxative and inhibits colonic bacterial growth. Clinically, these therapeutic goals can be achieved by titrating the dose of lactulose to have 2 to 4 soft bowel movements per day (15 to 30 mL of lactulose 4 to 6 hourly). Bowel decontamination can also be achieved with the use of poorly absorbable antibiotics such as neomycin or metronidazole. These antibiotics are as effective as lactulose alone in head to head comparison. In addition prolonged use of these antibiotics is associated with a small but significant risk of adverse effects such as renal failure with neomycin and painful neuropathy with metronidazole. Flumazenil, a CNS GABA receptor antagonist, has been used in those patients with acute HE secondary to benzodiazepine use but there are no data to support its routine use in all patients with HE. The 1-year mortality rate following HE is close to 40% and hence every effort should be made to refer those who are eligible to the nearest transplant center for OLT (Figure 2-4).

Coagulopathy

In cirrhosis, coagulopathy develops from decreased synthesis of factors II, V, VII, IX, and X. Spontaneous deep tissue hemorrhage is rarely a problem in these patients. Clinically, international normalized ratio (INR) is most useful parameter that is used to monitor the bleeding risk prior to invasive procedures in this subgroup of patients. An INR value of <1.4 is considered to be acceptable for performing most endoscopic procedures including sphincterotomies and polypectomies. In those that require invasive procedures acutely, current recommendations advise the use of fresh frozen plasma (FFP) to correct the coagulopathy. The drawbacks of FFP including volume overload can be avoided by the use of recombinant human factor VIIa (rFVIIa) which has been shown to produce a rapid correction of coagulopathy. However, widespread use of this product is limited by its high cost and is not recommended as an initial therapeutic option.

Thrombocytopenia and qualitative platelet dysfunction also contributes to the coagulopathy seen in cirrhotic patients. Platelet transfusion is recommended prior to high-risk therapeutic procedures when the platelet count is below 50,000 per µl. However, most low risk procedures such as mucosal biopsies can be done with plate-

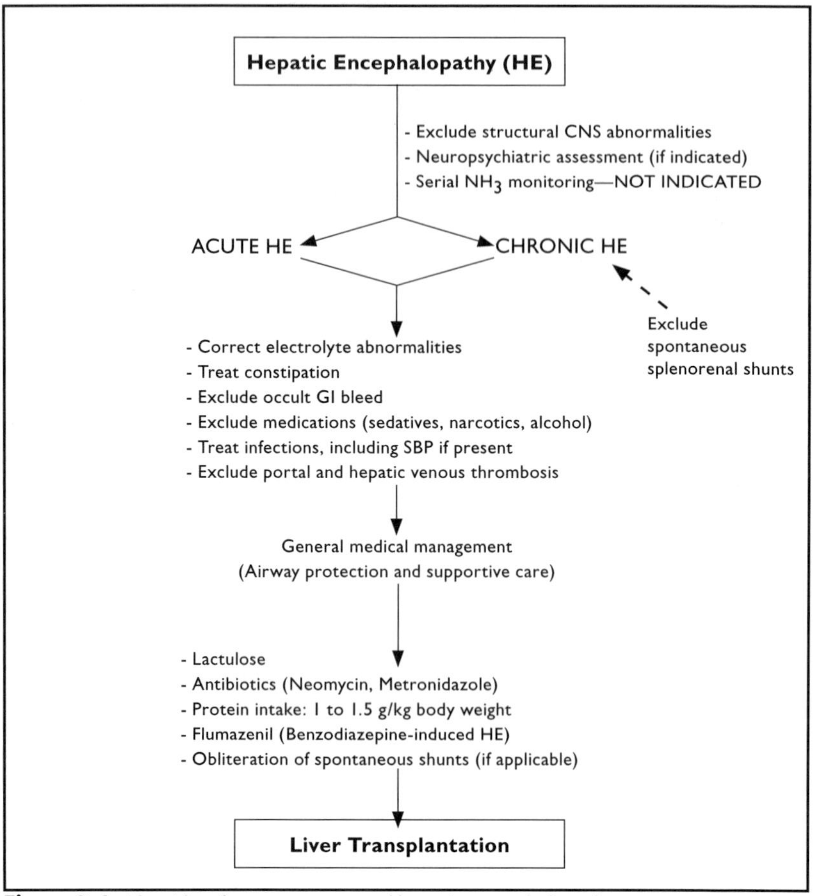

Figure 2-4. Algorithm for management of hepatic encephalopathy.

let counts of up to 20,000 per µL.[34] If qualitative platelet dysfunction is suspected, DDAVP (desmopressin) may be used.

In summary, cirrhosis is the end result of hepatic injury from a wide variety of causes. Early detection and aggressive treatment of various complications associated with cirrhosis forms the cornerstone of the management of this condition. Institution of prophylactic measures and lifestyle modifications, where applicable retards the development of deleterious complications and should be pursued aggressively. In addition, early referral of eligible patients for liver transplant has a major impact on the overall survival and should always form a part of the therapeutic algorithm.

This work is supported in part by two grants from the National Institute of Health (K 24 DK 02755-04 and T-32 DK 007150-27) to Dr. Sanyal

References

1. Wiesner R, Edwards E, Freeman R, et al. Model for end-stage liver disease (MELD) and allocation of donor livers. *Gastroenterology.* 2003;124(1):91-96.
2. de Dombal FT, Clarke JR, Clamp SE, et al. Prognostic factors in upper G.I. bleeding. *Endoscopy.* 1986;18 Suppl 2:6-10.
3. Smith JL, Graham DY. Variceal hemorrhage: a critical evaluation of survival analysis. *Gastroenterology.* 1982;82(5 Pt 1):968-973.
4. Soares-Weiser K, Brezis M, Tur-Kaspa R, Leibovici L. Antibiotic prophylaxis for cirrhotic patients with gastrointestinal bleeding. *Cochrane Database Syst Rev.* 2002;(2): CD002907.
5. Pauwels A, Mostefa-Kara N, Debenes B, Degoutte E, Levy VG. Systemic antibiotic prophylaxis after gastrointestinal hemorrhage in cirrhotic patients with a high risk of infection. *Hepatology.* 1996;24(4):802-806.
6. Soares-Weiser K, Brezis M, Tur-Kaspa R, et al. Antibiotic prophylaxis of bacterial infections in cirrhotic inpatients: a meta-analysis of randomized controlled trials. *Scand J Gastroenterol.* 2003;38(2):193-200.
7. Gimson AE, Westaby D, Hegarty J, Watson A, Williams R. A randomized trial of vasopressin and vasopressin plus nitroglycerin in the control of acute variceal hemorrhage. *Hepatology.* 1986;6(3):410-413.
8. Escorsell A, Ruiz dA, Planas R, et al. Multicenter randomized controlled trial of terlipressin versus sclerotherapy in the treatment of acute variceal bleeding: the TEST study. *Hepatology.* 2000;32(3):471-476.
9. Imperiale TF, Teran JC, McCullough AJ. A meta-analysis of somatostatin versus vasopressin in the management of acute esophageal variceal hemorrhage. *Gastroenterology.* 1995;109(4):1289-1294.
10. Grace ND. Diagnosis and treatment of gastrointestinal bleeding secondary to portal hypertension. American College of Gastroenterology Practice Parameters Committee. *Am J Gastroenterol.* 1997;92(7):1081-1091.
11. Gotzsche PC. Somatostatin or octreotide for acute bleeding oesophageal varices. *Cochrane Database Syst Rev.* 2000;(2):CD000193.
12. Planas R, Quer JC, Boix J, et al. A prospective randomized trial comparing somatostatin and sclerotherapy in the treatment of acute variceal bleeding. *Hepatology.* 1994;20(2):370-375.
13. Sung JJ, Chung SC, Lai CW, et al. Octreotide infusion or emergency sclerotherapy for variceal haemorrhage. *Lancet.* 1993;342(8872):637-641.
14. Besson I, Ingrand P, Person B, et al. Sclerotherapy with or without octreotide for acute variceal bleeding. *N Engl J Med.* 1995;333(9):555-560.
15. Primignani M, Andreoni B, Carpinelli L, et al. Sclerotherapy plus octreotide versus sclerotherapy alone in the prevention of early rebleeding from esophageal varices: a randomized, double-blind, placebo-controlled, multicenter trial. New Italian Endoscopic Club. *Hepatology.* 1995;21(5):1322-1327.
16. Villanueva C, Ortiz J, Sabat M, et al. Somatostatin alone or combined with emergency sclerotherapy in the treatment of acute esophageal variceal bleeding: a prospective randomized trial. *Hepatology.* 1999;30(2):384-389.
17. Hunt PS, Korman MG, Hansky J, Parkin WG. An 8-year prospective experience with balloon tamponade in emergency control of bleeding esophageal varices. *Dig Dis Sci.* 1982;27(5):413-416.

18. Laine L, Cook D. Endoscopic ligation compared with sclerotherapy for treatment of esophageal variceal bleeding. A meta-analysis. *Ann Intern Med.* 1995;123(4):280-287.
19. Saeed ZA, Stiegmann GV, Ramirez FC, et al. Endoscopic variceal ligation is superior to combined ligation and sclerotherapy for esophageal varices: a multicenter prospective randomized trial. *Hepatology.* 1997;25(1):71-74.
20. Sanyal AJ, Freedman AM, Luketic VA, et al. Transjugular intrahepatic portosystemic shunts for patients with active variceal hemorrhage unresponsive to sclerotherapy. *Gastroenterology.* 1996;111(1):138-146.
21. Westaby D, Polson RJ, Gimson AE, Hayes PC, Hayllar K, Williams R. A controlled trial of oral propranolol compared with injection sclerotherapy for the long-term management of variceal bleeding. *Hepatology.* 1990;11(3):353-359.
22. Runyon BA, Montano AA, Akriviadis EA, Antillon MR, Irving MA, McHutchison JG. The serum-ascites albumin gradient is superior to the exudate-transudate concept in the differential diagnosis of ascites. *Ann Intern Med.* 1992;117(3):215-220.
23. Runyon BA. Care of patients with ascites. *N Engl J Med.* 1994;330(5):337-342.
24. Runyon BA. Management of adult patients with ascites caused by cirrhosis. *Hepatology.* 1998;27(1):264-272.
25. Perez-Ayuso RM, Arroyo V, Planas R, et al. Randomized comparative study of efficacy of furosemide versus spironolactone in nonazotemic cirrhosis with ascites. Relationship between the diuretic response and the activity of the renin-aldosterone system. *Gastroenterology.* 1983;84(5 Pt 1):961-968.
26. Santos J, Planas R, Pardo A, et al. Spironolactone alone or in combination with furosemide in the treatment of moderate ascites in nonazotemic cirrhosis. A randomized comparative study of efficacy and safety. *J Hepatol.* 2003;39(2):187-192.
27. Li CP, Lee FY, Hwang SJ, et al. Treatment of mastalgia with tamoxifen in male patients with liver cirrhosis: a randomized crossover study. *Am J Gastroenterol.* 2000; 95(4):1051-1055.
28. Gines P, Arroyo V, Vargas V, et al. Paracentesis with intravenous infusion of albumin as compared with peritoneovenous shunting in cirrhosis with refractory ascites. *N Engl J Med.* 1991;325(12):829-835.
29. Sort P, Navasa M, Arroyo V, et al. Effect of intravenous albumin on renal impairment and mortality in patients with cirrhosis and spontaneous bacterial peritonitis. *N Engl J Med.* 1999;341(6):403-409.
30. Gines A, Escorsell A, Gines P, et al. Incidence, predictive factors, and prognosis of the hepatorenal syndrome in cirrhosis with ascites. *Gastroenterology.* 1993;105(1):229-236.
31. Akriviadis E, Botla R, Briggs W, Han S, Reynolds T, Shakil O. Pentoxifylline improves short-term survival in severe acute alcoholic hepatitis: a double-blind, placebo-controlled trial. *Gastroenterology.* 2000;119(6):1637-1648.
32. Moreau R, Durand F, Poynard T, et al. Terlipressin in patients with cirrhosis and type 1 hepatorenal syndrome: a retrospective multicenter study. *Gastroenterology.* 2002; 122(4):923-930.
33. Ortega R, Gines P, Uriz J, et al. Terlipressin therapy with and without albumin for patients with hepatorenal syndrome: results of a prospective, nonrandomized study. *Hepatology.* 2002;36(4 Pt 1):941-948.
34. Van Os EC, Kamath PS, Gostout CJ, Heit JA. Gastroenterological procedures among patients with disorders of hemostasis: evaluation and management recommendations. *Gastrointest Endosc.* 1999;50(4):536-543.

chapter **3**

Acute and Chronic Viral Hepatitis

Barbara A. Piasecki, MD, MSCE

Hepatitis A

Background

Hepatitis A (HAV) is spread by the fecal-oral route and is responsible for outbreaks of infectious hepatitis, and is an important public health issue today. Worldwide, approximately 1.4 million people are affected by hepatitis A each year. Infection with HAV is usually symptomatic and results in significant morbidity and economic costs. While it was probably responsible for epidemic jaundice going far back in history, it was first identified in 1973 by a group at the National Institutes of Health. Unlike some of the other hepatotrophic viruses, hepatitis A can be grown in cell culture. As a result, it was possible to develop a vaccination against hepatitis A that has been widely available for clinical practice since the early 1990s.

Hepatitis A is distinguished from the other hepatotrophic viruses by its fecal-oral transmission route and the fact that it usually causes only acute, self-limited hepatitis that may occur in individuals or on an epidemic scale. The hepatitis A virus is an effective pathogen that can be shed in the stool and resist environmental degradation. This promotes its survival and spread. HAV is usually spread through inter-personal contact with an infected individual. It is more prevalent among lower socioeconomic groups and institutionalized individuals, particularly children and mentally handicapped, where group-living and available sanitation and hygiene standards may facilitate spread. HAV has not been reported to spread from mother to fetus, and it is not usually spread sexually. Infection of water supplies may lead to contamination of shellfish and to larger community outbreaks of HAV.

Clinical Picture

HAV typically causes an acute, symptomatic hepatitis that is self-limited. The clinical picture of HAV may be very similar to that of acute hepatitis B (HBV) or hepatitis C (HCV). Symptoms may include jaundice, anorexia, fatigue, malaise, abdominal pain, nausea, vomiting, fever, and myalgias. Rarely, HAV may evolve into acute fulminant hepatitis. The spectrum of the clinical picture in HAV may be related to the age of the individual infected. Children are more likely to have a subclinical or less symptomatic course compared to adults who are more likely to develop jaundice and to have clearly identifiable symptoms.

After exposure to the virus the incubation period before symptoms develop is usually approximately 4 weeks. Jaundice usually peaks approximately 2 weeks after symptom onset, and the other symptoms usually abate by the time jaundice has fully developed. The course of HAV infection is likely to be more severe if there is concomitant other liver disease. It is for this reason that individuals known to have chronic liver disease, such as hepatitis C, are advised to get immunized against HAV because they are far less likely to tolerate the infection well.

HAV is not always an acute self-limited condition. Less commonly, HAV may cause prolonged cholestasis where jaundice lasts more than 12 weeks. This may be associated with protracted other symptoms. Cholestatic HAV may still resolve spontaneously and steroids have been used in such cases. Another unusual course is a relapsing hepatitis A infection. This has been reported to occur in 6% to 12% of cases where after initial remission there is a relapse of symptoms occurring approximately 4 to 15 weeks later. During these relapses, transaminases may be remarkably elevated, as during the initial infection. It is not entirely clear why this occurs.

Diagnosis

History

In cases of acute HAV, there may be history that contributes to making the diagnosis. This may include having contact with someone already known to have recent HAV infection, having contact with children or institutionalized individuals, a community outbreak of jaundice and hepatitis, or travel to an area where HAV is endemic. Regions in the US where HAV is more common include Southwestern states (ie, California, Nevada, New Mexico, Arizona), Washington, and Alaska.

Physical Examination

Physical examination of a person with acute HAV infection may reveal jaundice and hepatomegaly, which occurs in most individuals. Other physical exam findings may include splenomegaly, an evanescent rash, arthritis, cervical lymphadenopathy, and leukocytoclastic vasculitis.

Serologic Tests

Serologic tests play an important role in helping to make the diagnosis of acute HAV infection. The hallmark of acute HAV infection is the detection of anti-HAV immunoglobulin M (anti-HAV IgM). This antibody remains detectable in the blood for 4 to 6 months following exposure to HAV. As the anti-HAV IgM level decreases, the IgG form of the antibody (anti-HAV IgG) increases and remains detectable for decades (Figure 3-1).

In addition to antibody tests, it can be useful to examine other liver-associated laboratory tests to help make the diagnoses. The transaminases, alanine aminotrans-

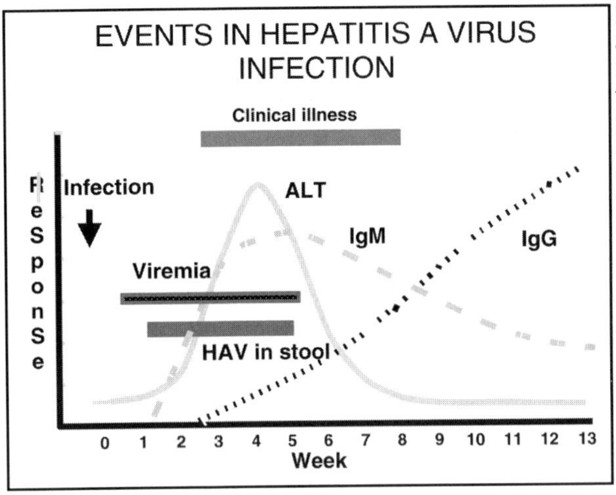

Figure 3-1. Serologic and clinical profile after infection with hepatitis A. (Reprinted with permission from the US Department of Health and US Sevices Centers for Disease Control and Prevention.)

ferase (ALT) and aspartate aminotransferase (AST) are usually greater than 1000 IU/dL with ALT usually higher than AST. The total and direct bilirubin levels may be elevated and may exceed 10mg/dL. Typically the transaminases elevations occur sooner than the hyperbilirubinemia.

The Role of Liver Biopsy

Liver biopsy is not usually required to make the diagnosis of acute HAV. This diagnosis can usually be made based on the history, clinical picture, and blood tests.

Management and Treatment

The main aspect of managing cases of acute HAV infection is supportive care. A minority of patients may require hospitalization. HAV infection is usually self-limited and most cases (~85%) will have full recovery within 3 months and nearly all will be recovered within 6 months.

Prognosis and Complications

The severity of HAV infection is dependent at least in part on the age of the individual. Fatalities due to HAV are more common with increasing age although the overall fatality rate for individuals above the age of 40 years of age is less than 2%. HAV infection may have a more severe course in individuals who have underlying chronic liver disease prior to infection with HAV.

Complications of HAV infection may include fulminant hepatitis occurring in 1% to 5%. The extrahepatic manifestations of HAV infection included vasculities, arthritis, aplastic anemia, red cell aplasia, optic neuritis, transverse myelitis, and thrombocytopenia.

Table 3-1

MEASURES TO TRY TO PREVENT THE TRANSMISSION OF HEPATITIS A

- Hygiene (eg, hand washing)
- Sanitation (eg, clean water sources)
- Hepatitis A vaccine (pre-exposure)
- Immune globulin (pre- and post-exposure)

Reprinted with permission from the US Department of Health and Human Services Centers for Disease Control and Prevention.

Table 3-2

RECOMMENDATIONS ON WHO SHOULD RECEIVE HEPATITIS A VACCINE

Advisory Committee on Immunization Practices of the CDC recommendations of persons at increased risk who should be routinely vaccinated with the hepatitis A vaccine:

- International travelers
- Men who have sex with men
- Illegal drug users
- Persons who have occupational risk for exposure—persons working with HAV infected primates or HAV in a research laboratory
- Persons who have clotting factor disorders and are administered clotting-factor concentrates
- Persons with chronic liver disease

PREVENTION AND POSTEXPOSURE PROPHYLAXIS

Prevention of HAV is possible because the virus is spread primarily by the fecal-oral route, and an effective and safe vaccine is available. Some general guidelines for preventing HAV have been proposed by the Centers for Disease Control (CDC)[1] (Table 3-1). The vaccine is an inactivated virus vaccine that is highly immunogenic leading to effective immunity in nearly 100% of cases after the 2 prescribed doses of the vaccine. This protective immunity is estimated to last approximately 20 years and booster vaccination is not recommended at this time. The Advisory Committee on Immunization Practices (ACIP) for the CDC has made recommendations on persons at increased risk for HAV who should be receive the vaccine (Table 3-2).

If an individual has had an exposure to an infected person then anti-HAV immunoglobulin (Ig) can be given to confer passive protective immunity immediately. This

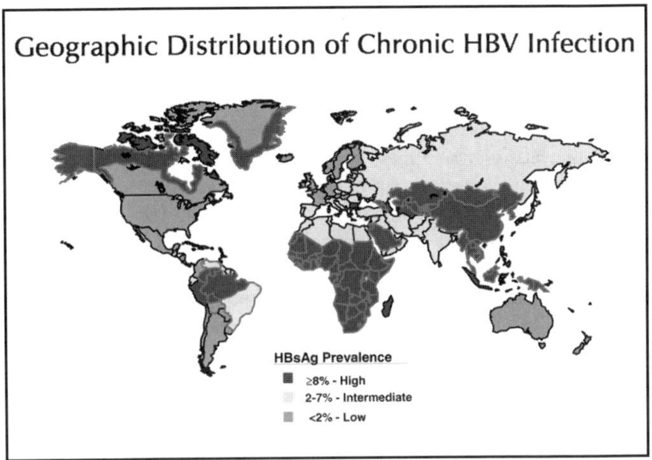

Figure 3-2. Geographic distribution of chronic hepatitis B infection. (Reprinted with permission from the US Department of Health and US Services Centers for Disease Control and Prevention.)

must be given within 2 weeks of the exposure. It is highly effective and may prevent infection in 85% to 95% of exposed persons. The disadvantage of using such post-exposure prophylaxis is the cost, injection site pain, the need for repeat dosing in order to maintain immunity beyond 3 to 6 months, and the risk associated with receiving a pooled blood product. The main individuals who are candidates of anti-HAV Ig are unvaccinated travelers to endemic areas and household contacts of known acute HAV cases. It is not necessary to confirm that these individuals are HAV IgG negative before administering the anti-HAV Ig because waiting on these serologic tests will simply delay treatment and decrease the benefits of preventing HAV in the negative cases since the Ig must be given in a timely fashion. In such cases, anti-HAV Ig should be given in combination with the HAV vaccine in order to allow for long-term immunity. In addition, improving sanitary conditions and encouraging hand washing can effectively decrease spread of the virus, since HAV depends on the fecal oral route.

Hepatitis B

Background

Hepatitis B (HBV) infection is a global public health problem. It is estimated that over 350 million individuals worldwide are chronically infected with HBV.[2] HBV is caused by a virus that is a 42 nm DNA virus, which belongs to the hepadnaviridae family. There are eight genotypes of the HBV that have been identified (A to H) based on a divergence of the HBV genome. These genotypes show geographical variation and the clinical significance of different genotypes is being investigated but is not yet clear. The prevalence of HBV is widely variable in different parts of the world. (Figure 3-2) Low prevalence areas include the United States, Canada, Western Europe, Australia, and New Zealand. Intermediate prevalence rates occur in Mediterranean countries, Japan, Central Asia, the Middle East, and Latin and South America. High prevalence areas include Southeast Asia, China, and sub-Saharan Africa. The mode of transmission of HBV varies and is related to the prevalence of the infection in an area of the world. In high prevalence areas, the most common mode of transmission tends to be perinatal infection. In areas with an intermediate prevalence of HBV, the primary mode of transmission appears to be horizontal transmission, particularly in early childhood. In lower prevalence areas, such as in the United States, the most common mode of transmission of HBV is unprotected sexual intercourse and intravenous drug use in adults. Importantly, infection with HBV can be prevented by the highly effective recombinant vaccination that that is available. If global vaccination practices could be implemented, HBV could be controlled and virtually eradicated.

Clinical Picture

Acute Hepatitis B Infection

HBV can cause an acute infection as well as a chronic infection. After exposure to the virus, the incubation period may last 1 to 4 months. The clinical spectrum of acute hepatitis B includes asymptomatic disease, cholestatic hepatitis, and fulminant hepatic failure. Of those individuals exposed to the virus, approximately 30% will develop a clinically apparent icteric hepatitis. The severity of acute HBV may vary although fulminant hepatitis is relatively rare occurring in only 0.1% to 0.5% of patients. After the incubation period a serum sickness-like syndrome may develop which may be followed by systemic symptoms including anorexia, fatigue, nausea, jaundice, and right upper quadrant discomfort. These symptoms usually resolve in a few months although patients may complain of fatigue lasting longer than this.

After acute hepatitis, the infection may resolve or become chronic. The likelihood of progressing to a chronic infection depends largely on the age at the time of infection and the immune status of the person. The risk of chronic infection is approximately 90% when HBV is acquired perinatally, it is approximately 20% to 50% for infections occurring between the age of 1 to 5 years, and it is less than 5% for HBV infection acquired in adulthood. Another important risk factor for progression to chronic infection is immunosuppression. Factors which decrease the immune response effectively decrease the probability of an effective immune response against the virus.

Chronic Hepatitis B Infection

Chronic infection with HBV if defined as having a persistently detectable HBV surface antigen (HBsAg) on at least two serologic tests taken at least 6 months apart in time. The infection is typically further characterized by the presence or absence of hepatitis e antigen (HBeAg), which is a marker of infectivity. In the majority of individuals identified as having chronic HBV infection, there is no history of acute hepatitis and many may in fact be asymptomatic at the time that chronic HBV is diagnosed. Those individuals that are most likely to be symptomatic are those who have already progressed to decompensated cirrhosis or those with extrahepatic manifestations of HBV.

HBV is a hepatotrophic virus, and through the immune-mediated mechanisms, it may lead to significant inflammation in the liver. Over time, this inflammation may lead to fibrosis and cirrhosis. The clinical complications of HBV cirrhosis are similar to other causes of cirrhosis including coagulopathy, variceal bleeding, ascites,

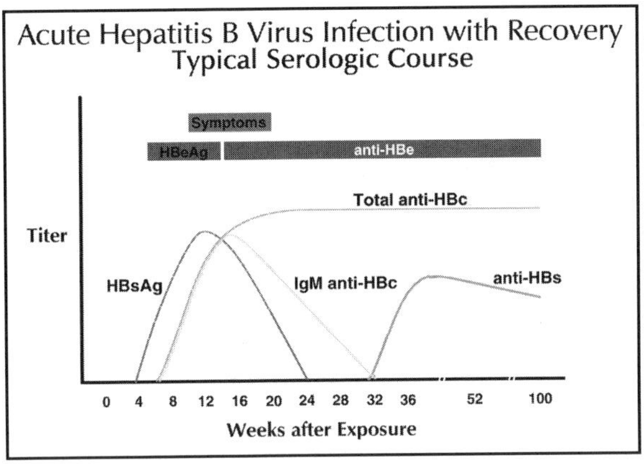

Figure 3-3. Serologic profile during acute hepatitis B infection with recovery. (Reprinted with permission from the US Department of Health and US Services Centers for Disease Control and Prevention.)

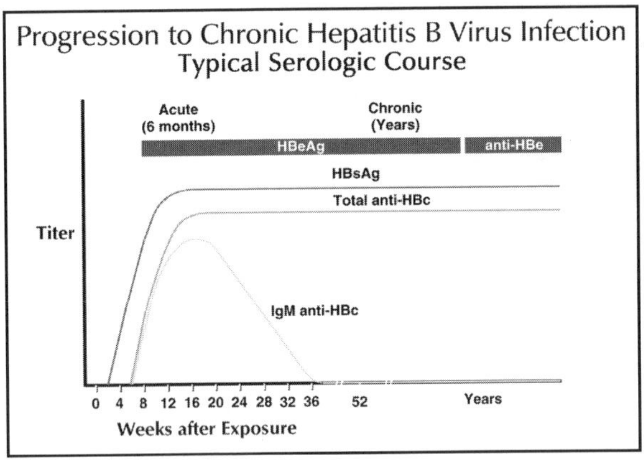

Figure 3-4. Serologic profile during acute hepatitis B infection with progression to chronic infection. (Reprinted with permission from the US Department of Health and US Services Centers for Disease Control and Prevention.)

and hepatic encephalopathy. The risk of hepatocellular carcinoma appears particularly high with HBV infection.

Chronic HBV infection may be associated with extrahepatic manifestations which are thought to be mediated mainly by circulating immune complexes. Such extrahepatic manifestations occur in approximately 10% to 20% of patients with chronic HBV infection. Extrahepatic manifestations may include a serum-sickness-like syndrome during acute hepatitis, polyarteritis nodosa, glomerular disease, mixed cryoglobulinemia, popular acrodermatitis (Gianotti's disease), and aplastic anemia.

Phases of Chronic HBV Infection

In chronic infection, there is a persistence of HBsAg, HBeAg, and HBV DNA (Figures 3-3 and 3-4). After the acute hepatitis resolves, serum transaminases levels usually fall but may remain abnormal. There may be a dectectable HBcAb IgM for the initial 6 months of infection that is later replaced by HBcAb IgG. Over time, there may be seroconversion as defined by a loss of HBeAg and development of HBeAb. Seroconversion is usually preceded by a marked decrease in serum HBV DNA.

Seroconversion may be associated with a flare in serum ALT levels but these levels typically decrease and normalize after seroconversion. In a minority of cases, there has been observed HBsAg seropositivity simultaneously with HBsAb.

Hepatitis B Mutants

HBV has a propensity for mutations to occur while it is replicating. The main reason for this is that the reverse transcriptase polymerase lacks a proofreading function. Mutations can occur in any of HBV's genes. There are several commonly identified mutations that may occur spontaneously or as a result of selective pressure due to antiviral therapy with lamivudine or adefovir. The most commonly encountered spontaneously occurring mutations are the precore mutants and the core promoter mutants. These mutations are characterized by the absence of HBeAg during replicative infection. These mutations tend to be less sensitive to antiviral treatment and may be associated with ALT elevations and high HBV DNA levels. When individuals with chronic HBV are given suppressive therapy with medications such as lamivudine or adefovir, these medications may exert a selective pressure on the wild type strain of the virus to develop mutations that will confer resistance to the drugs. The mutations associated with lamivudine antiviral therapy is the tyrosine-methionine-aspartate-aspartate (YMDD) mutation. The newer antiviral agent, adefovir, has the advantage of being much less likely to evoke mutations in HBV, but an adefovir-resistant mutation has been identified in a few individuals after 2 years of treatment. Fortunately, these mutations are not cross-resistant; therefore, switching medications or using combination therapy still appears to successfully suppress the virus.

Diagnosis

History

In addition to routine medical interviewing, the history should focus on risk factors for HBV exposure including travel history, family history of liver disease, occupation, and sexual history. Family history is important for any history of HBV, any chronic liver diseases, and hepatocellular carcinoma. It is important to ask questions about other causes of liver injury including alcohol consumption and prescription and non-prescription drug use. Individuals who should be considered for screening for HBV include persons born in endemic areas, men who have sex with men, injection drug users, pregnant women, dialysis patients, human immunodeficiency virus (HIV) positive patients, and household and sexual contacts of someone known to have HBV.[3]

Physical Examination

The physical examination should focus on any evidence of acute hepatitis such as jaundice or hepatomegaly. The exam should look for evidence of advanced chronic liver injury including ascites, spider angiomata, peripheral edema, and hepatic encephalopathy.

Serologic Tests

Routine blood work should be performed including complete blood count, comprehensive metabolic panel, and coagulation studies. It is also important to evaluate for other viruses that may contribute to the overall liver injury including HCV, HDV, and HIV. The fundamental way to diagnosis HBV includes serologic tests looking for the presence of HBV-specific antigens, antibodies, and viral DNA.

The laboratory findings in acute HBV include marked elevations in the serum transaminases up to 1000 to 2000 IU/L typically with ALT>AST. The bilirubin may also become elevated, although this does not occur in all case of acute HBV infection. The prothrombin time may also become elevated and this is an important prognostic marker to follow to assess the risk of fulminant hepatic failure. An elevated prothrombin time should prompt transfer of patients with acute HBV to medical centers with liver transplant programs. In cases of HBV that evolve into acute fulminant hepatic failure, expeditious liver transplantation is the only chance for saving the patient.

ALT in chronic HBV may be an important marker of necroinflammatory activity. For this reason, it is also considered in deciding treatment candidacy. Patients with normal ALT tend to have a decreased likelihood of responding to antiviral treatment.

In terms of the specific viral markers in early acute HBV one would expect to see a positive HBsAg, HBeAg, HBcAb IgM, and HBV DNA. In later-recovering acute HBV, the HBV panel would show a positive HBcAb IgG (anti-HBc IgG), HBsAb (anti-HBs), HBeAb (anti-HBe), and no HBV DNA (see Figure 3-3). In chronic HBV, one would expect to see persistent HBsAg, HBeAg, and HBcAb (anti-HBc). There is eventual loss of HBc IgM and possibly seroconversion (HBeAg lost with development of detectable HBeAb/anti-HBe) (see Figure 3-4).

Hepatitis B Surface Antigen

HBsAg is a marker of acute and chronic infection. When it persists beyond 6 months, it signifies chronic infection.

The disappearance of HBsAg is followed by the appearance of HBsAb is the hallmark of recovery. The window period is that short period of time (weeks) during which HBsAg has become undetectable, but before the HBsAb is detectable. If acute HBV is suspected, an HBcAb IgM should be checked to make the diagnosis although there are conditions in which the presence of HBcAb IgM does not signify acute infection. After exposure to HBV, a minority of individuals may be found to be positive for both HBsAg and HBsAb. It is believed that in these cases the HBsAb is not able to neutralize the HBsAg, and, therefore, the antigen remains detectable.

Hepatitis B Surface Antibody

As indicated above, HBsAb is the antibody directed against HBsAg. It is an important marker of recovery and of immunization. Isolated HBsAb is most commonly the profile seen in individuals that have been successfully immunized against HBV with the vaccination. In cases of recovery after natural infection, there is typically detectable HBsAb and HbcAb, although overtime the antibody levels may wane to the point that only HBsAb or HBcAb is detectable. In cases of immunization, there will never be detectable HBcAb.

Hepatitis B Core Antibody

HBcAb is an antibody directed against the core antigen of the HBV. While HBcAb is detectable throughout HBV infection (either IgM or IgG subclass), the core antigen is typically located intracellularly and cannot be detected in the routinely used assays that are currently widely available. Hepatitis B core antibody (HBcAb) is an important marker of natural exposure to the virus and distinguishes individuals who have had infection with the virus as opposed to those exposed only to the vaccination against HBV. It is detectable as IgM, which is usually a marker of more acute infection and as IgG in later infection. It should be noted, however, that detectable HBcAb

IgM does not always signify acute HBV infection. It may remain detectable for up to several years after the acute infection and may increase to detectable levels during exacerbations of hepatitis in cases of chronic HBV. Therefore, a detectable HBcAb IgM needs to be placed in the context of the individual. After natural infection with HBV, the HBcAb IgG remains detectable whether the individual recovers or develops chronic infection.

There are cases in which there may be only isolated HBcAb detected without detectable HBsAg or HBsAb. The explanations for such a HBV profile may include: the window period of acute HBV infection, years after recovery from HBV infection when the titer of HBsAb falls below detectable levels, and after years of chronic infection when the HBsAg levels drop below detectable levels but without neutralizing antibody (HBsAb) present. In cases of isolated HBcAb, there have been cases of positive HBV DNA and HBV transmission reported. The management of an isolated HBcAb case would include repeat testing of the HBsAb, HBsAg, HBcAb IgM, and IgG. It would also be reasonable to check HBV DNA, particularly if chronic liver disease is suspected.

Hepatitis E Antigen

HBeAg is a marker of HBV replication and infectivity. The absence of HBeAg does not ensure that there is no HBV replication or infectivity, however. The precore mutant strain of HBV does not produce HBeAg, but it still successfully replicates and can cause progressive liver damage.

Hepatitis E Antibody

The loss of HBeAg and the appearance of the HBeAb is called seroconversion. When seroconversion occurs, HBV DNA typically becomes undetectable and there may be remission in terms of liver disease, although this is not always there case. There have been cases of HBV infection described in which despite the loss of HBeAg with the appearance of HBeAb, there was continued persistence of HBV DNA with ongoing liver injury.

Hepatitis B DNA

HBV DNA can be measured by qualitative and quantitative assays. These assays vary in terms of the molecular techniques used and their lower limits of detection. The main techniques used in HBV DNA assays include hybridization assays, signal amplification branched DNA (bDNA) assay, and polymerase chain reaction (PCR) assays. The major role of HBV DNA assays is to assess HBV replication and appropriateness for antiviral therapy. Higher pretreatment HBV DNA levels may suggest a decreased likelihood of response to interferon therapy, although this is not so clearly predictable of a response to other antiviral therapies. HBV DNA measurements are also important in assessing response to therapy. It should be noted that in case of fulminant hepatic failure related to HBV infection, the HBV DNA assay may be crucial to identifying the etiology of hepatic failure. In these cases, HBsAg may be cleared by the time of presentation due to the overwhelming immune response against the virus, which is also related to the fulminant course of the infection.

HBV DNA level is an important factor in determining a patient's candidacy for antiviral treatment. Traditionally, a cut-off of >105 copies/mL has been used to decide if treatment is indicated. This cut off was decided on somewhat arbitrarily since this was the lower limit of detection of the older nonamplified HBV DNA assays. This is not necessarily the precise clinically relevant threshold at which a patient is likely to have progressive liver injury if untreated. Indeed, there may be ongoing injury at lower levels; however, the precise threshold is unknown. With the advent of PCR-based techniques, the sensitivity of HBV DNA assays has markedly increased and we are now able to measure lower levels. In the future the guidelines for treatment may be revised as we learn more about the clinical impact of various levels of HBV DNA. Recovery from HBV infection is usually associated with a loss of HBV DNA; however, despite clinical recovery the more sensitive polymerase chain reaction (PCR) assays may continue to detect low levels of HBV DNA. This finding is explained by the idea that HBV recovery may actually represent effective immune system control of the virus but not complete eradiation of the virus.

As mentioned previously, HBV can be classified into at least 8 genotypes. Genotypes differ in their DNA sequences and in geographic distribution. It is not common practice to test for the HBV genotype since the clinical relevance of has not yet been entirely elucidated. At this time, knowing the genotype would not affect treatment recommendations or yield clear prognostic information. In the future, as we learn more genotype testing may become a common part of HBV management.

Liver Biopsy

Liver biopsy may play an important role in assessing the degree of liver injury caused by chronic HBV infection. The typical pathologic findings include primarily mononuclear inflammatory infiltrates in the portal tracts and periportal necrosis as well as varying degrees of fibrosis. The degree of inflammation (grade) and amount of fibrosis (stage) can be assessed using the histology activity index (HAI) or the Metavir score. Immunostaining for HBsAg and HBcAg may be helpful. A characteristic finding on liver biopsy of HBV infection includes ground-glass appearing hepatocytes which are full of HBsAg. While it may be informative, the actual HBV antigen staining pattern is not correlated with disease severity, however.

Management and Treatment

Treatment of Acute Hepatitis B

Most cases of acute HBV infection are asymptomatic. Those cases that are symptomatic require mainly supportive treatment including intravenous fluids, antiemetics, and reassurance. In the more rare case of fulminant hepatic failure due to HBV, treatment will be require intensive care units monitoring at a medical center with a liver transplant program. While most patients do not develop acute liver failure, all patients identified as having acute HBV should be educated about the disease and the risk they pose in possibly transmitting this infection to other people. They should be counseled on using barrier protection during sexual intercourse for at least a number of months following infection and until recovery is documented. In addition, adults who acquire HBV should be offered testing for other viruses and infections that share transmission routes with HBV including HIV and HCV. Vertically transmitted HBV is less likely to occur with concomitant viruses, although the mother should be tested.

Contacts of infected individuals should be identified and contacted. Nonvaccinated close contacts of the individual should be offered post-exposure prophylaxis in the form of hepatitis B immunoglobulin (HBiG). All contacts should be offered vaccination against HBV. After the initial diagnosis of acute HBV, individuals should be monitored for loss of HBsAg and the development of HBsAb to document recovery or the persistence of HBsAg/HBeAg to document development of chronic infection.

Treatment of Chronic Hepatitis B

After a patient has been identified as having chronic HBV infection, there are several important aspects to managing this infection. Management focuses on preventing transmission of HBV to others, staging the amount of liver injury that is present at the time of diagnosis, minimizing other liver injury as from alcohol, and medications to eradicate or at least control the virus in order to limit progression of liver injury.

Patients should be educated about their infectivity and their contacts should be notified to receive HBV vaccination and possibly HBIG, if not previously vaccinated. Patients should be evaluated carefully to stage their degree of liver injury including serologic testing for hepatitis A and other causes of chronic liver disease, imaging such as ultrasound or MRI, and a careful history regarding alcohol and drug exposures to evaluate for possible concomitant hepatotoxin exposure, and possibly liver biopsy. Patients should be offered immunization against HAV if they are not already immune and they should be counseled about the importance of avoiding alcohol in order to minimize liver injury.

Currently, there are three FDA-approved medications for the treatment of chronic HBV. These include interferon alpha (IFN-alfa-2a), lamivudine, and adefovir. The goal underlying these medical therapies is to achieve sustained viral suppression and remission of liver disease. While eradication of the virus would be ideal, this is not usually achieved. The endpoints of treatment include normalization of serum ALT level, undetectable serum HBV dNA by an unamplified assay, loss of HBeAg with or without detection of anti-HBe, and improvement in liver histology (Lok and McMahon, 2001). Even after successful treatment with seroconversion, reduced amounts of HBV DNA are detectable in serum when the more sensitive PCR tests are used. Supression of HBV DNA without complete eradication can still confer a significant biochemical, histological, and clinical benefit. HBeAg seroconversion is usually associated with a marked reduction in the HBV DNA levels to <10,000 copies/mL. These medications differ in their efficacy and side-effects and the choice of treatment needs to be tailored to the individual patient. Treatment is not appropriate for everyone and specific factors need to be considered to predict the likelihood of a response to one of these treatments.

Factors that should be looked at in order to evaluate an individual patient's candidacy for receiving HBV treatment include have a persistently positive HBsAg (for >6 months, HBV DNA level >105 copies/mL, ALT level greater that 2 times the normal limit, and liver biopsy showing necroinflammatory injury.

Interferon

Interferons are endogenous antiviral factors with both immunomodulatory and antiviral effects. The following are factors considered to be associated with an increased chance of a favorable response to interferon therapy for chronic HBV infection: high pretreatment serum ALT level, low pretreatment HBV DNA level, acquisition of the infection in adulthood, active liver histology, female sex, no concomitant HIV infection, and being Delta virus antibody negative. Interferon is administered as a subcutaneous injection given either daily or three times/week. It can have side-effects that can be significant including flu-like symptoms, fatigue, leucopenia, and depression.

Lamivudine

Lamividuine works by inhibiting HBV DNA synthesis. It can result in suppression in HBV replication with histologic improvement, normalization of ALT, and seroconversion in a subset of patients. It is administered as an oral pill and generally well tolerated. The main disadvantage of lamivudine is this potential for resistant strains developing and the fact that long-term therapy is required to maintain viral suppression. If the medication is stopped, the virus is likely to increase replication and HBV DNA will increase. Therefore, although it can be highly efficacious in suppressing the virus, there is no clear endpoint in time for stopping the medication and this can be particularly problematic when managing HBV in younger patients.

Adefovir Dipivoxil

Adefovir dipivoxil is the prodrug of adefovir. It works by inhibiting HBV DNA polymerase at levels much lower than those needed to inhibit human DNA polymerases. It appears to have good efficacy in suppressing HBV DNA, ALT normalization, and HBeAg to HBeAb seroconversion. Adefovir is well tolerated with the main potential side-effect being nephrotoxicity. Adefovir is effective in suppressing both the wild type HBV virus, as well as the lamivudine-resistant HBV strains. Therefore, it may be very useful in cases of lamivudine resistance or possibly in combination therapy regimens. To date, adefovir appears much less likely to induce resistant strains compared to lamivudine, although a small number of cases of resistance have been reported.

Combination Therapy

It has been suggested that combination therapy may be a good option for some patients. This may be particularly true in patients in whom resistant strains develop. This is not yet standard of care, but there is great interest in designing trials to evaluate this.

Liver Transplantation

When HBV infection has caused decompensated cirrhosis, liver transplantation may be to only efficacious therapy. HBIg and antiviral therapy are often used in the peritransplant period in order to control the virus and prevent injury to the graft liver. Individual transplant centers may vary to some degree in the exact regimen used.

Prognosis And Complications

HBV can progress to cirrhosis and may cause portal hypertension and hepatocellular carcinoma. The risk of hepatocellular carcinoma is particularly high with HBV infection and chronically infected individuals need to undergo surveillance for the development of hepatocellular carcinoma with AFP and liver imaging examinations of the liver every 6 months. The risk or progression to cirrhosis and the associated complications may depend on multiple factors including the host's age, the host's immune system, concomitant liver disease or alcoholism, and geographic and genetic factors among others. Prolonged HBV replication appears to be a risk factor for a worse prognosis; thus, achieving HBeAg seroconversion to HBeAb is desirable and may have a positive impact on prognosis.

In addition to the common complications of cirrhosis and hepatocellular carcinoma, HBV is associated with extrahepatic complications including polyarteritis nodosa, glomerular disease, a serum sickness-like syndrome, mixed cryglobulinemia, popular acrodermatitis (Gianotti's disease), and aplastic anemia. These extrahepatic complications are mainly due to circulating immune complexes and may respond to antiviral treatments.

Prevention

Active Immunization

The HBV vaccine is widely available and very efficacious at inducing effective, long-term immunity against HBV infection. It is based on the HBsAg and can induce long-term protective immunity in 95% of children and 90% of adults. This immunity is usually long-term lasting up to 15 years. Booster immunization is not routinely recommended but may be appropriate for immunocompromised individuals or those with ongoing risk for HBV infection and titer below 10 IU/mL. There has been some media attention regarding potential risks of the HBV vaccination implicating an association with adverse reactions such as arthritis, autism, and demyelinating disease. Formal epidemiologic studies have failed to prove this association yet. The CDC has issued guidelines on a strategy to try to eliminate HBV transmission in the United States. This strategy calls for the vaccination of all infants, children in high-risk groups, all children if not vaccinated by age 11 to 12, vaccination of all adolescents with risk factors for HBV, and vaccination of adults in high-risk groups. Risk factors among adults that warrant HBV vaccination include occupational risk, such as health care workers and those who perform tasks involving contact with blood or body fluids; clients and staff of institutions for the developmentally disabled; hemodialysis patients; recipients of blood products, such as clotting-factor concentrates; household contacts and sex partners of HBV carriers; adoptees from countries where HBV is endemic; international travelers planning to spend more than 6 months in an endemic area; intravenous drug users; sexually-active homosexual or bisexual men; sexually-active men or women who have a history of other sexually transmitted diseases, prostitution or multiple partners; and inmates of long-term correctional facilities.

Passive Immunization

Passive immunization is appropriate for individuals who have been exposed to HBV and were not previously vaccinated or immune to the virus. Passive immunization consists of administering immunoglobulin that contains a high titer of HBsAb (anti-HBs) or HBIg. This is commonly given to babies born to HBsAg-positive mothers and for individuals with a significant exposure to and HBV-infected person, and to liver transplant patients with a history of HBV infection.

Hepatitis C

Background

The hepatitis C virus (HCV) is currently an important public health issue both in the United States and Worldwide. In the US, it is estimated that 2.7 million people are chronically infected with the virus.[4] Currently, HCV infection is the number one indication for liver transplantation. It only became possible to test for HCV after the genetic sequence of the virus was identified in 1989. Prior to this time HCV was clinically recognized as a form of hepatitis commonly occurring after blood transfusions.

Table 3-3

EXPOSURES KNOWN TO BE ASSOCIATED WITH HEPATITIS C INFECTION IN THE UNITED STATES

- Injecting drug use
- Transfusion, transplant from infected donor
- Occupational exposure to blood (mostly needle sticks)
- Iatrogenic (unsafe injections)
- Birth to HCV-infected mother
- Sex with infected partner (multiple sex partners)

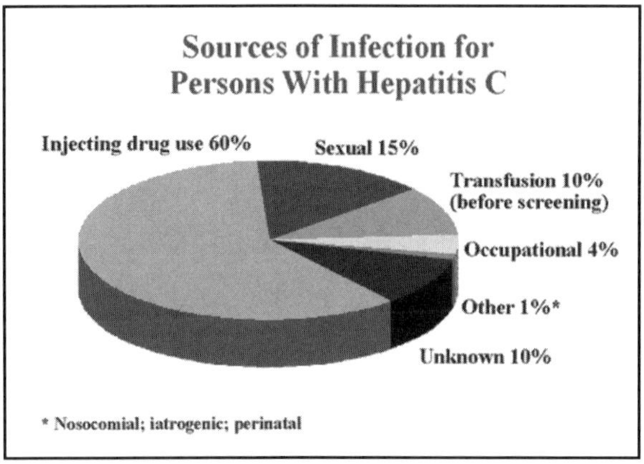

Figure 3-5. The main routes of hepatitis C infection in the United States. (Reprinted with permission from the US Department of Health and US Sevices Centers for Disease Control and Prevention.)

HCV is an RNA virus that has 6 major genotypes identified. The significance of HCV genotypes is that different genotypes may cluster geographically and demonstrate very different sensitivity to interferon and ribavirin treatment. The likelihood of successfully clearing the virus on interferon and ribavirin treatment may differ greatly depending on the genotype, and, therefore, this has implications when counseling patients on treatment options.

HCV is transmitted parenterally. Routes by which individuals may have been exposed to HCV include receiving of blood products or transplanted solid organs prior to 1992, transfusion of clotting factors prior to 1987, or a history of intravenous drug use (Table 3-3). Because HCV has been molecularly characterized, screening the blood supply and potential organ donors is possible and the risk associated with transfusions and transplants has markedly diminished. Intravenous drug use remains a very common way that people acquire HCV in the United States (Figure 3-5). In many cases, a clear risk factor or exposure is never identified. There appears to be a high prevalence of HCV among individuals with a history of alcoholism and in US Veterans. HCV can be transmitted sexually, but this is not a common route. In

Table 3-4

HOUSEHOLD TRANSMISSION OF HEPATITIS C

1. Rare, but not absent
2. Could occur through percutaneous/mucosal exposures to blood:
   - Contaminated equipment used for home therapies (eg, IV therapy, injections)
   - Theoretically through sharing of contaminated personal articles (eg, razors, toothbrushes)

fact, the risk of sexual transmission appears to be very low in monogamous couples in which one partner is HCV positive and the other is not. It does appear that as in the case of other sexually transmitted diseases male to female transmission may be more efficient. Sexual practices that may be associated with increased risk of HCV transmission include having multiple partners, other sexually-transmitted diseases, sex with trauma, and nonuse of condoms. HCV is not usually transmitted by routine household contact and patients and their families need to be informed of this. A few behaviors should be avoided including sharing razors, toothbrushes, and any practices in which the possibility of blood exposure is high (Table 3-4).

CLINICAL PICTURE

HCV may cause an acute icteric hepatitis, as well as a chronic hepatitis. Most commonly the acute phase of infection is asymptomatic, or at least unrecognized, and the infection is diagnosed once it is in the chronic phase.

Once a person has been exposed to HCV approximately 20% of individuals will recover completely while approximately 80% will go on to develop chronic infection with persistently detectable HCV RNA in the blood. Of this 80% developing chronic infection, approximately 20% to 30% will have severe progression of their liver disease and may develop cirrhosis and have an increased risk for hepatocellular carcinoma.[5]

Acute Hepatitis C

In most cases, HCV infection is not identified during the acute phase of infection, although HCV may cause a clinical acute hepatitis with symptoms similar to that seen in other forms of acute viral hepatitis. Patients may present with malaise, nausea, vomiting, right upper quadrant pain, and jaundice. These symptoms may last several weeks. The development of fulminant hepatic failure secondary to acute HCV infection is very rare. The risk for fulminant failure may be increased when acute HCV infection occurs in persons who already have chronic liver disease, such as chronic HBV infection. A small percentage of individuals who do develop symptomatic acute HCV may mount a successful immune response against the virus and clear the virus without interferon/ribavirin treatment. Indeed, the presence of symptoms such as jaundice may be due to a more vigorous immune response.

Chronic Hepatitis C

After exposure to HCV, most individuals will develop a chronic infection with persistent viremia (55% to 74%).[4,6] Most patients with chronic HCV infection will not have symptoms. Symptoms that may be associated with chronic HCV infection included fatigue, nausea, anorexia, myalgia, arthralgia, and weight loss. These symptoms are associated with HCV but are quite nonspecific; therefore, other causes must be considered. Chronic infection with HCV is often identified incidentally when an abnormality in the liver tests is noted such as a mild elevation in the transaminases. Chronic HCV may also be detected in patients initially presenting with complications of cirrhosis such as ascites, variceal bleeding, or encephalopathy in a person previously unknown to have liver disease. Once an individual is cirrhotic, it is far more likely that there will be lots of symptoms related to the liver failure.

Diagnosis

Diagnostic tests for HCV include serologic tests that are based on measuring the presence of an antibody response against the virus and molecular tests that are based on detecting the presence of viral proteins (RNA) in the bloodstream.[7] Since 1989, when HCV was molecularly characterized, the sensitivity and specificity of these HCV diagnostic tests has rapidly advanced. The diagnosis of HCV can be made based on the serologic and molecular blood tests for the virus, but fully characterizing the infection and assessing the extent of liver disease also includes taking a careful history, physical examination, other molecular tests (genotype testing), and often liver biopsy.

The CDC has published guidelines on risk factors that should prompt HCV testing (Table 3-5).

Serologic Tests

Serologic tests for detecting HCV antibodies can be divided into screening assays and supplemental tests for confirming infection. The screening assay is a multiantigen enzyme immunoassays (EIA). There have been several generations of HCV EIAs with improving sensitivity and specificity. Currently, the second- and third-generation EIAs are available in the United States. Although these are excellent assays for screening for the presence of HCV antibodies, the possibility of false positive and negative test results still exists. False negative test results may occur in individuals who are immunocompromised (eg, HIV, hypogammaglobulinemia), and, therefore, may not mount an adequate immunoglobulin response to be detectable by the assay.

Factors associated with false positive tests include: low prevalence situations where an individual does not have clear risk factors for exposure to HCV or the presence of high immunoglobulins as with other autoimmune disease. In cases where a false positive test is suspected a supplemental assay, the recombinant immunoblot assay (RIBA), can be used to sort out whether the screening assay was a true or a false positive result. RIBA is performed only on specimens in those cases where a positive EIA result is called into question as in low risk groups. It is not used as the primary screening test because it is more technically demanding. In patients with known risk factors for HCV with a positive screening test for HCV, it is not necessary to perform a RIBA test—rather, it is more informative to move directly to HCV RNA quantification and characterization (genotype) with molecular tests. RIBA is based on detecting HCV

Table 3-5

Hepatitis C Testing Recommendations

HCV Testing Routinely Recommended

Based on increased risk for infection:

- Ever injected illegal drugs
- Received clotting factors made before 1987
- Received blood/organs before July 1992
- Ever on chronic hemodialysis
- Evidence of liver disease

Based on need for exposure management:

- Health care, emergency, public safety workers after needle stick/mucosal exposures to HCV-positive blood
- Children born to HCV-positive women

Routine HCV Testing Not Recommended

Unless Risk Factor Identified:

- Health care, emergency medical, and public safety workers
- Pregnant women
- Household (nonsexual) contacts of HCV-positive persons
- General population

Routine HCV Testing of Uncertain Need

Not confirmed as risk factor/prevalence low or unknown:

- Recipients of transplanted tissue
- Intranasal cocaine or other noninjecting illegal drug users
- History of tattooing, body piercing

Confirmed risk factor but prevalence of infection low:

- History of STDs or multiple sex partners
- Long-term steady sex partners of HCV-positive persons

Reprinted with permission from US Department of Health and Human Services Centers for Disease Control and Prevention.

antibodies to specific multiple HCV antigens. If it is positive, it usually confirms previous exposure to HCV. If it is negative, it usually identifies a false-positive screening assay. It should be kept in mind, however, that a positive screening antibody test and a positive RIBA do not confirm that there is ongoing active infection with HCV. Individuals who have cleared HCV with interferon treatment or spontaneously after acute HCV infection may maintain a detectable antibody response for a long time afterwards. In order to assess the presence of active infection with HCV, it is necessary to perform molecular tests that can quantify the presence of HCV RNA. If a patient is found to have a positive screening antibody test, a positive RIBA, but a negative HCV

RNA, this suggests possible previous exposure to HCV with clearance of viremia. Given the availability and excellent technology of molecular tests for HCV, the utility of RIBA is limited mainly to resolving possibilities of false positive screening assays.

Molecular Tests

Molecular tests are based on detecting HCV RNA in serum samples. These tests have become very important in identifying and quantifying active infection at the time of diagnosis, as well as monitoring response to antiviral therapy such as with interferon and ribavirin. Molecular HCV RNA tests may be used to assess the viral load or the genotype of the HCV. There are two fundamental types of the viral load molecular tests the qualitative tests and the quantitative tests. The qualitative tests have a lower threshold of detection of HCV RNA and are very useful in confirming whether there is any evidence of active HCV infection or not. When a qualitative HCV RNA test is ordered, the result will be either positive or negative. This is particularly useful in following patients who have cleared the virus in order to confirm ongoing clearance with the most sensitive assay possible. When a quantitative HCV RNA test is ordered, the result will be expressed as an actual number (viral load). In the past, various units were used to express HCV viral load including copies/mL or genome equivalents for each assay but now results are being standardized to international units/mL (IU/mL).

Molecular tests also allow for identifying the genotype of the virus. There are at least six genotypes of the HCV virus. The genotype is relevant in cases when patients are considering treatment for their HCV infection with interferon and ribavirin. Certain genotypes (genotypes 2,3) are significantly more sensitive to the combination treatment compared to others (genotypes 1,4), and actually have a shorter course of treatment with a reduced dosage of ribavirin.

Liver Biopsy

Liver biopsy is not required in order to make the diagnosis of HCV infection, but it can be an integral part to staging the degree of liver injury and evaluating for other causes of liver disease. It can be difficult to predict the degree of liver fibrosis and injury on the basis of clinical and blood tests alone, therefore, liver biopsy may be an important adjunct in evaluating patients. Performing a liver biopsy can also help patients decide whether to undergo treatment of HCV or not, depending on the condition of their liver. When a person has clear evidence of fibrosis or evolving cirrhosis, it may be more important to aggressively pursue treatment in order to halt the progression of the disease. In persons with no significant fibrosis on liver biopsy and mild hepatitis, clinically deferring treatment may be a reasonable option.

Management and Treatment

A new diagnosis of HCV infection often causes significant stress for patients. Patients can become upset about the fact that they may have had this infection for a long period of time and were unaware of it and that it may have a significant impact on their long-term health. In addition, a diagnosis of HCV often causes stress or conflict in a patient's personal life as the people close to them are informed. There arise many questions about the potential long-term health impact, whether treatment should be pursued at this time, and what family, friends, and work colleagues should be told. Since the treatment for HCV can have significant side-effects, it often impacts daily life at home and in the office. It is important to recognize this psychosocial aspect of diagnosing and treating HCV. Educating patients as much as possible about the virus and its treatment empowers them to make the right decisions for themselves. Treatment for depression, counseling, and family meetings may be important before direct antiviral treatment is started.

In addition to the psychosocial aspect of treatment, it is important to counsel patients on avoiding the consumption of alcohol and other toxins that may contribute to the progression of liver disease. Patients should also be carefully evaluated and treated for any other causes of chronic liver disease that may also affect overall prognosis. If they are not already immune, vaccinations for HAV and HBV should be given.

The fundamental treatment for HCV currently consists of combination treatment with interferon and ribavirin.[8] Interferon is given as a subcutaneous injection and is available in a peglyated form, as well as nonpeglyated form. The pegylated form of interferon allows for dosing once weekly, whereas the nonpegylated interferon is generally administered 3 times per week. Ribavirin is given as a pill with weight-based dosing that is taken daily. The goal of treatment with interferon and ribavirin is to achieve a sustained virologic response (SVR), which is defined as the absence of detectable HCV RNA in the serum by an assay with a sensitivity of at least 100 copies (50 IU) per mL at the end of treatment and at least 6 months after the cessation of therapy. Studies have suggested that if a person has a negative qualitative HCV RNA for 6 months or longer after the end of interferon/ribavirin therapy, then there is a high probability that individual will remain nonviremic long-term. The specific likelihood that a person will respond to interferon/ribavirin with eradication of viremia depends on multiple factors. Factors that appear to be important include viral genotype, liver histology, and viral load. Patients with HCV genotype 1, which is the most common genotype in the US, are less likely to respond to interferon therapy (~40% to 50%) compared to patients with the less common genotypes 2 or 3 (up to 80% may respond). Patients with advanced liver fibrosis (cirrhosis) appear to be less likely to respond to interferon/ribavirin treatment and may not tolerate the treatment as well due to increased side-effects. Patients with a very high viral load also appear to be somewhat more resistant to interferon/ribavirin treatments. Of these factors, genotype has the clearest impact on likelihood of response and should always be considered when discussing treatment options and efficacy with patients.

Interferon and ribavirin therapy may have significant side-effects that must be considered before starting a patient on therapy. The most common side-effects from interferon include flu-like symptoms (fatigue, fever, headache, myalgia, arthralgia), gastrointestinal symptoms (nausea, vomiting, diarrhea, weight loss), hematologic symptoms (neutropenia, thrombocytopenia), and psychiatric symptoms (irritability, depression, insomnia). Patients must be carefully screened for a history of psychiatric disease. It is appropriate to defer initiation of treatment if a person has a history of significant or currently unstable psychiatric disease. Interferon has been known to be associated with worsened depression and suicide; therefore, this potential side-effect must be taken very seriously and patients monitored closely. Ribavirin has side-effects as well the most significant being dose-related hemolytic anemia. Because ribavirin is excreted through the urinary system it must be used with great caution in patients with renal insufficiency. This risk factor must also be considered seriously in patients with known coronary insufficiency or lung disease who might not tolerate anemia well at all. Careful monitoring with frequent blood tests is required throughout the duration of therapy and in particular initiation of therapy when anemia may first develop.

Given that interferon and ribavirin therapy achieves virus eradication in up to 50% of genotype 1 patients (up to 80% in the less common genotypes 2,3) and may have significant side-effects, the decision whether to start treatment or not must be individualized to each patient. The potential benefit must be weighed by the individual patient's risk for side-effects and their current psychosocial circumstances.

Acute Hepatitis C

Shortly after exposure, HCV may result in a symptomatic, icteric hepatitis, although most often acute infection with HCV is asymptomatic and the infection is not identified until it is in the chronic phase. If HCV is identified in the acute stage, either due to evident symptoms or a known exposure time, the clinical course may be quite different to that of chronic HCV. There appears to be spontaneous clearance viremia in acute HCV at a higher rate than in chronic HCV and the likelihood of clearing viremia with interferon is also much higher when given in the acute phase. There have been a number of studies looking at the immune response and natural history of acute HCV.[9-13] Since in most cases it appears that acute HCV infection will progress to chronic infection, there is great interest in treating patients early in the course of disease in an effort to prevent this progression. The studies on the treatment of acute HCV performed to date have often been small, heterogeneous, and uncontrolled. They have mainly looked at using interferon monotherapy rather than combination therapy with ribavirin. Interestingly, these studies have suggested that the ability to eradicate HCV viremia may be significantly higher when treated in the acute phase compared to the chronic phase. In addition, these studies have provided more observation into the natural history of acute HCV infection and a chance to try to observe how many individuals will naturally clear the infection by their innate immune response. While these studies don't yet provide clear guidelines on how to manage acute HCV infection, the current data suggests that is would be reasonable to treat acutely infected patients with interferon if they have persistently detectable HCV viremia 2 to 4 months after the exposure time. This window of time is suggested to allow for spontaneously clearance if it is likely to occur.[14]

Chronic Hepatitis C

The cornerstone for treatment of chronic HCV is pegylated interferon in combination with ribavirin. The major determinant of achieving a SVR is genotype. The response rates for patients with genotype 1 is 40% to 50%, while it is nearly 80% for patients with genotypes 2 or 3.[8] When the decision has been made to pursue combination treatment for chronic HCV, the actual regimen will also vary depending on the genotype. Those patients with genotype 1 will receive combination therapy for 48 weeks with a ribavirin dosage of 1000 to 1200 mg depending on weight (1000 mg if ≤75 kg; 1200 mg if >75 kg). Those patients with genotype 2 or 3 will receive combination therapy for a shorter course (only 24 weeks) with a reduced dosage of ribavirin (800 mg/day).

During treatment with interferon and ribavirin it is necessary to monitor patients regularly with frequent blood test (CBC, metabolic panel, TSH) and clinically with office visits to assess for side-effects. Dose modification of the interferon or ribavirin may be necessary particularly if hematologic suppression is observed. For genotype 1 patients, it is recommended to assess a viral load at 12 weeks of therapy. The expectation is that there will be at least a 2 $\log_{10}$ units drop or the virus will be undectectable at this point in time in order to continue forward with the full 48 weeks of treatment.

If at 12 weeks, there is not at least a 2 $\log_{10}$ units drop in the viral load, then therapy should be discontinued as it is not likely to result in a sustained virologic response.[15] This early stopping rule is based on two large multicenter treatment trials. It may not apply to populations not studied in these trials such as children, elderly, cirrhotics, or patients coinfected with the HIV. Such rules may need to be modified in different cases.

Prognosis and Complications

The natural history of HCV infection is not clearly defined. This is based largely on the nature of the infection and the observational studies available to date. Because the infection if rarely identified in the acute phase and it may have a long asymptomatic course, it can be difficult to assess natural history. Previously, it was believed that at least 20% of individuals with chronic HCV would progress to cirrhosis and the associated complications with a subset of this group developing hepatocellular carcinoma. More recent studies have suggested that the rate of spontaneous clearance may be higher than previously thought and that the percentage progressing to cirrhosis may be lower. These studies focused on younger populations of infected individuals but nonetheless called into question the real natural history of HCV infection.[16] There are likely multiple and variable determinants of HCV progression to cirrhosis. These may include viral concentration, genotype, patient age/sex/ethnicity, behavioral factors (alcohol, environmental exposures) and co-morbid conditions (HIV, HBV, other chronic liver disease).

Complications of chronic HCV infection include cirrhosis and extrahepatic manifestations of HCV. Cirrhosis is associated with hepatocellular carcinoma, as well as the complications of portal hypertension including variceal bleeding, hepatic encephalopathy, ascites, and hepatorenal syndrome. Currently, HCV infection is the main indication for liver transplantation in the United States. Extrahepatic manifestations of HCV include autoimmune disease (thyroiditis), dermatologic diseases (porphyria cutanea tarda and lichen planus), renal disease (membranoproliferative glomerulonephritis), hematologic disease (lymphoma and cryoglobulinemia), and possibly diabetes mellitus.

Prevention and Prophylaxis

The fundamental way to avoid exposure to HCV is to avoid those risk factors known to be associated with HCV (see Table 3-3). Patients known to have HCV should be advised to minimize the risk of exposing others to the virus (Table 3-6). There is no postexposure prophylaxis available. If a known exposure to HCV has occurred, as in the case of health care workers with a percutaneous injury from a known HCV positive patient, interferon therapy has been used. In these cases, interferon therapy when administered during the acute phase of infection can result in an excellent prognosis for clearing the infection. In cases of infants born to mothers known to be HCV positive, there is no immediate treatment of the infant recommended and there is no need to alter the mode of delivery or plan for breastfeeding. The estimated risk for transmission in these cases is approximately 1% to 5% in non-HIV infected women and higher in HIV infected women (14% to 19%). It is appropriate to recommend testing the infant for HCV but not until they are at least 15 to 18 months old in order to minimize the risk for maternal antibodies and an immature immune system affecting the results (Table 3-7).

Table 3-6

PREVENTING HEPATITIS C TRANSMISSION TO OTHERS

Avoid Direct Exposure to Blood

1. Do **not** donate blood, body organs, other tissue or semen
2. Do **not** share items that might have blood on them:
    - Personal care (eg, razor, toothbrush)
    - Home therapy (eg, needles)
    - Cover cuts and sores on the skin

Reprinted with permission from US Department of Health and Human Services Centers for Disease Control and Prevention.

Table 3-7

MOTHER TO INFANT TRANSMISSION OF HEPATITIS C

1. Postexposure prophylaxis not available
2. No need to avoid pregnancy or breastfeeding:
    - Consider bottle feeding if nipples cracked/bleeding
3. No need to determine mode of delivery based on HCV infection status
4. Test infants born to HCV-positive women:
    - >15 to 18 months old
    - Consider testing any children born since woman became infected
    - Evaluate infected children for CLD

Reprinted with permission from US Department of Health and Human Services Centers for Disease Control and Prevention.

HEPATITIS D

BACKGROUND

The hepatitis delta virus (HDV) is a defective RNA virus. Its most distinctive feature is that it cannot survive without the HBV, which provides it with its outer envelope (HBsAg). For this reason, HDV infection can be found only in the setting of concurrent or pre-existing infection with HBV. HDV does depend on HBV for its survival, but interestingly, the geographic distribution of HDV does not exactly parallel that of HBV (Figure 3-6). The differences in the geographic distribution between HDV and HBV have been attributed to differences in their efficiency of transmission. HDV is not common the United States and in other developed countries. The pattern of distribution of HDV has also been changing in recent years due to public health measures in different parts of the world aimed at reducing HBV and HIV transmis-

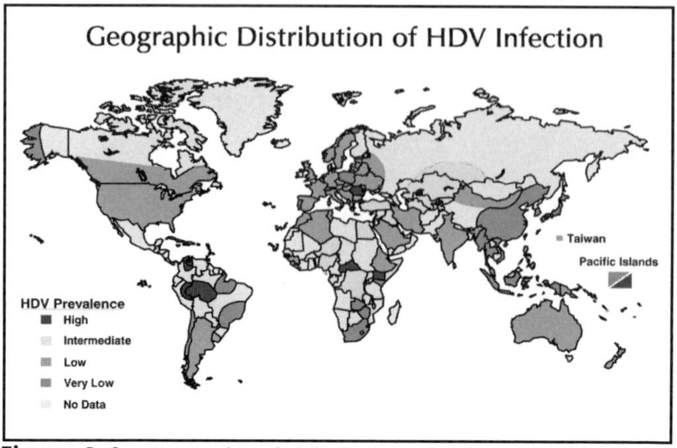

Figure 3-6. Geographic distribution of the hepatitis delta virus. (Reprinted with permission from the US Department of Health and US Services Centers for Disease Control and Prevention.)

sion. The important routes of transmission for HDV include sexual, parenteral, and household. The HDV virus does display different genotypes that cluster geographically and may have an impact on the clinical course of the HDV infection.

Clinical Picture

Infection with HDV always occurs in the setting of HBV infection. HDV may be acquired at the same time as HBV (coinfection) or it may occur in persons already chronically infected with the HBV (superinfection). The clinical picture of HDV may depend on whether it occurs as a coinfection or as a superinfection. When HDV is acquired at the same time as HBV (coinfection), the clinical picture is identical to that of acute HBV monoinfection. It may clinically look like an acute, icteric hepatitis. It is usually transient and self-limited. It may be associated with liver failure as acute HBV monoinfection may be. The incidence of chronic HBV infection is not increased if HBV is acquired with coinfection with HDV. Obviously, if the HBV infection is self-limited, the HDV infection will also be self-limited because HDV relies on the HBsAg production for its own survival.

In the case of superinfection where HDV is acquired in the setting of pre-existing chronic HBV infection, the clinical picture will be that of hepatitis exacerbation in a person previously known to have HBV or it may be the initial diagnosis of chronic HBV. In this scenario progression to chronic HDV infection is almost uniform since chronic HBV infection is already set up and can sustain support HDV. Interestingly, when there is chronic HBV/HDV infection, the replication of HBV DNA is often suppressed.

Diagnosis

History

It is important to consider HDV infection in individuals known to have chronic HBV and who present with a flare of hepatitis or in those with acute hepatitis and possible risk factors for HDV including travel to endemic countries of high-risk behaviors.

Physical Examination

The physical findings of HDV infection may include jaundice and the other findings typical of acute hepatitis.

Serologic Tests

Serologic tests for HDV include testing for anti-HDV antibodies (IgM and IgG). These tests are available in the United States. It is also important to test of other causes of hepatitis especially HBV. Testing for HBV will yield information about the phase of HBV infection to try to figure out whether the current infection represents co-infection or super-infection. This is important in predicting the clinical course and likelihood of chronic infection.

The Role of Liver Biopsy

Tissue markers of HDV infection include hepatitis D antigen (HDAg) and HDV RNA. The detection of intrahepatic HDAg has been proposed as the gold standard for the diagnosis of current HDV infection. It should be noted, however, that the yield of liver biopsy for making a diagnosis of HDV appears to decrease over time. Detecting HDV RNA is possible but technically challenging.

Management and Treatment

The management and treatment of HDV is linked to that of HBV. Treating HBV essentially treats HDV since it cannot survive without HBV. In cases of decompensated liver disease, liver transplantation may be necessary. The prognosis for transplantation of HBV/HDV cirrhosis carries a better prognosis than that of transplantation for other forms of viral hepatitis.

Prognosis and Complications

There is a risk of fulminant hepatitis with HDV infection. This risk appears to be increased when HDV infection occurs simultaneously with HBV infection (coinfection). There is also the risk of progressive liver cirrhosis with the associated complications of portal hypertension and hepatocellular carcinoma. The risk of hepatocellular carcinoma appears to be similar to that of HBV infection alone.

Prevention and Postexposure Prophylaxis

Since HDV cannot survive without HBV, vaccination against HBV is effective for preventing HDV as well.

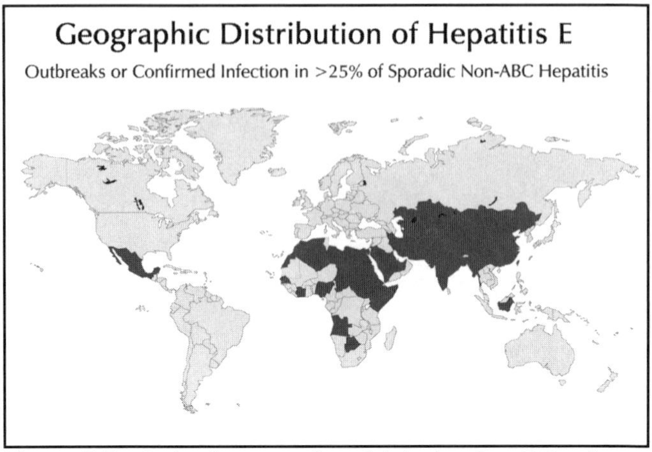

Figure 3-7. Outbreaks or confirmed infection in >25% of sporadic non-ABC hepatitis. (Reprinted with permission from the US Department of Health and US Services Centers for Disease Control and Prevention.)

Hepatitis E

Background

The hepatitis E virus (HEV) is an RNA virus that is enterically transmitted usually in contaminated water. HEV is similar to HAV in that both of these viruses are transmitted by the fecal-oral route, however, HEV is mainly transmitted by contaminated water, is not usually spread by interpersonal contact, and has a smaller worldwide distribution compared to HAV. The regions in the world where HEV is endemic include: Asia, Central America, Africa, Middle East, India, and Southeast Pacific (Figure 3-7). HEV is not endemic in the United States and the majority of cases identified in the US will have a history of travel to an endemic region. Historically, HEV is associated with pregnant women because of it high mortality and morbidity when it affects pregnant women. HEV may be responsible for large outbreaks of hepatitis in communities. This is usually following heavy rains and floods that increase the potential for contamination of the community water supply with feces. HEV is not readily spread by person-to-person contact perhaps due to it inability to survive in the environment.

Clinical Picture

HEV typically causes an acute, self-limited hepatitis. The symptoms are similar to that of acute hepatitis from other causes including jaundice, malaise, anorexia, nausea, vomiting, abdominal pain, and fever. Symptoms may last a few weeks. Although HEV is usually self-limited it does have an overall high fatality rate (0.5% to 4%). Fulminant hepatic failure has been reported with HEV infection, and appears to be more common when it infects pregnant women, particularly in the third trimester of pregnancy.

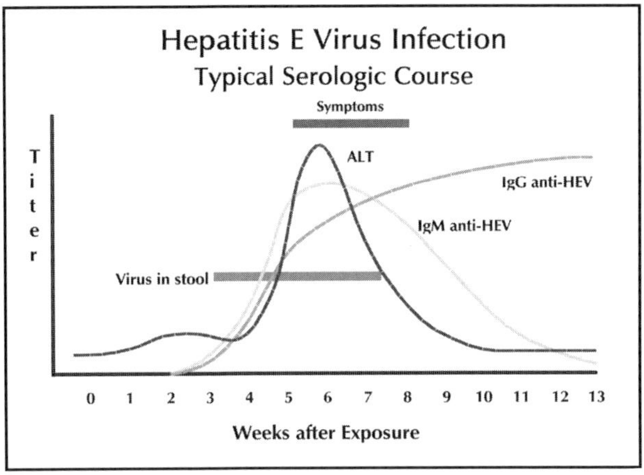

Figure 3-8. Typical serologic profile after infection with heaptitis E. (Reprinted with permission from the US Department of Health and US Services Centers for Disease Control and Prevention.)

Diagnosis

History

An important piece of the history would be residence or recent travel to an area where HEV is endemic. This will raise the level of suspicion for this infection. This should also be considered in a pregnant patient since it could have significant impact causing morbidity and mortality.

Physical Examination

Relevant features of the physical examination may include jaundice and hepatomegaly.

Serologic Tests

There is usually elevation of the transaminases and total bilirubin (Figure 3-8). Jaundice often sets in after the peak of the transaminases. There are serologic tests to identify antibodies against HEV and to directly detect HEV antigens, however, these tests are largely for research purposes and will not be available in most labs in the United States. An important part of making a diagnosis of acute HEV infection includes excluding the other causes of acute hepatitis serologically including hepatitis A, B, C, D, as well as cytomegalovirus (CMV) and Epstein-bar virus (EBV).

Liver Biopsy

Liver biopsy is usually not required in cases of HEV infection unless the cause of hepatitis is very unclear.

Management and Treatment

The mainstay of the management of cases of acute HEV infection is supportive care. If fulminant hepatic failure develops then expeditious transfer to an liver transplant center is imperative. It is not necessary to treat household contacts since this is not a common route of transmission of HEV.

Prognosis and Complications

HEV is usually associated with complete recovery, however, fulminant hepatic failure can develop and this may result in a significant fatality rate. The prognosis in pregnant women also appears to be significantly worse than in non-pregnant individuals.

Prevention

An important measure to try to prevent HEV infection is good sanitation. Boiling water does appear to inactivate HEV. For those who travel to areas where HEV is endemic, it is important to avoid drinking water and beverages with ice of unknown purity, and eating uncooked shellfish and unpeeled or uncooked fruits and vegetables. There is no vaccine against HEV at this time, and there is no clear evidence that the administration of anti-HEV immunoglobulin is beneficial in decreasing transmission.

Other Potential Hepatotrophic Viruses

In addition to the well-known hepatotrophic viruses discussed in this chapter, there are several viruses that may affect the liver. These include the hepatitis G virus (HGV) (also called GBV-C), the transfusion-transmitted virus (TTV), the SEN virus, as well as a number of viruses that may be associated with hepatitis.

HGV, or the GBV-C virus, has been described as a putative hepatotrophic virus. It is an RNA virus and is structurally similar to HCV. It is transmitted parenterally through blood transfusions, intravenous drug use, possibly sexually, and vertically from mother to infant. Although HGV/GBV-C has been identified, it is controversial whether this virus is truly hepatotrophic and whether it causes hepatitis or liver disease at all. It is not definitively associated with either acute or chronic hepatitis.

The "transfusion-transmitted virus" (TTV) has been suggested as a cause of non-A through E hepatitis. While there has been interest in identifying and characterizing this family of viruses, it is not yet clear that they play a pathogenic role in causing hepatitis in humans. The SEN virus similarly was linked to transfusion-associated non-A through E hepatitis. There is no proof that this virus actually causes hepatitis.

Other viruses that may be associated with hepatitis included the Epstein-Barr virus, yellow fever, Ebola, Marburg virus, adenoviruses, influenza, enteroviruses, and Rift Valley fever. These viruses should be considered in persons presenting with hepatitis with appropriate exposures or travel that might put them at risk for these viruses.

References

1. ACIP. Prevention of hepatitis A through active or passive immunization: recommendations of the Advisory Committee on Immunization Practices (ACIP). *MMWR.* 1999;48(RR12):1-37.
2. Lee W. Hepatitis B virus infection. *N Engl J Med.* 1997;337:1733-1745.
3. Lok AS, McMahon BJ. (2001). Chronic hepatitis B. *Hepatology.* 2001; 34(6):1225-1241.
4. Alter M, Kruszon-Moran D, et al. The prevalence of hepatitis C virus infection in the United States, 1988 through 1994. *N Engl J Med.* 1999;341(8):556-562.
5. Seef LB. Pathogenesis, natural history, treatment and prevention of hepatitis C. *Ann Intern Med.* 2000;132(4):299-300.

6. Kenny-Walsh E. Clinical outcomes after hepatitis C infection from contaminated anti-D immune globulin. *N Engl J Med.* 1999;340(16):1228-1233.
7. Gretch DR. Diagnostic tests for hepatitis C. *Hepatology.* 1997;26(3):43S-47S.
8. DiBisceglie A, Hoofnagle J. Optimal therapy of hepatitis C. *Hepatology.* 2002;36(5 Suppl 1):S121-127.
9. Diepolder H, Zachoval R, et al. Possible mechanism involving T-lymphocyte response to non-structural protein 3 in viral clearance in acute hepatitis C virus infection. *Lancet.* 1995;346(8981):1006-1007.
10. Missale G, Bertoni R, et al. Different clinical behaviors of acute hepatitis C virus infection are associated with different vigor of the anti-viral cell-mediated immune response. *J Clin Invest.* 1996;98(3):706-714.
11. Rehermann B, Chang K, et al. Differential cytotoxic T-lymphocyte responsiveness to the hepatitis B anc C viruses in chronically infected patients. *J Virol.* 1996; 70(10):7092-7102.
12. Lechner F, Wong D, et al. Analysis of successful immune responses in persons infected with hepatitis C virus. *J Ex Med.* 2000;191(9):1499-1512.
13. Chang K, Thimme R, et al. Differential CD4(+) and CD8(+) T cell responsiveness in hepatitis C virus infection. *Hepatology.* 2001;33:267-276.
14. Alberti A, Boccato S, et al. Therapy of acute hepatitis C. *Hepatology.* 2002;36(5 Suppl 1): S195-200.
15. Davis GL. Monitoring of viral levels during therapy of hepatitis C. *Hepatology.* 2002;36(5 Suppl 1):S150.
16. Seef LB. Natural history of chronic hepatitis C. *Hepatology.* 2002;36(5 Suppl 1):S35-46.

chapter **4**

Primary Biliary Cirrhosis and Primary Sclerosing Cholangitis

Mical S. Campbell, MD and Thomas Faust, MD

Introduction

Primary biliary cirrhosis (PBC) is a chronic cholestatic liver disease that predominantly affects middle-aged women. It is an autoimmune disease, and antimitochondrial antibodies are found in the majority of patients. Granulomatous destruction of bile ducts within the liver is characteristic of PBC. Over time fibrosis, cirrhosis, and complications of portal hypertension and cholestasis may develop. Ursodeoxycholic acid has been shown to improve cholestatic liver associated enzymes. It appears to improve transplant-free survival, though the effect is not certain. In addition to PBC-specific treatment, therapies should also be directed towards complications of portal hypertension and prolonged cholestasis. Liver transplantation is the treatment of choice for patients with advanced PBC.

Primary sclerosing cholangitis (PSC) is a chronic cholestatic liver disease that primarily affects young to middle-aged men, who typically have concurrent inflammatory bowel disease. Strictures with intervening normal or dilated segments produce the beading characteristic on cholangiography. PSC patients are at risk for bacterial cholangitis, cholangiocarcinoma, and complications of liver failure and cholestasis. There is no proven therapy specific for PSC. Medical therapies should be directed towards complications of portal hypertension and progressive cholestasis. Liver transplantation is the only option that has been clearly shown to improve patient survival.

Primary Biliary Cirrhosis

Epidemiology

Women outnumber men by a ratio of 9:1. PBC can be seen in patients between 30 and 70 years of age, and most present during middle age. PBC accounts for 2% of worldwide deaths from chronic liver disease. The highest incidence and prevalence of PBC have been reported from Northern Europe and the United States. Data from the United Kingdom show a recent increase in incidence and prevalence of PBC, possibly reflecting better detection and awareness. Data from Minnesota, USA reveal a constant incidence of PBC over the past 25 years.

Familial clustering of PBC has been reported, though the disease is not inherited in a simple recessive or dominant fashion. Patients with PBC have a family history of PBC at a rate of 1% to 6%. One study showed a 0.72% prevalence of PBC among first degree relatives, 1.2% prevalence in offspring, and 2.3% prevalence in female offspring.[1]

A recent American study showed that PBC is associated with increasing number of pregnancies. Other variables independently associated with PBC include presence of extrahepatic autoimmune disease, having ever smoked, and history of a genitourinary infection.[2]

Clinical Features

Forty to 60% of PBC patients are asymptomatic at the time of diagnosis. Patients are commonly identified after the incidental discovery of abnormal liver associated enzymes. Most patients will progress over time to develop symptoms and complications from PBC, though the asymptomatic phase may last for up to 20 years.

Fatigue occurs in up to 85% of PBC patients. Fatigue does not correlate with severity of liver disease or age. In one study, 85% of PBC patients were fatigued. Unexpectedly 45% of patients were also diagnosed with depression, and depression was shown to correlate with fatigue.[3]

Pruritus (25% to 70%) is more frequently seen with early disease and may improve as PBC progresses. Occasionally, pruritis may prove debilitating and refractory to medical therapy. Liver transplantation may be required.

Jaundice (10% to 30%) is an important indicator of advanced PBC. Concluding that jaundice is a result of advanced PBC should be made after considering alternative possibilities, including Gilbert's syndrome, common bile duct stones, and a toxic medication effect.

Hepatosplenomegaly, right upper quadrant pain, and hyperpigmentation are present in 15% to 70% of patients. Xanthelasmas (cholesterol deposits around the eyes) and xanthomata (cholesterol deposits in tendon sheaths, bones, and nerves) are not uncommon in PBC. They may or may not be associated with hypercholesterolemia. Xanthomata may spontaneously disappear with disease progression.

Up to 85% of PBC patients may demonstrate hyperlipidemia. Despite often markedly elevated cholesterol levels, available data do not demonstrate increased risk of atherosclerosis and cardiovascular events among PBC patients; therefore, treatment recommendations for hyperlipidemia are controversial. A recent large study of 400 PBC patients showed that both HDL and LDL tended to be lower in more advanced disease. No significant difference in cardiovascular events from the general age and sex matched population were noted.[4]

Malabsorption and steatorrhea are typically seen only with advanced PBC. Concomitant pancreatic insufficiency and celiac disease must be considered in the differential diagnosis. Deficiencies of fat soluble vitamins A, D, E, and K may occur in advanced PBC, but are rarely symptomatic.

Metabolic bone disease is common in PBC. Osteomalacia, characterized by decreased bone mineralization, is uncommon in PBC. Typically associated with vitamin D deficiency, treatment emphasizes normalization of plasma calcidiol (25-hydroxyvitamin D) levels. Osteoporosis (33%) is more common than osteomalacia and may account for an increased risk of vertebral and rib fractures before and after liver transplantation. Some, but not all, reports have shown that severity of liver disease correlates with increased risk of osteoporosis. Other predictors of osteoporosis include age and body mass index. On the other hand, a recent large study of osteoporosis in 272 PBC patients showed osteoporosis to be no more common in PBC than in similar patients without PBC.[5] The study included patients who had relatively less advanced PBC. It is possible that a high background rate of osteoporosis in a predominantly female and postmenopausal group of patients swamped any effect on bone density from early PBC.

Variceal hemorrhage has been observed in PBC patients without cirrhosis, due to presinusoidal portal hypertension. More commonly, bleeding from esophageal or gastric varices reflects the preterminal phase of PBC, which lasts approximately 2 years and is associated with hepatic synthetic dysfunction and complications of portal hypertension. Variceal hemorrhage, intractable ascites, refractory encephalopathy, and malnutrition may develop and are indications for liver replacement.

Patients with advanced disease are at risk for hepatobiliary malignancies. Hepatocellular carcinoma can develop in 6% of patients with stage III or IV PBC, and may be more prevalent in males. Cholangiocarcinoma has also been reported but is rare. Patients with PBC are not at increased risk for nonhepatobiliary cancers, including breast cancer.[6]

Up to 70% of patients with PBC may develop a variety of extrahepatic, primarily autoimmune disorders. Thyroid disease is present in 15% to 20% of patients. Hashimoto's thyroiditis is much more common than Graves' disease. Autoimmune thyroid disorders often predate PBC and are frequently associated with the production of antithyroid antibodies. Thyroid function tests should be checked in all patients with PBC. CREST syndrome, scleroderma, systemic lupus erythematosus, and rheumatoid arthritis are present in 5%, 15%, 5%, and 10% of patients respectively. Raynaud's phenomenon and polymyositis may also develop in 10% of patients. Seventy percent of patients with PBC complain of xerophthalmia, xerostomia, dysphagia, and dyspareunia consistent with the sicca syndrome. Proximal or distal renal tubular acidosis and membranous or focal proliferative glomerulonephritis can develop in 50% and 5% of patients respectively. Other rare extrahepatic manifestations of PBC include celiac disease, gallstones, autoimmune warm and cold hemolytic anemia, immune thrombocytopenia, inflammatory bowel disease, fibrosing alveolitis, pulmonary interstitial fibrosis, myasthenia gravis, vitiligo, and hypertrophic pulmonary osteoarthropathy.

Diagnosis

Biochemical Tests

The serum alkaline phosphatase is greater than 3 to 4 times the upper limits of normal in most patients. Alkaline phosphatase levels do not correlate with disease severity and are not prognostically important. Most patients with PBC have elevations in the transaminases, usually below 3 times the upper limit of normal. Markedly elevated values in PBC patients suggest other conditions including viral hepatitis, drug-induced hepatotoxicity, or an overlap syndrome with autoimmune hepatitis. The bilirubin of patients with early PBC is usually normal. With disease progression, bilirubin will increase. The rise in serum bilirubin is a sign of poor prognosis and may indicate the need for liver transplantation. Prolongation of the prothrombin time and hypoalbuminemia are also suggestive of impaired hepatic reserve. Hypercholesterolemia is a common finding, though it is not a marker for increased risk of atherosclerotic complications in PBC patients.

Serology

Antimitochondrial antibodies (AMA) are the serologic hallmark of PBC. Titers ≥1:40 are significant and are present in 95% of patients with PBC. The sensitivity and specificity of AMA for diagnosis approaches 95%. For patients with significant AMA titers and normal liver associated enzymes, annual biochemical liver tests should be performed; most patients have histologic injury compatible with PBC and will develop symptomatic disease over time. ANA and/or ASMA are present in low titer in one-third and two-thirds, respectively, of PBC patients. Antithyroid, antiacetylcholine receptor, antiplatelet, antihistone, and anticentromere antibodies have also been identified with PBC in isolated cases. Patients with PBC typically have elevated immunoglobulin M in serum.

AMA-negative PBC, or autoimmune cholangiopathy, is diagnosed in patients with clinical, biochemical, and histologic features compatible with a diagnosis of PBC in patients who do not develop antimitochondrial antibodies. Such patients may have high titers of ANA or ASMA and elevated immunoglobulin G in serum. The natural history for patients with AMA-negative disease is similar to that of classic PBC.

Medical Imaging

Medical imaging does not serve an important role for the diagnosis of PBC. Ultrasound, computed tomography (CT), and magnetic resonance imaging (MRI) are primarily used to exclude biliary obstruction and malignancy. In early disease, CT may demonstrate a normal or large liver. Patients with advanced disease may have a small heterogenous liver with intraabdominal collaterals, splenomegaly, ascites, and portacaval or portahepatic adenopathy. Hepatocellular carcinoma may also be detected. The "periportal halo sign" may be a specific MR sign of PBC; low intensity signals around enhancing intrahepatic portal branches represent cellular drop out and fibrosis. Cholangiography is generally not required in the evaluation of patients with suspected PBC unless extrahepatic disease is suspected.

Histology

Liver biopsy may not be necessary for diagnosis in patients with AMA titers ≥1:40, typical symptoms and signs of PBC, and cholestatic liver indices. Liver biopsy plays a key diagnostic role if the AMA is negative, if an overlap syndrome with autoimmune hepatitis is possible, or if diagnostic uncertainty exists.

In addition to diagnosis, liver biopsy provides important staging and prognosis information. Four stages of PBC have been described. Stage 1 (portal stage) demonstrates granulomatous destruction of bile ducts (the florid duct lesion) with infiltration of the portal tracts by lymphocytes and plasma cells. The florid duct lesion is identified in only 10% of liver biopsies. Bile duct loss in association with periportal hepatitis represents stage 2 (periportal stage). Septal fibrosis between adjacent portal tracts is observed in stage 3. Established cirrhosis with regenerative nodule formation represents stage 4. Granulomatous destruction of bile ducts is pathognomonic for PBC.

Table 4-1

DIFFERENTIAL DIAGNOSIS OF PRIMARY BILIARY CIRRHOSIS

- Choledocholithiasis
- Biliary stricture
- Pancreaticobiliary malignancy
- Medications (estrogens, androgenic steroids, phenothiazines)
- Sarcoidosis
- Granulomatous hepatitis
- Small duct variant of PSC
- Autoimmune hepatitis and autoimmune hepatitis/PBC overlap

Nodular regenerative hyperplasia (nodules of hepatocytes without fibrosis) can be seen with early disease and may account for presinusoidal portal hypertension in patients without cirrhosis.[7]

DIFFERENTIAL DIAGNOSIS

Many diseases associated with intrahepatic and extrahepatic cholestasis require exclusion before a diagnosis of PBC can be made (Table 4-1). Choledocholithiasis, isolated biliary strictures, and pancreaticobiliary neoplasms can produce extrahepatic obstruction with cholestasis. Noninvasive imaging or cholangiography is usually required to exclude these conditions. Although PSC typically has characteristic cholangiographic signs of biliary duct dilation and structuring, the small duct variant of PSC can be confused with PBC.

Many medications (eg, estrogens, androgenic steroids, and phenothiazines) can produce intrahepatic cholestasis. Autoimmune hepatitis can occasionally be confused with PBC, especially if an overlap syndrome exists. Patients with autoimmune hepatitis and PBC overlap have high titers of AMA as well as antinuclear or anti-smooth muscle antibody; histology is consistent with both autoimmune hepatitis and PBC.

HCV may show granulomatous bile duct destruction, but AMA is negative and HCV antibody is positive. Sarcoidosis is associated with granulomatous portal inflammation and intrahepatic cholestasis. Ninety percent of patients with sarcoidosis have abnormal chest radiographs.

NATURAL HISTORY AND PROGNOSIS

In most cases, PBC is a progressive disease. Survival of patients with asymptomatic disease is less than that of age, race, and gender-matched controls; however, asymptomatic patients live longer than patients with symptomatic disease. One study of 91 asymptomatic patients showed that 36% of patients became symptomatic during study observation (median follow-up 61 months), and that median survival was 14 years, (less than that for age and gender matched controls). No prognostic feature identified those initially asymptomatic patients who would develop progressive disease.[8]

Numerous models have been developed which aid the clinician to predict prognosis in PBC. The Mayo Clinic model is the most popular and well validated. It uses five variables (age, serum total bilirubin, albumin, prothrombin time, and edema). The Mayo model does not take into account histological stage, variceal hemorrhage, the development of hepatocellular carcinoma, and quality of life parameters. Bilirubin is the single most important variable in predicting disease severity and the need to consider liver transplantation.

Treatment

Because survival of asymptomatic and symptomatic PBC patients is inferior to that of a control population, all patients may benefit from treatment. Unfortunately, no medical treatment has been shown to stop disease progression and obviate the need for liver transplantation. Ursodeoxycholic acid is currently the only US Food and Drug Administration-approved (FDA) medication for PBC. The overall goals of treatment are to slow disease progression and to treat symptoms and complications resulting from both cholestasis and portal hypertension.

Medical Therapy of PBC

A number of immunosuppressive medications have been studied for the treatment of PBC. Unfortunately, no immunomodulatory agent is clearly effective. Systemic corticosteroids may improve symptoms, cholestatic liver function tests, and histology in some patients, but there is no improvement in overall survival. Furthermore, corticosteroids may worsen osteopenia. Budesonide has also been studied in small trials and has not been shown to be effective. Azathioprine, penicillamine, cyclosporine, colchicine, and chlorambucil have not improved mortality in PBC, though many of the studies were too small to expect a survival benefit. Although pilot studies suggest possible benefit from methotrexate, potential methotrexate hepatic toxicity is concerning. Mycophenolate mofetil has shown some initial promising results and is currently under study. Combination therapy with immunosuppressive medications and ursodeoxycholic acid will require further study.

Ursodeoxycholic acid (UDCA) is the most effective and only FDA-approved medication for patients with PBC. UDCA at 13 to 15 mg/kg/day leads to improvement in symptoms and cholestatic liver indices. The drug is safe and well tolerated; the most common side effect is diarrhea. Some, but not all, studies have shown other positive effects, including a mortality benefit, improvement of transplant free survival rate, improvement of histologic stage, and a reduction in the risk of developing esophageal varices. UDCA has a variable effect on pruritis, and it has not been shown to improve osteoporosis or fatigue. A meta-analysis of three randomized controlled trials with adequate dosing of UDCA (13 to 15 mg/kg/day) and long-term follow-up (4 years) showed improved survival without liver transplantation compared to placebo.[9] Studies that have not shown a mortality benefit from UDCA have been criticized for their small size, low dose of UDCA (lower than 13 to 15 mg/kg/day), and follow-up for only 2 years or less. Regardless of the benefits that may accrue from taking UDCA, most treated patients will ultimately progress to end-stage liver disease and require liver replacement.

Liver Transplantation

Liver transplantation is indicated for patients with advanced PBC and evidence of impaired hepatic reserve. Progressive hyperbilirubinemia and a Mayo risk score between 7.5 and 8 are poor prognostic signs and important indicators of the need to consider transplantation. Patients with intractable pruritus and severe osteoporosis with nontraumatic bone fractures may also benefit from liver replacement.

Cadaveric transplantation is standard of care for patients with decompensated cirrhosis, but adult to adult living donor transplantation is another option for carefully selected patients. Patients considered for live donation should be reasonably well compensated and have a low Mayo risk score. One and 5-year survival rates after transplantation are excellent, approximately 92% and 85% respectively. Even though UDCA has been shown to delay timing of liver transplantation, outcome after transplantation for patients taking UDCA is not negatively affected.

Antimitochondrial antibodies persist after transplantation, but there is no correlation between the antibody titer and the risk of histologic recurrence of PBC. Liver biopsy is the gold standard to diagnose PBC recurrence and should reveal granulomatous bile duct destruction. Moreover, exclusion of acute and chronic rejection, medication effects, viral hepatitis, and graft vs host disease is important. Ten to 30% of patients transplanted for PBC may develop recurrence of PBC within the graft after 3 to 10 years. Patients who receive tacrolimus may be at higher risk for recurrence compared to patients who receive cyclosporine.[10] Fewer than 10% of PBC patients undergo retransplantation.

Portal Hypertension

Portal hypertension can develop either as a consequence of the development of cirrhosis or as a result of nodular regenerative hyperplasia in patients without cirrhosis. AASLD guidelines recommend that upon diagnosis of PBC, patients should undergo upper endoscopy to screen for varices, though there are no convincing supportive data. Patients should continue to undergo endoscopy every 2 to 3 years until varices are found. Standard treatment with nonselective β-blockers can be administered to prevent a first variceal bleed once medium to large sized varices are documented. Standard therapy, including endoscopic sclerotherapy, band ligation, or nonselective β-blockers, is appropriate for patients with a history of variceal bleeding. For patients with variceal bleeding refractory to endoscopic therapy and β-blockers, distal splenorenal shunts are appropriate for patients with well-preserved hepatic synthetic function, whereas transjugular intrahepatic portosystemic shunts (TIPS) are advised for patients with decompensated liver disease awaiting liver transplantation.

Sodium-restricted diets, spironolactone, and furosemide are recommended for patients with volume overload and ascites. Therapeutic paracentesis or TIPS is appropriate for patients with ascites refractory to sodium restriction and diuretics. Lactulose, neomycin, and diets enriched with branched-chain amino acids are standard therapies for patients with hepatic encephalopathy.

Management of Complications Associated With PBC

Osteoporosis (T score >2.5 SD below the mean for normal young adults) is more common than osteomalacia. Dual-energy x-ray absorptiometry (DEXA) demonstrates decreased bone mineral density in patients with osteoporosis. The role of DEXA in screening for osteoporosis in PBC patients, in both early and late stage PBC, is not well established, although current AASLD guidelines recommend that DEXA be performed upon diagnosis of PBC and every 2 years thereafter. Questions remain whether patients with PBC truly have a higher rate of osteoporosis than the general population and whether current therapies for osteoporosis are effective in PBC patients.

Though evidence of benefit is lacking, all osteoporotic PBC patients should receive enough supplemental calcium so that total intake is at least 1500 mg/day. Vitamin D 800 IU/day may also be given. Furthermore, all patients are encouraged to stop smoking and exercise in moderation. Estrogen replacement, selective estrogen receptor modulators, and parathyroid hormone have not been adequately studied in PBC patients. Calcitonin has not been shown to improve osteoporosis associated with cholestatic liver disease. Contradictory results have so far been obtained from the use of bisphosphonates (alendronate and etidronate) in PBC patients with osteoporosis.

Liver transplantation is recommended for patients with severe osteoporosis and non-traumatic bone fractures. Even though bone density decreases shortly after OLT, bone density (T scores) approach that of healthy controls approximately 2 years after transplantation as a result of improved hepatic function, corticosteroid reduction, and increased mobility.

Pruritus is a significant problem in many patients with PBC. Antihistamines, phenobarbital, and UDCA are not consistently effective. Pruritus improves in 90% of patients who receive cholestyramine (4 g before and after breakfast). Cholestyramine impairs absorption of other oral drugs, and no other medication should be given within four hours of cholestyramine administration. For patients who do not respond to cholestyramine, rifampicin (300 to 600 mg/day) has been shown to be effective within 1 month of administration. Endogenous opioid antagonists (naloxone, nalmaphene, and naltrexone) may also be effective in selected patients with PBC and disabling pruritus who do not respond to the above measures. Liver transplantation is reserved for patients with intractable and debilitating pruritis.

Fat-soluble vitamin deficiency (vitamins A, D, E, and K) is uncommon in PBC. Deficiencies are more likely among patients with more advanced liver disease. One study of 180 patients with PBC showed that testing patients with a Mayo risk score of 5 or more maximizes sensitivity and specificity of identifying vitamin A deficiency (the most common deficiency). The authors recommend that all patients with a Mayo risk score of 5 or greater be screened for fat-soluble vitamin deficiencies.[11]

Thirty percent of patients with PBC have vitamin A deficiency, but most patients are asymptomatic and do not have night blindness. Vitamin A replacement (10,000 to 25,000 units daily or 25,000 to 50,000 units, 2 to 3 times weekly) is recommended and follow-up of serum levels is required. Vitamin D deficiency is seen in 13% of patients with PBC, but osteomalacia is rare. Vitamin D deficiency is detected by testing serum calcidiol (25-hydroxy-vitamin D) levels. Replacement dosing of vitamin D is 25,000 to 50,000 IU 2 to 3 times per week, given with supplemental calcium. Close follow-up of serum vitamin D levels is required. Vitamin E deficiency is rarely seen in the adult population, but significant deficiency is associated with reduced proprioception and gait disturbance. Daily doses between 400 and 1000 IU are usually sufficient for treatment. Prolongation of the prothrombin time in patients without cirrhosis is usually the result of vitamin K malabsorption, which corrects after parenteral vitamin K administration.

Although up to 85% of PBC patients may have *hypercholesterolemia*, patients do not appear to be at risk for an increased rate of cardiovascular events. UDCA has been shown to reduce LDL and increase HDL. The role of standard anticholesterolemic agents, such as statins, has not been established.

Steatorrhea is not uncommon in patients with advanced PBC. Decreased bile acid delivery, pancreatic insufficiency, celiac disease, and bacterial overgrowth (either alone or in combination) may play a role in fat malabsorption. Low fat diets with or without medium chain triglyceride supplementation is recommended for patients with luminal bile acid deficiency, whereas pancreatic enzyme supplementation is appropriate for patients with impaired pancreatic function. Gluten-free diets and antibiotic therapy are recommended for PBC patients with celiac disease and bacterial overgrowth respectively.

Table 4-2 further illustrates the various complications.

Primary Sclerosing Cholangitis

Epidemiology

Unlike PBC, up to 70% of patients with PSC are men. The mean age of presentation is 40 years. A population-based study in Minnesota showed that the incidence and prevalence of PSC are approximately one-third of those for PBC. More than half of patients are asymptomatic at diagnosis.[12]

Clinical Features

The majority of patients with PSC are asymptomatic at diagnosis. The diagnosis should be considered in patients with unexplained abnormal liver associated enzymes, particularly an elevated alkaline phosphatase in a patient with inflammatory bowel disease. With time, most patients will develop symptoms associated with progressive disease including fatigue, jaundice (Table 4-3), and pruritus. Fever and abdominal pain may be symptoms of bacterial cholangitis. Jaundice may indicate advanced PSC, sepsis from bacterial infection, or mechanical obstruction (gallstones, dominant stricture, or cholangiocarcinoma). Endoscopic therapy of common bile duct stones (present in up to one-third of patients with PSC) or a dominant biliary stricture may lead to resolution of jaundice. Other possible manifestations of PSC include hepatosplenomegaly and hyperpigmentation.

As for patients with PBC, PSC patients may be diagnosed with steatorrhea, fat soluble vitamin deficiencies, hypercholesterolemia, and metabolic bone disease. In one study of fat soluble vitamin deficiency and hyperlipidemia, up to 80% of PSC patients undergoing liver transplantation evaluation were deficient in Vitamin A (though no night blindness reported), and 57% were deficient in Vitamin D. Lower levels of fat soluble vitamin deficiency were noted among patients with less advanced PSC. Hypercholesterolemia was noted in 40% of PSC patients undergoing a randomized controlled trial of ursodeoxycholic acid.[13]

Although patients with PSC are more likely to have osteoporosis than the general population, the rate of osteoporosis appears to be lower than in PBC (10% vs 33%). Osteoporosis has been shown to correlate with more advanced PSC.[14] After liver transplantation, one third of patients with osteopenia will develop nontraumatic fractures.

Patients with decompensated cirrhosis are at risk for portal hypertensive complications. In particular, PSC patients who have undergone total colectomy for inflammatory bowel disease may bleed from peristomal varices.

Table 4-2

Complications Associated With Primary Biliary Cirrhosis

Complication	*Screening*	*Treatment*
Osteoporosis	??DEXA at diagnosis and every 2 years thereafter	Calcium (1500 mg/day), vitamin D (800 IU/day), ??Bisphosponates
Pruritis	Clinical history	Cholestyramine (8 g/day), rifampicin (300 to 600 mg/day), naltrexone (50 mg/day)
Fat soluble vitamin deficiency	If advanced PBC (Mayo risk score ≥5), check serum vitamin A, 25-hydroxyvitamin D, vitamin E, prothrombin time	Vitamin A (10,000 to 25,000 U/day), Vitamin D (25,000 to 50,000 IU 2 to 3 times/week), vitamin E 1000 IU/day, vitamin K (10 mg IV)
Hypercholesterolemia	No proven role for cholesterol screening	No treatment needed, ??role of statins
Malabsorption and diarrhea	Stool fecal fat; evaluate for celiac disease, bacterial overgrowth, and pancreatic insufficiency	Low-fat diet, gluten-free diet for celiac disease, antibiotics for overgrowth, pancreatic enzymes if insufficient
Variceal bleeding	??EGD to screen for medium to large varices upon diagnosis of PBC, follow-up EGD's depend on findings	Nonselective β-blockers to prevent first bleed; β-blockers, sclerosis, or banding to prevent recurrent variceal bleeding

The lifetime risk of cholangiocarcinoma in PSC patients is up to 33%. Patients with malignancy can present with progressive jaundice, anorexia, weight loss, and abdominal pain. Patients at highest risk are those with long-standing ulcerative colitis and cirrhosis. Ultrasound and CT scanning are insensitive tests for early disease, but may identify metastatic disease. Based on cholangiography, cholangiocarcinoma may be difficult to distinguish from a benign dominant biliary stricture. Patients with a dominant stricture or a suspected cholangiocarcinoma should have biliary duct brushings performed, though cytology is only 40% to 60% sensitive for cancer. A CA 19-9 threshold of 100 U/mL has been shown to be 89% sensitive and 86% specific for

Table 4-3

DIFFERENTIAL DIAGNOSIS OF JAUNDICE IN PSC

- Advanced PSC
- Sepsis from bacterial infection
- Choledocholithiasis
- Dominant stricture
- Cholangiocarcinoma

diagnosing cholangiocarcinoma. At present, the role of positron emission tomography (PET) in the evaluation of suspected cholangiocarcinoma is unclear.

PSC can coexist with other autoimmune liver diseases. Autoimmune hepatitis and PSC overlap is predominantly seen in children and young adults. Patients with an overlap syndrome typically have cholangiography consistent with PSC as well as features associated with autoimmune hepatitis including elevated transaminases, positive ANA, positive antismooth muscle antibody, and liver biopsy showing necroinflammatory activity within portal tracts.

Patients with PSC frequently have other autoimmune-based diseases. Inflammatory bowel disease (IBD) is present in 75% to 90% of patients with PSC, and PSC is present in 2% to 7% of patients with IBD. Eighty-seven percent of patients with PSC and IBD have ulcerative colitis and 13% of patients have Crohn's colitis. IBD in PSC patients is usually a quiescent pancolitis. Colonoscopy may appear normal, and IBD will only be demonstrated on random colonoscopic biopsies of normal appearing colonic mucosa. Patients with PSC and ulcerative colitis have a greater risk of developing colon adenocarcinoma when compared to patients who have colitis alone. There is no relationship between the clinical course of IBD and that of PSC. Proctocolectomy should not be performed with the intent of altering the natural course of biliary tract disease. If a colectomy is required for IBD refractory to medical therapy, the ileoanal pouch procedure is preferred to avoid the risk of peristomal variceal formation associated with ileostomy.

Acute and chronic pancreatitis, diabetes mellitus, the sicca syndrome, autoimmune thyroid disease, retroperitoneal fibrosis, celiac sprue, autoimmune hemolytic anemia, immune thrombocytopenic purpura, systemic lupus erythematosus, rheumatoid arthritis, vasculitis, and systemic sclerosis can also be seen. Polymyositis, ankylosing spondylitis, myasthenia gravis, angioimmunoblastic lymphadenopathy, and membranous glomerulonephritis are rarely observed.

DIAGNOSIS

Biochemical and Serologic Tests

Liver associated enzymes reveal a cholestatic pattern. As in PBC, the alkaline phosphatase is usually greater than 3 to 5 times the upper limit of normal, whereas the transaminases are more commonly less than 3 times the upper normal limit. The serum bilirubin may be normal or elevated with early disease, but it usually rises steadily with disease progression. A variety of autoantibodies may be observed in PSC patients, but they serve little role in diagnosis. Antineutrophil cytoplasmic antibodies (ANCA) are present in up to 80% of patients, whereas ANA and ASMA can be seen in low titer in 20%. As with other forms of chronic liver disease, impaired hepatic reserve is associated with a fall in albumin and prolongation of the prothrombin time.

Medical Imaging

Cholangiography remains the gold standard for diagnosis of PSC. Endoscopic retrograde cholangiopancreatography (ERCP) is preferred to percutaneous transhepatic cholangiography, which should be reserved for patients in whom ERCP cannot be successfully accomplished. At the time of cholangiography, brushings for cytology, and balloon dilation with stenting of dominant strictures can also be performed. Magnetic resonance cholangiography (MRC) is a noninvasive imaging test that is 88% sensitive and 97% specific for detecting PSC. MRC has been used increasingly as an initial diagnostic test for PSC, including in children. The accuracy of MRC for detecting cholangiocarcinoma has not been determined.

Cholangiography shows diffuse strictures of the intrahepatic and/or extrahepatic bile ducts in approximately 90% of patients. Short segments of normal or dilated ducts may be seen between biliary strictures, giving a classic beaded appearance. The gallbladder and cystic duct are involved in 15% of patients. Ten to 20% of patients may develop a dominant biliary stricture. Patients typically have associated biliary obstruction, possibly with jaundice and ascending cholangitis. A dominant stricture can be difficult to distinguish from cholangiocarcinoma, which may appear as a mass or stricture, possibly with markedly dilated ducts and metastases.

Histology

Liver biopsy is complementary to cholangiography in the evaluation of patients with suspected PSC. Even though cholangiography is the gold standard for diagnosis, biopsy is useful for determining stage and prognosis. As with PBC, four histologic stages have been described. Stage 1 (portal stage) shows inflammation in the portal tracts. Onion skin lesions (concentric layers of connective tissue) may surround bile ducts. Periportal inflammation with ductopenia and mild fibrosis around the portal triads characterize stage 2 (periportal stage). Portal to portal septal fibrosis define stage 3 (septal stage), whereas stage 4 (cirrhotic stage) is associated with regenerative nodules and biliary cirrhosis. Liver biopsies are subject to sampling error and are not generally required for a diagnosis of PSC.

Differential Diagnosis

A diagnosis of PSC requires that a number of other diseases with similar cholangiographic appearance be excluded (Table 4-4). AIDS cholangiopathy, choledocholithiasis, congenital biliary tract disease, previous biliary tract surgery, biliary malignancy (unless a previous diagnosis of PSC has been established), and ischemic bile duct injury can produce cholangiographic findings similar to that of PSC. Hepatic arterial chemotherapy with fluoxuridine, cirrhosis not related to PSC, submassive hepatic necrosis, amyloidosis, metastatic carcinoma, and hepatic infiltration with leukemia or lymphoma can also resemble PSC.

Up to 5% of patients with PSC have small duct sclerosing cholangitis. These patients have normal cholangiograms, but they have liver biopsy results consistent

Table 4-4

DIFFERENTIAL DIAGNOSIS OF PRIMARY SCLEROSING CHOLANGITIS

- AIDS cholangiopathy
- Choledocholithiasis
- Congenital biliary disease
- Complications of prior biliary surgery
- Biliary malignancy
- Ischemic bile duct injury
- Metastatic cancer
- Leukemia, lymphoma
- PSC with autoimmune hepatitis overlap

with PSC. Liver associated enzymes (particularly alkaline phosphatase) are elevated, and inflammatory bowel disease is often present. It is important to perform liver biopsy on patients who clinically appear to have PSC, but demonstrate normal cholangiography because biopsy may show small duct sclerosing cholangitis. One recent report of 32 such patients shows a generally benign clinical course. Only 15% developed cholangiographic findings of typical PSC during follow-up.[15]

Natural History and Prognosis

As with PBC, PSC is a slowly progressive cholestatic liver disease. Over 75% of asymptomatic patients develop symptoms. Survival of patients with asymptomatic and symptomatic disease is shorter than healthy controls matched for age, gender, and race. The median survival of patients with PSC from the time of diagnosis is 10 to 15 years without transplantation. The revised Mayo risk score incorporates age, serum bilirubin, serum albumin, serum AST, and history of variceal bleeding. The risk score has been validated to correlate well with survival and helps guide timing of liver transplantation. Unlike other prognostic indices, the score does not incorporate findings from liver biopsy. Since diagnosis can be accurately made by cholangiography and prognosis is based on an index that does not use biopsy results, one group questions the need for liver biopsy in most PSC patients. Among 79 patients who underwent liver biopsy after cholangiography, in only one patient did biopsy change management (PSC/autoimmune overlap shown on biopsy), and one patient had a complication from liver biopsy (bile leak).[16]

Treatment

Medical Therapy of Primary Sclerosing Cholangitis

Many different medications have been tried without clear benefit to the progression of PSC. Colchicine, cyclosporine, methotrexate, penicillamine, tacrolimus, corticosteroids, azathioprine, pentoxifylline, nicotine, and budesonide have not demonstrated efficacy for treating PSC. Ursodeosycholic acid (UDCA) at a dose of 13 to 15 mg/kg/day for 6 years led to improvement in biochemical parameters, but did not improve histologic stage, time to death, or transplantation when compared to placebo. High dose (20 to 30 mg/kg) UDCA has shown promise in small studies to improve not only biochemical liver indices, but also histologic stage, cholangiographic appearance, and Mayo risk score. Large randomized controlled trials are required before high dose UDCA can become standard of care for PSC.

UDCA shows promise as a colon cancer chemopreventive agent. A recent analysis of a randomized controlled UDCA study in PSC patients with ulcerative colitis showed that patients assigned to UDCA 13 to 15 mg/kg/day had a relative risk of 0.26 (0.06 to 0.92) for developing colorectal dysplasia or cancer.[17]

Medical Treatment of Complications

Patients with cholestasis may have dominant strictures of the common bile and common hepatic ducts that are amenable to endoscopic or radiologic dilation and stenting. Patients with dominant strictures require careful assessment to exclude cholangiocarcinoma. Patients with PSC and symptomatic cholelithiasis and choledocholithiasis may require cholecystectomy and sphincterotomy with stone extraction respectively. Patients who present with symptoms and signs consistent with bacterial cholangitis require either endoscopic or radiologic biliary drainage in conjunction with broad-spectrum antibiotics (eg, ciprofloxacin, amoxicillin, or trimethoprim-sulfamethoxazole). Long-term antibiotic prophylaxis is justified for patients with recurrent bacterial infections.

Complications of steatorrhea, osteomalacia, pruritis, and fat-soluble vitamin deficiency occurring in PSC patients are treated as they are for PBC patients (as seen previously). For PSC patients with osteoporosis, no therapy has proven efficacy. Bisphosphonates (eg, alendronate or risedronate) may be tried, particularly in patients who have other standard risk factors for osteoporosis, but there is no evidence that they will be effective. In the absence of proven therapies for osteoporosis in PSC patients, routine DEXA for all PSC patients cannot yet be recommended.

Treatment of portal hypertensive complications in patients with PSC is the same as for PBC (see above). PSC patients who have had ileostomies after total colectomy may develop peristomal varices. If the varices bleed, transjugular intrahepatic portosystemic shunt (TIPS) placement or in some cases decompressive surgical shunts may be useful. Better yet is avoidance of ileostomy in PSC patients requiring colectomy; ileoanal pouch anastamosis is preferred.

Biliary Reconstruction

Biliary bypass surgery for dominant strictures is generally not recommended for patients who are transplant candidates, but may be considered in patients with good hepatic synthetic function. Surgery carries a risk of postoperative infection. Furthermore, scarring from surgery may complicate future liver transplantation. The impact of biliary reconstruction on transplant-free survival and the development of cholangiocarcinoma is not clear.

CHOLANGIOCARCINOMA

There are insufficient data to recommend any screening algorithm at this time. Some physicians perform yearly MRC or ERCP with biannual CEA and CA 19-9, but there is no evidence demonstrating benefit from such a program. Emerging data suggest that endoscopic ultrasonography may visualize cholangiocarcinomas and provide diagnostic tissue by fine-needle aspiration even when ERCP brushings are unrevealing. Intraductal ultrasonography requires biliary cannulation for probe placement and may also prove useful for cholangiocarcinoma detection. Therapeutic options for patients with cholangiocarcinoma are limited and include resection, systemic chemotherapy, and radiation. Long-term survival is poor after liver transplantation for patients with PSC and cholangiocarcinoma. Consequently, cholangiocarcinoma is a contraindication to liver replacement.

Liver Transplantation

Liver transplantation with Roux-en-Y choledochojejunostomy is standard of care for PSC patients with decompensated cirrhosis, complications of portal hypertension or cholestasis, and recurrent bacterial cholangitis. One- and 5-year patient survival are 97% and 88%, respectively. PSC may recur in the allograft in up to 20% of patients, but medium-term patient and graft survival are excellent. Before a diagnosis of recurrent PSC can be made, other causes for post-transplant biliary strictures must be excluded including hepatic arterial occlusion, ABO incompatibility between donor and recipient, prolonged cold ischemia time, chronic rejection, and infections.

After liver transplantation, the rate of colon cancer in ulcerative colitis patients with PSC appears to be increased. Annual colonoscopy with random biopsies to assess for colon cancer and dysplasia is recommended for patients with ulcerative or Crohn's colitis after transplantation.

SUMMARY

PBC and PSC are common causes of liver disease. There are some important differences between the two diseases (Table 4-5). PBC occurs in middle-aged women. PSC occurs more commonly in younger men who typically have either ulcerative colitis or less commonly Crohn's colitis. PSC is one third as prevalent as PBC. The diagnosis of PBC can reliably be made by serology; almost all cases are antimitochondrial antibody positive. PSC is diagnosed by cholangiography, which typically demonstrates a beaded appearance. Ursodeoxycholic acid is the cornerstone of therapy for PBC, whereas in PSC urodeoxcycholic acid at high doses shows some promise but no proven efficacy. PBC is not associated with any cancers (apart from hepatocellular carcinoma which can develop in cirrhosis of any cause). PSC is associated with an increased risk for colon cancer among IBD patients. Furthermore, cholangiocarcinoma may develop in up to one third of PSC patients and is a contraindication to liver transplantation.

On the other hand, PBC and PSC share a number of features in common. They are both chronic cholestatic liver diseases that are thought to be disorders of immune regulation. In both PBC and PSC, other autoimmune disorders are common. Pruritis, fatigue, hypercholesterolemia, metabolic bone disease, steatorrhea, and fat-soluble vitamin deficiencies are all potential complications of both PBC and PSC. Both conditions are typically slowly progressive and may result in cirrhosis with complications from portal hypertension. Finally, liver transplantation successfully treats advanced liver disease resulting from either PBC or PSC.

Table 4-5

Comparison of Primary Biliary Cirrhosis and Primary Sclerosing Cholangitis

Feature	*PBC*	*PSC*
Age	Middle-aged	Young to middle-aged
Gender	Female	Male
Association with IBD	Uncommon	Very common
Association with cancer	Hepatocellular carcinoma	Hepatocellular carcinoma Cholangiocarcinoma Colon cancer (with IBD)
Antibodies present	AMA (>95%), ANA (33%), ASMA (66%)	pANCA (80%), ANA (20%), ASMA (20%)
Diagnosis	AMA positive	Cholangiography (beading)
Atypical variant	AMA negative (requires biopsy to diagnose)	Small duct variant (normal cholangiography, requires biopsy to diagnose)
Disease-specific treatment	Ursodeoxycholic acid (13 to 15 mg/kg/day) standard	Ursodeoxycholic acid (20 to 30 mg/kg/day) possibly
Prognostic model	Mayo Risk score (age, bilirubin, albumin, prothrombin time, edema)	Modified Mayo Risk score (age, bilirubin, albumin, AST, variceal bleeding)

Bibliography

1. Jones DEJ, Watt FE, Metcalf JV, et al. Familial primary biliary cirrhosis reassessed: a geographically-based population study. *J Hepatol.* 1999;30:402-407.
2. Parikh-Patel A, Gold E, Utts, J, et al. The association between gravidity and primary biliary cirrhosis. *Ann Epidemiol.* 2002;12:264-272.
3. Huet PM, Deslauriers J, Tran A, et al. Impact of fatigue on the quality of liver of patients with PBC. *Am J Gastroenterol.* 2000;95:760-767.
4. Longo M, Crosignani A, Battezzati PM, et al. Hyperlipidemic state and cardiovascular risk in PBC. *Gut.* 2002;51:265-269.

5. Newton J, Francis R, Prince M, et al. Osteoporosis in PBC revisited. *Gut.* 2001;49:282-287.
6. Nijhawan PK, Therneau TM, Dickson ER. Incidence of cancer in PBC: the Mayo experience. *Hepatology.* 1999;29:1396-1398.
7. Colina F, Pinedo F, Solis JA. Nodular regenerative hyperplasia of the liver in early histological stages of PBC. *Gastroenterology.* 1992;102:1319-1324.
8. Springer J, Cauch-Dudek K, O'Rourke K, et al. Asymptomatic primary biliary cirrhosis: a study of its natural history and prognosis. *Am J Gastroenterol.* 1999;94:47-53.
9. Poupon RE, Lindor KD, Cauch-Dudek K, et al. Combined analysis of randomized controlled trials of ursodeoxycholic acid in primary biliary cirrhosis. *Gastroenterology.* 1997;113:884-890.
10. Sanchez EQ, Levy MF, Goldstein RM, et al. The changing clinical presentation of recurrent primary biliary cirrhosis after liver transplantation. *Transplantation.* 2003;76: 1583-1588.
11. Philips JR, Angulo P, Petterson T, et al. Fat-soluble vitamin levels in patients with primary biliary cirrhosis. *Am J Gastroenterol.* 2001;96:2745-2750.
12. Bambha K, Kim WR, Talwalkar J, et al. Incidence, clinical spectrum, and outcomes of primary sclerosing cholangitis in a United States community. *Gastroenterology.* 2003;125: 1364-1369.
13. Jorgensen RA, Lindor KD, Sartin JS, et al. Serum lipid and fat-soluble vitamin levels in primary sclerosing cholanigitis. *J Clin Gastroenterol.* 1995;20:215-219.
14. Angulo P, Therneau TM, Jorgensen RA, et al. Bone disease in patients with primary sclerosing cholangitis: prevalence, severity, and prediction of progression. *J Hepatol.* 1998;29:729-735.
15. Broome U, Glaumann H, Lindstom E, et al. Natural history and outcome in 32 Swedish patients with small duct primary sclerosing cholangitis (PSC). *J Hepatol.* 2002;36:586-589.
16. Burak KW, Angulo P, Lindor KD. Is there a role for liver biopsy in primary sclerosing cholangitis? *Am J Gastroenterol.* 2003;98:1155-1158.
17. Pardi DS, Loftus EV, Kremers WK, et al. Ursodeoxycholic acid as a chemopreventive agent in patients with ulcerative colitis and primary sclerosing cholangitis. *Gastroenterology.* 2003;124:889-893.

Bibliography

Angulo P, Lindor KD. Primary sclerosing cholangitis. *Hepatology.* 1999;30(1):325-332.

Lee YM, Kaplan MM. Management of primary sclerosing cholangitis. *Am J Gastroenterol.* 2002;97:528-534.

Talwalkar JA, Lindor KD. Primary biliary cirrhosis. *Lancet.* 2003;362:53-61.

chapter 5

Autoimmune Hepatitis

Stanley Martin Cohen, MD

Introduction

Autoimmune hepatitis is a condition of unresolving liver inflammation primarily affecting young women. It is characterized by elevated liver enzymes, hypergammaglobulinemia, serum autoantibodies, interface hepatitis (piecemeal necrosis), and plasma cell infiltrates on liver biopsy, extrahepatic manifestations, and steroid responsiveness.

This chapter will cover all aspects of the disease, with an emphasis on diagnosis and treatment. Overlap syndromes (such as those occurring between autoimmune hepatitis and primary biliary cirrhosis or primary sclerosing cholangitis) will not be discussed.

Historical Perspective

Hepatitis of unclear etiology associated with hypergammaglobulinemia in young women was first described by Waldenström in 1950. The disorder has been given several different names including chronic active liver disease, autoimmune chronic active hepatitis, and lupoid hepatitis due to its association with the lupus erythematosus prep test. The presence of serum autoantibodies was initially linked to autoimmune hepatitis in the mid-1960s, and immunosuppressive agents were used to treat the condition at that time. Prednisone was shown to improve survival in the early 1970s.

Epidemiology

Autoimmune hepatitis affects 100,000 to 200,000 persons in the United States, with a mean annual incidence of 1.9 per 100,000. Caucasian Northern Europeans are more susceptible than other groups. The majority of patients are women (70%), and 50% of them are 40 years of age or younger.

Table 5-1

Subclassifications of Autoimmune Hepatitis

Features	*Type 1*	*Type 2*	*Type 3*
Autoantibodies	ANA, SMA	Anti-LKMI	Anti-SLA/LP
Age onset (mean)	40	25	35
% women	70	90	90
Extrahepatic immune disorders	15% to 30%	40%	Unknown
Autoantigen	Unknown	Cyt P450 IID6	50 kD protein
Steroid response	70% to 80%	40% to 70%	90% to 100%
Progression to cirrhosis	40%	80%	Unknown

Autoimmune hepatitis can occasionally occur in multiple family members. Relatives can also demonstrate hypergammaglobulinemia and/or the presence of autoantibodies.

Pathogenesis

The precise cellular and humoral mechanisms involved in initiating and propagating the liver cell damage are unknown. Presumably, a genetically-predisposed individual is exposed to a stimulus that triggers an autoimmune process directed at the liver.

Genetic predisposition focuses on the major histocompatibility complex (MHC) class II genes in the human leukocyte antigen (HLA)-DR locus. Type 1 autoimmune hepatitis is associated with HLA-DR3 and/or HLA-DR4 in 85% of cases. Patients with HLA-DR3 are younger and have a worse clinical course with higher rates of treatment failure, relapse after drug withdrawal, and subsequent need for liver transplantation. On the other hand, patients with HLA-DR4 are typically older, have other concurrent autoimmune disorders, and respond better to steroid therapy. Type 2 autoimmune hepatitis has also been associated with specific HLA haplotypes, but these associations have not yet been established for type 3 disease.

The exact stimuli that trigger the onset of the illness are unknown. Infections with hepatitis A, Epstein-Barr virus, and rubella have been implicated. Medications, such as interferon and minocycline, may also play a role.

Actual hepatic cellular damage appears to involve the interplay of two separate mechanisms under the control of various cytokines: 1) cell-mediated antibody-dependent cytotoxicity, and 2) cytotoxic T-lymphocytes. The specific autoantigens targeted vary by the different disease subtypes (Table 5-1).

Natural History and Prognosis

The natural history of this disease is largely based on the histology at the time of presentation. The 3-year survival of patients with untreated, severe autoimmune hepatitis is only 50%, with a 10-year survival of 10% to 30%. However, in patients with mild histologic disease, the rate of progression is less than 20%, with a 5-year survival comparable to that of age- and gender-matched controls.

The natural history of autoimmune hepatitis is dramatically altered in those patients who respond to therapy. Life expectancy in treated patients approximates that of age- and sex-matched controls; however, 40% will progress to cirrhosis despite appropriate treatment.

The prognosis depends on the severity of inflammation at the time of presentation, presence or absence of cirrhosis, underlying medical conditions, and the patient's HLA haplotype. Patients with AST and ALT >10 times the upper limit of normal, or >5 times the upper limit of normal plus gamma globulin levels >2 times the upper limit of normal have a worse prognosis. Furthermore, patients with bridging necrosis, cirrhosis, or HLA-DR3 have an inferior outcome compared to patients without these parameters.

Clinical Features

Subclassifications

Three types of autoimmune hepatitis have been proposed based on different autoantibody patterns (see Table 5-1). Approximately 13% of cases fail to be classified into a specific subtype and are considered cryptogenic.

The most common form of the disease is Type 1 (classic or lupoid) autoimmune hepatitis, representing approximately 80% of all cases. Seventy percent of the patients are women less than 40 years of age, and 15% to 30% have concurrent autoimmune diseases.

Type 2 autoimmune hepatitis is much less common (4% of cases), and affects mostly children. These patients frequently present with severe acute or fulminant disease. This type also tends to progress more commonly to cirrhosis despite medical therapy. Approximately 40% of patients have other extrahepatic autoimmune diseases.

Type 3 autoimmune hepatitis is the least understood form of the disease. It represents only 3% of cases in the United States. This diagnosis may play an important role in helping to define the specific etiology of patients who were previously categorized as cryptogenic hepatitis or cirrhosis (see the following section).

Clinical Presentation

The clinical presentation of autoimmune hepatitis is extremely variable, ranging from an asymptomatic condition to fulminant hepatic failure. Although generally a disease of insidious onset in young women, approximately 25% present with an acute onset of hepatitis. Approximately 25% of all patients are already found to be cirrhotic at the time of presentation.

Table 5-2 outlines the common symptoms and physical findings at initial presentation. Fatigue is the most common presenting symptom and affects up to 85% of patients. Amenorrhea occurs frequently in young women and appears to correlate with the severity of disease. Return of regular menstrual cycles often occurs with successful treatment.

Physical findings frequently include hepatomegaly and splenomegaly. Spider angiomata, jaundice, ascites, and hepatic encephalopathy are commonly seen in patients with severe, long-standing, or histologically-advanced disease.

Table 5-2

Clinical Features of Autoimmune Hepatitis

Symptoms	*Frequency*
Fatigue	50% to 85%
Amenorrhea	50% to 75%
Jaundice	50%
Right upper quadrant pain	30% to 50%
Polymyalgias/arthralgias	20% to 30%
Anorexia	30% to 40%
Pruritus	20% to 40%
Diarrhea	20% to 30%
Physical Findings	
Hepatomegaly	50% to 80%
Splenomegaly	25% to 45%
Jaundice	50% to 75%
Spider angiomata	30% to 60%
Ascites	20%
Encephalopathy	10% to 15%

Concurrent autoimmune disorders are seen in 40% of patients with autoimmune hepatitis. Table 5-3 outlines some of these extrahepatic manifestations. The most common conditions include autoimmune thyroid disease, rheumatoid arthritis, and chronic ulcerative colitis. Thyroid disorders affect approximately 60% of these patients. Hashimoto's thyroiditis and Grave's disease are the most commonly observed conditions. Patients with HLA-DR4 have concurrent autoimmune diseases more commonly than those lacking this genetic marker (65% vs 31%).

Biochemical Tests

The predominant laboratory abnormality at presentation is elevation of the aminotransferases, with up to 16% of patients having AST and/or ALT levels exceeding 1000 U/L. More than 85% of patients will also have polyclonal hypergammaglobulinemia. Elevated bilirubin levels are extremely common but only exceed 3 mg/dL in 46% of patients. Minor elevations in alkaline phosphatase are also common, but values exceeding 2 times and 10 times the upper limit of normal are seen in only 33% and 10% of patients, respectively.

Serology

There are many autoantibodies associated with autoimmune hepatitis. Although these autoantibodies are used to define the various subtypes of the condition, they are not disease- or liver-specific, and do not appear to be directly pathogenic. In addition, their levels do not tend to correlate with disease activity.

Table 5-3

ASSOCIATED EXTRAHEPATIC CONDITIONS IN AUTOIMMUNE HEPATITIS

- Autoimmune thyroid disease
- Ulcerative colitis
- Synovitis
- Autoimmune thrombocytopenia purpura
- Rheumatoid arthritis
- Lichen planus
- Diabetes mellitus
- Vitiligo
- Alopecia
- CREST syndrome
- Nail dystrophy

Antinuclear antibodies (ANA) are found in approximately 75% of patients with Type 1 autoimmune hepatitis. The median titer at presentation is 1:320, with either a homogeneous or speckled pattern. The speckled pattern occurs in younger patients and is associated with higher AST and ALT levels. Elevated ANA titers may also be seen in other liver conditions including primary biliary cirrhosis, primary sclerosing cholangitis, viral hepatitis, and drug-induced hepatitis. However, the titers are generally lower in these conditions.

Smooth muscle antibodies (SMA) are seen in 87% of patients with type 1 autoimmune hepatitis. They occur alone in 25% to 35% of cases, or in association with a positive ANA in 85% to 90% of cases. The median titer at presentation is 1:160. Antiactin antibodies (a subset of anti-SMA) have been associated with a poorer prognosis.

Perinuclear antineutrophil cytoplasmic antibodies (pANCA) are present in 50% to 92% of patients with type 1 autoimmune hepatitis.

Type 2 autoimmune hepatitis is characterized by antibodies to liver-kidney-microsome 1 (LKM1). Only 4% of US adults with autoimmune hepatitis demonstrate anti-LKM1; however, this entity is seen in up to 20% of cases in Europe. Anti-LKM1 is also seen in up to 10% of patients with hepatitis C. Anti-LKM2 is associated with drug-induced hepatitis, and anti-LKM3 is associated with hepatitis D.

Type 3 autoimmune hepatitis is associated with antibodies against soluble liver antigen (SLA) and liver-pancreas (LP). Anti-SLA/LP can also be detected in 11% of patients with type 1 disease. Fourteen percent of patients previously diagnosed as cryptogenic hepatitis or cirrhosis have also been found to be anti-SLA/LP positive. The major clinical role of these antibodies may be in the evaluation and reclassification of some patients with cryptogenic hepatitis or cirrhosis.

Antibodies to asialoglycoprotein receptors (ASGPR) are present in all types of autoimmune hepatitis. Over 80% of patients with type 1 are anti-ASGPR positive.

Unlike the other autoantibodies, titers of anti-ASGPR correlate with activity and may rise in the face of impending relapse.

Pathology

The hallmark pathologic findings of autoimmune hepatitis are interface hepatitis (previously known as piecemeal necrosis), plasma cell infiltrates, and lobular inflammation. Various stages of fibrosis can also be seen. Up to 25% of patients will have cirrhosis at the time of initial presentation. These pathologic findings are not absolutely specific for the diagnosis of autoimmune hepatitis and can be seen in other conditions including hepatitis C. Overall, biopsy specimens are approximately 80% specific with a positive predictive value of 70% for making a definitive diagnosis.

Bile duct pathology can also be seen in autoimmune hepatitis. Up to 26% of patients exhibit evidence of cholangitis and/or bile duct loss; however, these features are more frequently associated with overlap syndromes.

Diagnosis

The diagnosis of autoimmune hepatitis is based on clinical, biochemical, serologic, and histologic criteria, and requires a high degree of clinical suspicion. Definitive diagnosis requires exclusion of other types of liver disease that can mimic autoimmune hepatitis. Table 5-4 shows a diagnostic scoring criteria that was established by the International Autoimmune Hepatitis Group in 1993,[1] and subsequently revised in 1999.[2] These diagnostic criteria allow the clinician to classify patients as having "probable" or "definite" autoimmune hepatitis based upon objective data. The scoring system can be used before or after the initiation of therapy. A pretreatment score of >15 is defined as "definite", whereas a score of 10 to 15 is defined as "probable" for the diagnosis. A post-treatment score of >17 is defined as "definite," and a score of 12 to 17 is defined as "probable."

This diagnostic scoring system has been validated and shown to have a sensitivity of 97% to 100%, and specificity up to 92% in those with "definite" disease. The scoring system is not as accurate in patients with "probable" autoimmune hepatitis or overlap syndromes.

Differential Diagnosis

Establishing the diagnosis of autoimmune hepatitis requires a strong index of clinical suspicion. Table 5-5 lists several hepatic diseases which need to be excluded prior to establishing the diagnosis. Extensive review of historical features, biochemical liver indices, serologies, and possibly liver biopsy are often required. Furthermore, overlap syndromes can be extremely difficult to separate from pure cases of autoimmune hepatitis.

Treatment

The goals of treatment are to slow the progression of the disease, prevent the complications of cirrhosis, and postpone the need for liver transplantation. Treatment endpoints include remission, incomplete response, failure to induce remission, clinical deterioration despite therapy, or development of drug toxicity.

Table 5-4

Scoring Criteria for the Diagnosis of Autoimmune Hepatitis

Criterion		Score
Female sex		+2
Alk phos – AST (ALT) ratio:		
	>3	-2
	<1.5	+2
Gammaglobulin or IgG levels (ng)		>2
	+3	
	1.5 to 2	+2
	1 to 1.4	+1
Antimitochondrial antibodies		-4
ANA, SMA, or anti-LKM1:		
	>1:80	+3
	1:80	+2
	1:40	+1
	<1:40	0
Viral serologies:		
	Positive	-3
	Negative	+3
Hepatotoxic drugs:		
	Yes	-4
	No	+1
Alcohol use:		
	<25 grams/day	+2
	>60 grams/day	-2
HLA-DR3 or HLA-DR4		+1
Concurrent autoimmune disease		+2
Other liver-related autoantibodies		+2
Interface hepatitis		+3
Plasmacytic infiltrate		+1
Rosettes		+1
No characteristic biopsy features		-5
Biliary changes on biopsy		-3
Other biopsy features (eg, fat, etc)		-3
Treatment response		+2
Treatment relapse		+3

Definite diagnosis *prior to* treatment >15 points
Probable diagnosis *prior to* treatment 10 to 15 points
Definite diagnosis *after* treatment >17 points
Probable diagnosis *after* treatment 12 to 17 points

Table 5-5

Differential Diagnosis of Autoimmune Hepatitis

- Acute/chronic viral hepatitis
- Medication-induced hepatitis:
    - α-methyldopa
    - Minocycline
    - Isoniazid
    - Nitrofurantoin
    - Oxyphenisatin
    - Propylthiouracil
- Alcoholic liver disease
- α-1-antitrypsin deficiency
- Hemochromatosis
- Nonalcoholic steatohepatitis
- Primary biliary cirrhosis
- Wilson's disease

The indications for treatment of autoimmune hepatitis focus on those patients with incapacitating clinical symptoms, relentless clinical progression, or laboratory and histologic features suggesting poorer outcomes. The standard laboratory indications include sustained abnormalities in the aminotransferases alone (≥10 times the upper limit of normal), or in association with elevations of serum gamma globulin (AST and ALT ≥5 times the upper limit of normal, AND gamma globulin ≥2 times the upper limit of normal). The presence of active bridging necrosis with interface hepatitis on liver biopsy is an absolute indication for treatment. The treatment of patients with more benign histologic abnormalities, mildly elevated liver function tests, or inactive cirrhosis is controversial.

Medical Therapy of Autoimmune Hepatitis

Three randomized, controlled trials in the early 1970s established corticosteroids and azathioprine as the mainstays of acute (induction) therapy.[3-5] In patients with significant autoimmune hepatitis, corticosteroids have been shown to improve the clinical signs and symptoms, hepatic inflammation and fibrosis,[6-8] and survival. Life expectancy in treated patients is equivalent to age- and sex-matched controls. Patients with histologically-active cirrhosis respond as well as those without cirrhosis, but have a higher risk of relapse. Patients with inactive cirrhosis do not tend to show improvement with therapy.

Treatment regimens using corticosteroids, with or without azathioprine, are equally effective and should be used as first-line or induction therapy. Various dosing regimens can be utilized. One possible regimen for therapy is shown in Table 5-6. An overall treatment course algorithm is outlined in Figure 5-1.

Table 5-6

INDUCTION THERAPY FOR AUTOIMMUNE HEPATITIS

	Prednisone Monotherapy	*Combination Therapy*
Induction	40 to 60 mg daily (Taper to 15 to 20 mg daily over 4 to 6 months)	Prednisone 20 to 30 mg daily (Taper or withdraw prednisone over 1 to 3 months) Azathioprine 0.5 to 1.0 mg/kg daily Titrate azathioprine to 1 to 2 mg/kg daily
Maintenance	15 to 20 mg daily	Prednisone 0 to 10 mg daily Azathioprine 1 to 2 mg/kg daily

Regimens using prednisone monotherapy are appropriate if a short course of therapy is contemplated, the patient is or may become pregnant, or the patient has contraindications to azathioprine (eg, cytopenia, active malignancy, or thiopurine methyltransferase deficiency). However, high-dose prednisone alone is associated with a higher risk of complications than combination therapy (44% vs 10%). Prednisone monotherapy is generally begun at doses of 40 to 60 mg daily and tapered over a 4- to 6-week period to a maintenance dose of 15 to 20 mg daily. Patients should be monitored for evidence of hyperglycemia, hypertension, cataracts, and glaucoma. Patients requiring long-term corticosteroids should be monitored for osteopenia and osteoporosis with annual bone density evaluations.

Combination regimens can begin with either prednisone alone followed by the addition of azathioprine, or with the initiation of the two agents simultaneously. As azathioprine can rarely cause cholestatic hepatitis, some experts prefer to begin the azathioprine after the patient begins to show clinical improvement on corticosteroids. The prednisone dosage is started between 20 to 30 mg daily, with azathioprine started at 0.5 to 1 mg/kg daily. Prednisone is withdrawn over a 1- to 3-month period, or tapered to a maintenance dose of 5 to 10 mg daily. Azathioprine is subsequently increased to a maintenance dose of 1 to 2 mg/kg daily. Patients should be monitored for leukopenia, thrombocytopenia, or evidence of pancreatitis.

Prednisone and azathioprine can induce clinical, biochemical, and histologic remission in 70% to 80% of patients with type 1 autoimmune hepatitis within 2 years of the initiation of therapy. Response rates for patients with type 2 disease are less (40% to 70%). Despite biochemical remission, histologic improvement may take up to 6 months. Therapy should, therefore, be continued at least 3 to 6 months beyond the time of biochemical remission. This approach decreases the chance of relapse upon drug withdrawal.

To minimize long-term side effects, and due to the fact that some patients will be able to maintain a long-term remission off medication, most experts advocate attempts at complete withdrawal of immunosuppression. These withdrawal trials should probably only be attempted in patients who have demonstrated sustained remission for at

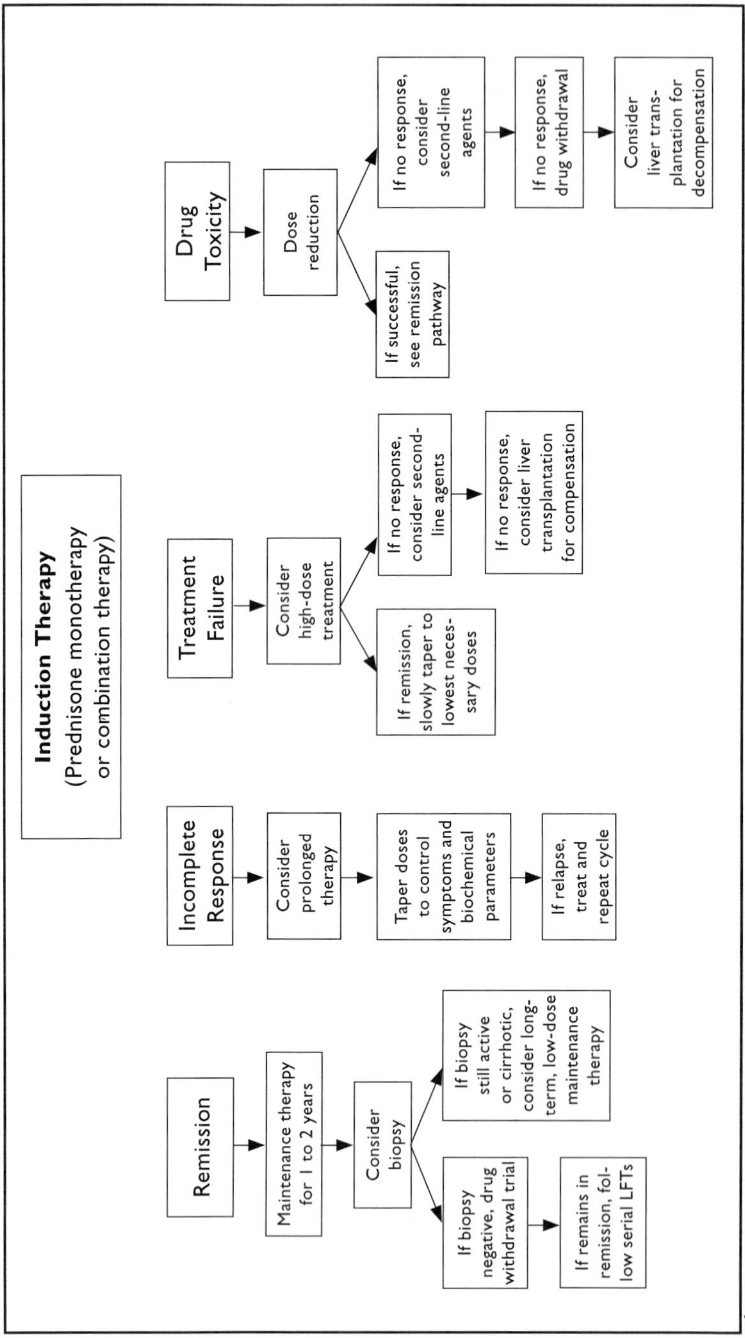

Figure 5-1. Induction therapy logorithm.

least 12 to 24 months. Liver biopsy should be considered prior to these trials as histology may be helpful in predicting risk of disease recurrence. Patients with normalization of the inflammatory component of their biopsy have only a 20% risk of recurrence upon medication withdrawal, whereas patients with active portal inflammation have a 50% risk of recurrence. Patients who are cirrhotic at the onset of therapy or develop cirrhosis during therapy have an 87% to 100% risk of hepatitis recurrence after medications are discontinued; withdrawal trials may not be warranted in this group.

Treatment withdrawal strategies vary depending on the type of maintenance therapy. For patients on prednisone monotherapy, the dosage should be reduced by approximately 2 to 2.5 mg every 3 months. For patients maintained on azathioprine, the dosage should be reduced by approximately 25 mg every month. Both groups should be followed with monthly liver profile testing.

Unfortunately, complete and sustained remission of autoimmune hepatitis is uncommon, occurring in only 17% of patients. The major problem is disease relapse following withdrawal of therapy. Fifty percent of patients will develop recurrent disease within 6 months of stopping therapy, and 70% will experience recurrance within 36 months. Reinstitution of therapy generally induces another remission but relapse is common in these patients upon further withdrawal attempts. Patients who relapse should probably be maintained on the lowest dose of prednisone alone, azathioprine alone, or combination therapy necessary to keep biochemical and clinical parameters in the normal to near-normal range. Although any of these regimens can be expected to give an 80% to 90% remission rate, azathioprine monotherapy offers the advantages of prospectively-studied success, and a steroid-sparing effect.[9] Additional attempts to discontinue immunosuppressive medications should be considered after a longer treatment course.

Side-effects necessitating dose reduction or discontinuation of immunosuppression occur in approximately 13% of patients, and are more frequently encountered in patients with cirrhosis (25%) compared to those without cirrhosis (8%). Steroid-related complications generally occur in patients on prolonged courses at prednisone doses exceeding 10 mg/day.

Despite therapy, up to 40% of patients develop cirrhosis within 10 years of diagnosis. Cirrhosis most commonly occurs in those patients with multiple relapses requiring retreatment. Patients who exhibit sustained remission after withdrawal of therapy have only a 5% chance of developing cirrhosis.

Incomplete Responders and Treatment Failures

Incomplete response, defined as improvement in biochemical and clinical parameters without histologic improvement, occurs in approximately 13% of patients. A longer treatment schedule generally does not increase the rate of remission, but should probably be used to control the clinical and biochemical features of the disease. Using the lowest possible medication doses is prudent to minimize side effects.

Treatment failures despite therapy with conventional doses of corticosteroids or corticosteroids and azathioprine occur in 9% to 15% of patients. Using higher doses of prednisone (30 to 60 mg/day), with or without azathioprine (in doses up to 2 mg/kg/day), can induce biochemical remission in more than 60% of these patients within 2 years, however, histologic remission occurs in only 20%. The benefit of increased immunosuppression must be weighed against the risk of significant side effects. The goal of therapy in these patients is to taper medications to the lowest doses needed to maintain biochemical and clinical improvement.

Several medications have been evaluated for the treatment of refractory autoimmune hepatitis, including cyclosporine, 6-mercaptopurine, cyclophosphamide, methotrexate, ursodeoxycholic acid, budesonide, mycophenolate mofetil, tacrolimus, and 6-thioguanine. Despite their appeal, none of these agents has been conclusively proven effective in controlled clinical trials.

Liver Transplantation

Liver transplantation is recommended for patients who develop end-stage liver disease (ESLD) despite medical therapy. Indications include refractory variceal bleeding, hepatic encephalopathy, intractable ascites, spontaneous bacterial peritonitis, hepatorenal syndrome, and early hepatocellular carcinoma. ESLD due to autoimmune hepatitis accounts for approximately 6% of liver transplants in the United States. The 5-year patient and graft survival rates exceed 80% in many centers.

Autoimmune hepatitis recurs in the transplanted graft in approximately 20% of cases.[10,11] Most recurrences are mild, but on occasion, patients can present with aggressive disease. These patients may benefit from more intensive post-transplant immunosuppression. Techniques such as switching from cyclosporine to tacrolimus, or adding additional agents such as mycophenolate mofetil are undergoing evaluation in clinical trials.

Complications

Patients with autoimmune hepatitis are susceptible to all of the standard complications of cirrhosis and portal hypertension. However, patients with autoimmune cirrhosis receiving immunosuppressive therapy have fewer portal hypertensive complications and enjoy better long-term survival when compared to patients with cirrhosis from other etiologies. Esophageal varices occur less frequently in autoimmune cirrhotics (15% vs 66% to 90% in all cirrhotics), and the probability of variceal hemorrhage in this cohort is <10% (vs 30% to 40% in all cirrhotics). Five- and 10-year survival rates of 90% are not uncommon in most long-term series of patients with cirrhosis from autoimmune hepatitis.

Hepatocellular carcinoma develops in 7% of autoimmune hepatitis patients with cirrhosis. The risk is 311 times higher than an age- and sex-matched control group. Patients with at least 5 years of cirrhosis are most susceptible to malignant degeneration. Similar to any other patient with cirrhosis, periodic screening for hepatocellular carcinoma with imaging and alpha-fetoprotein is recommended.

Complications due to immunosuppressive therapy can also occur. Steroid-induced osteopenia is the most common iatrogenic side effect. Other adverse effects are outlined in the treatment section above.

Summary

In summary, autoimmune hepatitis is primarily a disease of young women associated with abnormal liver tests, hypergammaglobulinemia, pathology showing interface hepatitis, the presence of autoantibodies, and the presence of extrahepatic manifestations. Diagnosis requires a high index of clinical suspicion, as several liver conditions can mimic autoimmune hepatitis. Most patients respond to immunosuppressive medications with improvement in clinical symptoms, biochemical liver tests, hepatic histology, and patient survival, however, relapse is the rule. A significant proportion of patients (up to 40%) will progress to cirrhosis despite therapy. These patients have a better prognosis than cirrhotics from other etiologies. Liver transplantation is reserved for those patients with decompensated liver disease.

References

1. Johnson PJ, McFarlane IG. Meeting report: International Autoimmune Hepatitis Group. *Hepatology.* 1993;18:998-1005.
2. Alvarez F, Berg PA, Bianchi FB, et al. International Autoimmune Hepatitis Group report: review of criteria for diagnosis of autoimmune hepatitis. *J Hepatol.* 1999;31:929-938.
3. Cook GC, Mulligan R, Sherlock S. Controlled prospective trial of corticosteroid therapy in chronic active hepatitis. *Quart J Med.* 1971;158:159-185.
4. Soloway RD, Summerskill WHJ, Baggenstoss AH, et al. Clinical, biochemical, and histological remission of severe chronic active liver disease: a controlled study of treatments and early prognosis. *Gastroenterology.* 1972;63:820-833.
5. Murray-Lyon IM, Stern RB, Williams R. Controlled trial of prednisone and azathioprine in active chronic hepatitis. *Lancet.* 1973;1:735-737.
6. Czaja AJ, Carpenter HA. Progressive fibrosis during corticosteroid therapy of autoimmune hepatitis. *Hepatology.* 2004;39:1631-1638.
7. Czaja AJ, Carpenter HA. Decreased fibrosis during corticosteroid therapy of autoimmune hepatitis. *J Hepatol.* 2004;40:646-652.
8. Malekzadeh R, Mohamadnejad M, Nasseri-Moghaddam S, et al. Reversibility of cirrhosis in autoimmune hepatitis. *Am J Med.* 2004;117:125-129.
9. Johnson PJ, McFarlane IG, Williams R. Azathioprine for long-term maintenance of remission in autoimmune hepatitis. *N Engl J Med.* 1995;333:958-963.
10. Hubscher SG. Recurrent autoimmune hepatitis after liver transplantation: diagnostic criteria, risk factors, and outcome. *Liver Transpl.* 2001;7:285-291.
11. Gonzalez-Koch A, Czaja AJ, Carpenter HA, et al. Recurrent autoimmune hepatitis after orthotopic liver transplantation. *Liver Transpl.* 2001;7:302-310.

Additional Selected Readings

Al-Khalidi JA, Czaja AJ. Current concepts in the diagnosis, pathogenesis, and treatment of autoimmune hepatitis. *Mayo Clin Proc.* 2001;76:1237-1252.

Heneghan MA, McFarlane IG. Current and novel immunosuppressive therapy for autoimmune hepatitis. *Hepatology.* 2002;35:7-13.

Manns MP, Strassburg CP. Autoimmune hepatitis: clinical challenges. *Gastroenterology.* 2001;120:1502-1517.

Czaja AJ, Menon N, Carpenter HA. Sustained remission after corticosteroid therapy for type 1 autoimmune hepatitis: a retrospective analysis. *Hepatology.* 2002;35:890-897.

Czaja AJ, Homburger HA. Autoantibodies in liver disease. *Gastroenterology.* 2001;120:239-249.

Czaja AJ, Freese DK. Diagnosis and treatment of autoimmune hepatitis. *Hepatology.* 2002;36:479-497.

Homberg J-C, Abuaf N, Bernard O, et al. Chronic active hepatitis associated with anti-liver/kidney microsome antibody type 1: a second type of "autoimmune" hepatitis. *Hepatology.* 1987;7:1333-1339.

Czaja AJ, Bianchi FB, Carpenter HA, et al. Treatment challenges and investigational opportunities in autoimmune hepatitis. *Hepatology.* 2005;41:207-215.

chapter 6

Nonalcoholic Fatty Liver Disease

John C. Sun, MD and Anne Burke, MD

Introduction

Since its first description by Ludwig et al in 1980,[1] our knowledge of nonalcoholic steatohepatitis (NASH) has evolved from a newly described but poorly-defined disease into a spectrum of findings now known as nonalcoholic fatty liver disease, or NAFLD (Table 6-1). Despite much research into its epidemiology, pathogenesis and treatment, NAFLD remains an incompletely understood entity. In the simplest terms, NAFLD is the presence of either steatosis or steatohepatitis on liver biopsy specimen in patients with little or no alcohol use. This chapter will first define the clinicopathologic spectrum of NAFLD, then proceed to review the important epidemiological data, and finally conclude with a discussion of the practical approach to the diagnosis and management of this disease.

Defining Nonalcoholic Fatty Liver Disease

NAFLD is defined as hepatic fat accumulation greater than 5% to 10% by weight, often estimated as the percentage of fat-laden hepatocytes visualized on light microscopy.[2] The most widely accepted histologic grading and staging system was proposed by Brunt, and is described in Table 6-2.[3]

Clinicopathologic criteria for the diagnosis of NASH were also proposed by Powell, et al in 1990:[3]

1. Liver biopsy results—moderate to gross macrovesicular fatty change with portal or lobular inflammation, with or without Mallory bodies, fibrosis, or cirrhosis. NASH cannot be differentiated from alcoholic hepatitis based on these findings alone.
2. Evidence of less than 40 g of ethanol consumption per week:
    - Detailed history independently obtained by three physicians.

Table 6-1

OTHER TERMS PREVIOUSLY USED TO DESCRIBE NONALCOHOLIC FATTY LIVER DISEASE

- Alcohol-like hepatitis
- Fatty liver hepatitis
- Steatonecrosis
- Diabetic hepatitis
- Pseudoalcoholic hepatitis
- Nonalcoholic Laennec's disease

- Confirmation through questioning of family members and health care providers.
- Random laboratory tests negative for ethanol.

3. No serologic evidence for hepatitis B or hepatitis C infection.

It may be impractical to obtain detailed patient information from three physicians, family and health care providers; instead, the focus should be on reliably excluding substantial alcohol use or abuse.

The amount of alcohol that is considered "risky" has been debated. Though the Powell criteria use a cutoff of 40 g of alcohol per week, other centers have used levels ranging from 10 g/day, up to 20 to 40 g/day in men and 20 g/day in women. Most clinicians would find two drinks per day or less an acceptable value.[2]

In regards to hepatitis B infection, some clinicians have proposed that NASH should not be excluded as a potential diagnosis in patients with prior infection and evidence of effective immunity (HBsAg negative, HBsAb positive).

A useful system has been developed to correlate the histologic findings with the clinical course of NAFLD.[2,4]

1. Class 1: Steatosis alone.
2. Class 2: Steatosis with lobular inflammation.
3. Class 3: Steatosis with lobular inflammation and ballooning hepatocytes.
4. Class 4: Class 3, with the addition of Mallory bodies or fibrosis.

Together, Class 3 and Class 4, where the histology reflects hepatocyte injury, comprise the clinical entity NASH. The prognosis of Class 3 and 4 NAFLD is worse than Class 1 or 2 (see below).

EPIDEMIOLOGY

Estimates from liver biopsy series suggest that the disease is present in 1.2% to 9% of patients.[5] Although the true prevalence of NAFLD is unknown, the actual values may be even higher than these estimates suggest. NAFLD is also felt to be the most common cause of abnormal liver-associated enzymes in the asymptomatic patient, accounting for up to 90% of elevated aminotransferase levels in this population.[6] The

Table 6-2

Grading and Staging System for NASH Proposed by Brunt

Grade 1, Mild

- Steatosis: Mainly macrovesicular, range from less than 33%, up to 66% of the lobules
- Ballooning: Occasionally in zone 3 hepatocytes
- Lobular inflammation: Scattered, mild acute and chronic inflammation with neutrophils and mononuclear cells, respectively
- Portal inflammation: None to mild

Grade 2, Moderate

- Steatosis: Any degree, mixed macrovesicular and microvesicular
- Ballooning: Present in zone 3
- Lobular inflammation: Neutrophils may be associated with ballooned hepatocytes, and/or pericellular fibrosis, with or without mild chronic inflammation
- Portal inflammation: None, mild to moderate

Grade 3, Severe (Florid steatohepatitis)

- Steatosis: Usually greater than 66% (zone 3 or panacinar), mixed steatosis common
- Ballooning: Marked, and predominantly in zone 3
- Lobular inflammation: Scattered acute and chronic inflammation; neutrophils concentrated in zone 3 areas of ballooning and perisinusoidal fibrosis
- Portal inflammation: Mild or moderate, but not marked.

Staging: Requires Masson trichrome or equivalent stain

- Stage 1: Zone 3 perivenular, perisinusoidal, or pericellular fibrosis; focal or extensive
- Stage 2: Stage 1, with focal or extensive portal fibrosis
- Stage 3: Bridging fibrosis, focal or extensive
- Stage 4: Cirrhosis with or without residual perisinusoidal fibrosis

disease tends to occur in the fifth to sixth decades of life,[1,5,7] with 65% to 83% of cases occurring in females.[1,3,7]

In certain high-risk populations, the disease prevalence is significantly greater. Studies have found an association between NAFLD and diabetes mellitus, obesity, and hyperlipidemia (Table 6-3).

Table 6-3

RISK FACTORS AND CONDITIONS ASSOCIATED WITH NONALCOHOLIC FATTY LIVER DISEASE

Metabolic

Obesity*

Type II Diabetes Mellitus*

Hyperinsulinemia*

Rapid weight loss, including starvation and bypass surgeries

TPN

Lipodystrophy

Medications

Cardiac:

- Amiodarone
- Calcium channel blockers
- Aspirin

Steroids:

- Glucocorticoids
- Synthetic estrogens

Antimicrobials:

- Tetracycline
- Antivirals, such as zidovudine and didanosine

Other:

- Tamoxifen
- Valproic acid
- Methotrexate
- Cocaine

Other Conditions

Inflammatory bowel disease

Small intestinal diverticulosis with bacterial overgrowth

HIV infection

Bacillus cereus toxin

*major risk factors

MAJOR RISK FACTORS

The major risk factors for NAFLD are obesity, Type II diabetes mellitus, and hyperlipidemia; all three are part of the so-called metabolic syndrome. These three factors predispose to NAFLD through the development of insulin resistance and increased hepatic accumulation of fatty acids (Table 6-4).

Table 6-4

EPIDEMIOLOGY OF MAJOR RISK FACTORS FOR NONALCOHOLIC FATTY LIVER DISEASE

Risk Factor	*Percent of Subjects With Risk Factor Who Have NAFLD*	*Percent of Subjects With NAFLD Who Have Risk Factor*
Obesity	57.5 to 74	30 to 100
Type II Diabetes Mellitus	75	34 to 75
Hyperlipidemia	?	20 to 81

Obesity

The prevalence of NAFLD ranges from 57.5% to 74% in obese patients.[3] An autopsy study found steatosis in 70% of obese patients and 35% of lean patients, and NASH in 18.5% of obese patients and 3.5% of lean patients.[8]

In addition, among patients with NAFLD, obesity is quite prevalent, with estimates ranging between 30% to 100%. In one study, 40 of 42 patients with biopsy-proven NASH were considered obese.[3]

Diabetes

Thirty-four to 75% of patients with NASH have Type 2 diabetes mellitus.[5] Of the 42 patients followed by Powell and associates, 15 (37%) were found to have hyperglycemia.[3] Other studies have also found a high prevalence of diabetes in patients with NASH.[1,7,8] The prevalence of NAFLD among patients with type II diabetes mellitus is estimated to be 75%.[2]

Hyperlipidemia

Hyperlipidemia has been found in 20% to 81% of patients with NASH.[5] In Powell and collegues' study of 42 patients, 26 (61%) were found to have hyperlipidemia.[3]

OTHER RISK FACTORS

Rapid weight loss and jejuno-ileal bypass are also risk factors for NAFLD. Wanless and Lentz found an association between fatty liver disease and weight loss shortly before death, as well as jejuno-ileal bypass surgery.[8] McFarland and collegues, in a review of jejuno-ileal bypass surgery, found that 40% of patients status-postjejuno-ileal bypass for weight loss had evidence of liver dysfunction.[9] Approximately 2.2% to 6% of patients undergoing rapid weight loss have evidence of liver dysfunction within the first 12 to 18 months.[5]

Medications that may cause NAFLD include amiodarone, glucocorticoids, tamoxifen, tetracycline, and antiviral medications such as zidovudine. Also, the administration of total parenteral nutrition or IV glucose may result in NAFLD.

A Different Epidemiologic Finding

Bacon and associates published a series in 1994 that painted a different epidemiological picture of NASH.[10] In their series of 33 patients, the mean age was 47, 58% of the patients were men, 61% were nonobese, 79% had normal glucose levels, and 79% had normal lipid profiles. Normal glucose levels, normal lipid levels, and lack of obesity were all present in 42% of the patients. Of 33 patients, 13 had increasing fibrosis, of which 5 had cirrhosis. In these 13 patients with more severe disease, 8 were female, 8 were obese, 4 were glucose intolerant, and 3 were hyperlipidemic.

Nonalcoholic Fatty Liver Disease and Cryptogenic Cirrhosis

Until recently, both the lack of awareness of NASH and the loss of hepatic steatosis in the cirrhotic liver lead to an underappreciation of NAFLD as an important cause of cryptogenic cirrhosis. A case-control study of 70 patients with cryptogenic cirrhosis (diagnosed by exclusion of alcohol use, autoimmune and viral hepatitis) demonstrated that a significantly larger percentage of patients with cryptogenic cirrhosis were found to have either diabetes and/or obesity than were found to have hepatitis C (HCV) infection or primary biliary cirrhosis.[11] Another case-control study of 49 patients with cryptogenic cirrhosis compared with age-matched controls (with cirrhosis secondary to alcohol use, chronic viral hepatitis, autoimmune hepatitis, PBC and PSC) showed that the cryptogenic cirrhosis group had a higher percentage of Type 2 diabetes mellitus (47% vs 22%), obesity (55% vs 24%), or both (23% vs 5%).[12]

Nonalcoholic Fatty Liver Disease and Hepatocellular Carcinoma

NASH is now thought to be the underlying disease that causes many cases of cryptogenic cirrhosis. Through this association, NASH may also predispose to hepatocellular carcinoma (HCC). Recently, two studies have looked at this problem.

Bugianesi and colleagues performed a case-control study to compare 23 patients with hepatocellular carcinoma and cryptogenic cirrhosis with a control group of patients with hepatocellular carcinoma and either viral or alcohol-induced cirrhosis.[13] The prevalence of obesity, diabetes, and hyperlipidemia was significantly higher in the cryptogenic cirrhosis group than the matched control group, suggesting an association between hepatocellular carcinoma arising in the setting of cryptogenic cirrhosis, and underlying NASH.

Marrero and associates investigated 105 consecutive patients with HCC, and found that cryptogenic cirrhosis was present in 29% of the cases. Of the patients with HCC and cryptogenic cirrhosis, half had histologic or clinical findings suggestive of NAFLD. Overall, NAFLD may account for at least 13% of cases of HCC[14] (Figure 6-1).

Natural History

Because there are few longitudinal studies of patients with NAFLD, a clear understanding of the natural history of NAFLD remains elusive. The estimated 5-year and 10-year survival for patients with NASH are 67% and 59%, respectively; however, it is difficult to separate death due to liver disease from death due to coexistent conditions, such as diabetes mellitus.[2,4] Compiled data from different studies also suggest

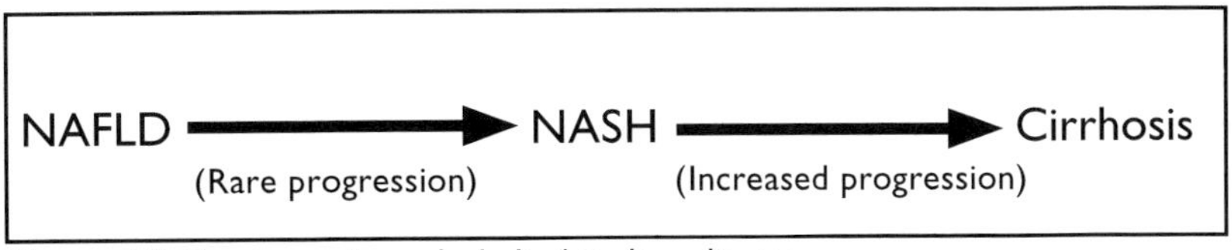

Figure 6-1. Spectrum of nonalcoholic fatty liver disease.

that patients with NASH have a 25% chance of developing fibrosis, and 15% chance of developing cirrhosis within 5 years.[2]

Powell and associates followed 42 patients for a median of 4.5 years, and found that 18 patients had fibrosis, 2 patients had marked fibrosis with disturbed architecture, and 1 patient had cirrhosis on the initial liver biopsy. During follow-up, one patient progressed from fibrosis to cirrhosis, and one patient with cirrhosis died from hepatocellular carcinoma. The two patients with marked fibrosis evolved to inactive cirrhosis.[3]

Lee's study followed 39 patients with NASH for a mean of 3.8 years, and found that one patient died of hepatic decompensation. After an average of 3.5 years, 13 patients underwent repeat histologic examination, which found progression of fibrosis in 5 patients, and cirrhosis in 2 patients.[7]

By contrast, in the placebo arm of a randomized controlled trial of ursodeoxycholic acid for the treatment of NASH, although no change was seen in the group as a whole, improvement in steatosis was seen in 37% and improvement in fibrosis was seen in 22% of subjects.[15] Furthermore, preliminary data from a longitudinal population study, suggests that although overall mortality is increased compared to the general population, (standardized mortality ratio 1.55), over a 7.6 year follow up period, only 3% of the NASH patients developed cirrhosis and only 1.7% had a liver-related death.[16] Thus although patients with NASH are at increased risk of death particularly from cardiovascular disease, the risk of progressive liver disease may be less than previously surmised.

Pathophysiology

Despite recent research, the precise pathophysiologic mechanisms that result in NAFLD remain unknown. However, a "two hit" theory implicates both insulin resistance and oxidative stress as potential factors leading to steatohepatitis, and, eventually, fibrosis and cirrhosis (Figure 6-2).

Fatty acid accumulation in the liver (the "first hit") may occur secondary to an imbalance between fatty acid delivery to and export from the liver. As fatty acid retention increases, steatosis develops. The mechanism by which steatosis progresses to steatohepatitis, and subsequently to fibrosis is unclear, but oxidative stress has been proposed as the "second hit." Mitochondrial injury, leading to ATP depletion, reactive oxygen species generation, lipid peroxidation, and cytokine induction may mediate hepatocyte injury.

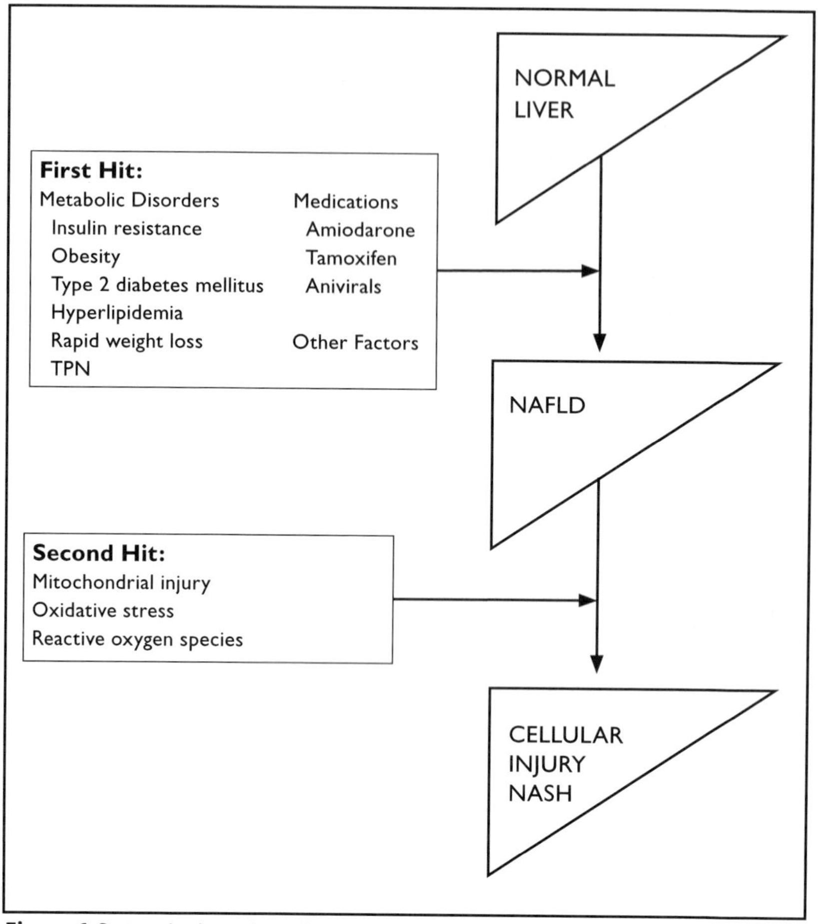

Figure 6-2. Two hit hypothesis for nonalcoholic fatty liver disease.

Insulin Resistance

Insulin resistance and hyperinsulinemia has been indirectly implicated as a factor in NAFLD through the high association between NAFLD and both impaired glucose tolerance or diabetes mellitus and the metabolic syndrome.

Often, altered glucose tolerance and hyperinsulinemia are found in patients with NAFLD, in the absence of clinically apparent diabetes. Pagano and collegues investigated 19 patients with a BMI of 26 + 2, with histologically documented NASH and 19 age- and gender-matched controls in a case-control study.[17] Plasma glucose, insulin, and C-peptide levels were measured during both an oral and intravenous glucose tolerance test. Although none of the subjects with NASH were found to be diabetic, they did have lower insulin sensitivity and higher total insulin secretion. In addition, 6 of the 19 NASH subjects had some degree of impaired glucose tolerance, and 9 of the 19 subjects had 2 criteria consistent with the metabolic syndrome.

Marchesini and associates found an interesting association between NAFLD and insulin resistance independent of both diabetes and obesity.[18] Forty-six persons with increased serum transaminases, "bright" liver on ultrasound, and normal glucose tolerance test were studied. Insulin resistance index and insulin secretion were measured using the homeostasis model assessment (HOMA) method, and compared to 92 age and gender-matched controls. Patients with NAFLD were found to have fasting and glucose-induced hyperinsulinemia and insulin resistance. Exclusion of overweight and obese persons did not alter the findings.

The association between NAFLD and the metabolic syndrome was explored in another study by Marchesini and colleagues, who studied 163 patients with biopsy proven NAFLD without diabetes. Waist circumference, HDL, glucose, triglyceride levels, and arterial pressure were used as criteria for the metabolic syndrome. Of the 73.6% of the patients were found to have NASH, 88% had a metabolic syndrome (compared with 53% with pure fatty liver only). They found that the presence of the metabolic syndrome is associated with an increased risk of progression to NASH (odds ratio 3.2) and fibrosis (odds ratio 3.5).[19]

Certainly, these studies have demonstrated an association between obesity, hyperlipidemia and particularly glucose intolerance with the development of NAFLD and progression to NASH. The specific pathway by which insulin resistance and hyperinsulinemia lead to the development of NAFLD remain unclear; however, the process appears to involve multiple molecular targets, including Rad, PC-1, leptin, and TNF-a.

Insulin resistance and hyperinsulinemia result in excess lipolysis, leading to higher levels of circulating fatty acids. Increased hepatic uptake of fatty acids, and the resulting overload of mitochondrial beta-oxidation, causes fatty acid accumulation within hepatocytes, and the entity known as NAFLD.[6]

Oxidative Stress

It is unclear why some patients develop NAFLD alone without hepatocyte injury, and other patients develop NASH, hepatic fibrosis and cirrhosis. Many postulate that increased oxidative stress may be the common pathway that results in hepatocyte damage.

The mitochondria is thought to be the major source of reactive oxygen species, which may cause steatohepatitis through lipid peroxidation and cytokine induction. Sanyal and collegues, in a small study, found evidence of insulin resistance and increased oxidative stress in NAFLD, but only patients with NASH were found to have structural mitochondrial defects, such as loss of mitochondrial cristae.[20]

Mitochondrial swelling and damage may also result in impaired ATP resynthesis and ATP depletion.[6] Cortez-Pinto and collegues performed a small case-control study, finding that recovery from hepatic ATP depletion is severely impaired in patients with obesity related NASH.[21]

In addition, inflammation and hepatocyte damage may cause inflammatory cell recruitment, cytokine induction, and generation of additional reactive oxygen species from macrophages and neutrophils.[2]

Altered Cytokine Milieu

Adipose tissue, particularly visceral adipose secretes both tumor necrosis factor alpha (TNFα) and adiponectin. These have opposing actions increasing obesity is associated with increased TNFα and decreased adiponectin levels. Adiponectin levels are strongly correlated with both peripheral and hepatic insulin sensitivity. Levels of adiponectin are decreased in patients with NASH compared to patients with simple steatosis.[22] This area has been reviewed by Diehl et al.[23]

Evaluation and Diagnosis

Table 6-5 summarizes the symptoms, signs, and other clinical and laboratory features of NAFLD.[5]

History and Physical Examination

Most patients with NAFLD are asymptomatic. Of the patients with symptoms, the most common are fatigue, malaise, and vague right upper quadrant discomfort.[10] The history should focus on identifying risk factors for both NAFLD as well as other potential explanations for the patient's symptoms (if present) or abnormal liver function tests. Risk factors for viral hepatitis, family history of liver disease (hemochromatosis, α-1 antitrypsin deficiency, or Wilson's disease), questioning for alcohol use, and a careful medication history are all important to rule out other hepatic disorders.

The most frequent finding on physical examination is hepatomegaly. Occasionally, patients may present with stigmata of chronic liver disease or cirrhosis, including spider angiomas, splenomegaly, and caput medusa.

Laboratory Tests and Imaging Studies

The levels of AST and ALT are usually less than two to three times the upper limit of normal, with the AST to ALT ratio less than one. This latter finding helps to distinguish NAFLD from alcoholic liver disease.[24] Less than 50% of patients will have an elevated alkaline phosphatase level, which is mildly increased at best. About 10 to 15 percent of patients will have a direct hyperbilirubinemia. Tests for liver synthetic function, such as the prothrombin time and serum albumin level, will be normal unless there is development of cirrhosis.

Exclusion of other liver disease is important. Chronic hepatitis B (HBV) and HCV infection should be ruled out. Other reasonable tests to order include serum iron studies, antinuclear antibodies, antismooth muscle antibodies, antimitochondrial antibodies, α-1 antitrypsin levels, and serum ceruloplasmin.

Substantial alcohol use can be assessed by laboratory testing if the information gathered through history alone is questionable. Random serum alcohol tests may be considered. A ratio of desialylated transferrin to total transferrin greater than 0.013 has an 81% sensitivity and 98% specificity in diagnosing current alcohol use,[25] depending on amount of alcohol intake.

Ultrasound, CT scan and MRI may all be able to detect fatty liver, but cannot distinguish between steatosis and steatohepatitis.

Table 6-5

CLINICAL FEATURES OF NONALCOHOLIC FATTY LIVER DISEASE

History

Age: 5th to 6th decade

Sex: More commonly female

Risk Factors:

- Obesity
- Type II diabetes mellitus
- Hyperlipidemia
- Rapid weight loss
- Medications (see Table 6-3)

Symptoms:

- Common:
    - Usually asymptomatic
    - Fatigue, malaise
    - Right upper quadrant discomfort.
- Less Common:
    - Complications of chronic liver disease or cirrhosis (eg, hepatic encephalopathy, ascites, jaundice)

Physical Examination

Hepatomegaly is common.

Stigmata of chronic liver disease or cirrhosis are less common.

Laboratory and Diagnostic Testing

Liver function tests:

- Mild increases in transaminases, usually less than 1.5 times the upper limit of normal, although values up to 10 times the upper limit of normal are possible.
- Usually, ALT is greater than AST, unless fibrosis or cirrhosis is present, in which case AST may be greater than ALT.
- Bilirubin, alkaline phosphatase, and GGT are usually normal, or mildly elevated.

Diagostic Imaging:

- Ultrasound, MRI, and CT scans may show hepatic steatosis, but cannot determine the presence or absence of hepatocyte injury.

Liver Biopsy

Liver biopsy is the gold standard for diagnosis of NAFLD. It provides both diagnostic and prognostic information by assessing the presence of hepatocyte injury and fibrosis or cirrhosis. Studies show a correlation between fibrosis and the following:

1. Age >45
2. Obesity
3. Type 2 diabetes mellitus.
4. Hypertriglyceridemia greater than or equal to 1.7 mmol/L.
5. ALT concentration greater than twice the upper limit of normal.

Patients with the above factors, or with cytopenia, splenomegaly, stigmata of chronic liver disease, or abnormal iron studies should be considered for biopsy.

In young patients who are only obese, without the other indicators mentioned, a trial period of exercise and weight loss may be attempted first.[2]

Treatment

No standard therapy for NAFLD has been formulated. Diet and exercise to achieve weight loss, and tight control of metabolic factors should form the cornerstone of any therapeutic plan. We describe various therapies for NAFLD below (see Table 6-6 for a summary).

Weight Loss

Diet and exercise should form the basis of any therapeutic plan. Exercise may positively alter insulin sensitivity; however, only about one third of patients will achieve sufficient levels of exercise.[2] Other studies have shown that the combination of diet and exercise result in biochemical improvement, but effects on histology are variable. One study by Kugelmas and collegues examined the effects of a step 1 American Heart Association diet and aerobic exercise on 16 patients with biopsy-proven NASH. Significant improvements in liver function tests, lipid profiles and body mass index were noted following 6 weeks of therapy.

It is important to set realistic diet and exercise goals for the patient. Loss of 1 to 2 pounds per week is reasonable, and weight loss should not exceed 1.6 kg/week, as this may result in a worsening of biochemical and histologic markers of NAFLD. Patients should be counseled on balanced nutritional intake, caloric contents of food, and appropriate duration of aerobic exercise. Referral to a nutritionist should be considered.

Alcohol

The effect of continued alcohol use is uncertain, but for patients with fibrosis, abstinence may be preferred.

Anti-Diabetic Medications

Due to the importance of insulin sensitivity in the pathogenesis of NAFLD, medications that act to improve insulin sensitivity, metformin and the thiazolidinediones, such as pioglitazone and rosiglitazone, have potential therapeutic value in NAFLD. Although these medications show promise, their use has not, as of yet, been examined with large scale randomized controlled trials.

Table 6-6

Treatment of Nonalcoholic Fatty Liver Disease

Treatment	*Dosing*	*LFT Effects*	*Histological Effects*	*Type of Study*
Diet alone	Not more than 1.6 kg per week	No change to improvement	Variable to improved	Unblinded studies and case series
Diet and exercise	Not more than 1.6 kg per week weight loss. Consider AHA Step 1 program.	Improved	Improved	Unblinded studies and case series
Ursodeoxycholic acid	13 to 15 mg/kg/day for 12 months	Improved	No change	Randomized controlled trial
Vitamins E + C	1000 IU+1g/day for 6 months	Improved	No change	Randomized controlled trial
Metformin	500 mg PO TID	Improved	Improved	Not a randomized controlled trial
Thiazolidinediones	Rosiglitazone 4 mg PO BID	Improved	Improved	Single arm, open label

Thiazolidinediones

Caldwell and associates examined the effects of troglitazone on both biochemical (normalization of ALT) and histologic improvement in 10 females with biopsy-proven NASH.[26] Troglitazone was administered at a dose of 400 mg daily for up to 6 months. Seventy percent (7 of 10 patients) had normal ALT levels at the end of therapy. Histologic improvement was less impressive; all follow-up biopsies had evidence of NASH, with only minimal improvement in four patients.

Most recently, Neuschwander-Tetri and collegues examined the effect of rosiglitazone on 22 patients with biopsies consistent with NASH by published criteria.[27] After 48 weeks of therapy with rosiglitazone 4 mg twice daily, histologic response was assessed with repeat biopsy. Liver function tests were assessed throughout the treatment course as well as during post-treatment follow-up. Biochemical markers improved significantly during treatment, with decreases in ALT, AST, alkaline phosphatase, and gamma-glutamyl transferase. However, the liver function tests increased towards pretreatment values during the 24 weeks of post-treatment follow-up. Histologic improvement was noted in 8 patients, no change in histology was seen in 11 patients, and 3 patients had worsening of their necroinflammatory score. The major side effect was weight gain.

Metformin

Another medication that may improve insulin sensitivity, metformin, was evaluated by Marchesini and associates.[28] Twenty patients with steatohepatitis were treated with metformin 500 mg three times daily for 4 months. Six noncompliant patients were used as controls. After therapy, normalization of transaminases was noted in 50% of patients. Metformin use in patients with NAFLD appears to be quite safe.

Other Medications

A pilot study of 40 patients with biopsy-proven NASH found that ursodiol, given in a dose of 13 to 15 mg/kg/day for 12 months had both a biochemical and histologic improvement.[25] However, a follow up RCT failed to show any benefit.[15]

Vitamin E alone was associated with a reduction in transaminases, and in combination with pioglitazone, resulted in histologic improvement;[26] however, in a follow-up placebo controlled trial, vitamin E in combination with vitamin C failed to improve histology.[29] In another small pilot study of 10 patients, betaine was found to improve both serum aminotransferase levels and liver histology.[30]

However, these are small-scale studies, and their findings need to be validated in larger, randomized controlled trials.

Summary

NAFLD is the most common cause of abnormal liver function tests in the asymptomatic adult. Although its true prevalence is unknown, it constitutes an important entity that may have severe consequences, including liver failure.

The major risk factors for NAFLD include diabetes mellitus, obesity, and hyperlipidemia. These pre-existing conditions predispose to hyperinsulinemia, insulin resistance, and fatty acid retention in hepatocytes. When combined with increased oxidative stress, inflammation and hepatocyte injury ensue, leading to steatohepatitis, fibrosis, and possibly cirrhosis.

Symptoms, when present, include fatigue, malaise, and right upper quadrant discomfort. Hepatomegaly is the most common physical finding; signs of chronic liver disease may be present as well. Laboratory investigation may reveal increased levels of transaminases, with an AST to ALT ratio less than one. Imaging may reveal fatty liver, but cannot distinguish between steatosis and steatohepatitis. Other causes of liver disease, such as viral hepatitis, hemochromatosis, autoimmune hepatitis, primary biliary cirrhosis, primary sclerosing cholangitis, Wilson's disease, and α-1 antitrypsin deficiency should be considered, and excluded if necessary. Liver biopsy remains the gold standard for diagnosis, and should be considered for patients older than 45 years of age, with diabetes, obesity or hyperlipidemia, as these constitute risk factors for fibrosis.

Diet and exercise remain the cornerstone of therapy. Weight loss should not exceed 1.6 kg per week, however, because this may lead to a flare of NASH. Tight control of metabolic factors, such as diabetes mellitus and hyperlipidemia should be instituted.

Insulin-sensitizing agents, including metformin and the thiazolidinediones, may be used in patients with diabetes mellitus or impaired glucose tolerance. Ursodiol and vitamin E have potential roles in the therapy of NAFLD, but large scale randomized controlled trials are lacking.

References

1. Ludwig J, Viggiano TR, McGill DB, Oh BJ. Nonalcoholic steatohepatitis: Mayo Clinic experiences with a hitherto unnamed disease. *Mayo Clinic Proceedings.* 1980;55(7):434-438.
2. Neuschwander-Tetri B, Caldwell S. Nonalcoholic steatohepatitis: summary of an AASLD Single Topic Conference. *Hepatology.* 2003;37(5):1202-1219.
3. Powell EE, Cooksley WG, Hanson R, Searle J, Halliday JW, Powell LW. The natural history of nonalcoholic steatohepatitis: a follow-up study of forty-two patients for up to 21 years. *Hepatology.* 1990;11(1):74-80.
4. Matteoni CA, Younossi ZM, Gramlich T, Boparai N, Liu YC, McCullough AJ. Nonalcoholic fatty liver disease: a spectrum of clinical and pathological severity. *Gastroenterology.* 1999;116(6):1413-1419.
5. Sheth SG, Gordon FD, Chopra S. Nonalcoholic steatohepatitis. *Ann Intern Med.* 1997;126(1):137-145.
6. Angulo P. Nonalcoholic fatty liver disease.[see comment]. [Review] [95 refs]. *N Engl J Med.* 2002;346(16):1221-1231.
7. Lee RG. Nonalcoholic steatohepatitis: a study of 49 patients. [Review] [33 refs]. *Human Pathology.* 1920;(6):594-598.
8. Wanless IR, Lentz JS. Fatty liver hepatitis (steatohepatitis) and obesity: an autopsy study with analysis of risk factors. *Hepatology.* 1990;12(5):1106-1110.
9. McFarland RJ, Gazet JC, Pilkington TR. A 13-year review of jejunoileal bypass. *Brit J Surg.* 1985;72(2):81-87.
10. Bacon BR, Farahvash MJ, Janney CG, Neuschwander-Tetri BA. Nonalcoholic steatohepatitis: an expanded clinical entity. *Gastroenterology.* 1994;107(4):1103-1109.
11. Caldwell SH, Oelsner DH, Iezzoni JC, Hespenheide EE, Battle EH, Driscoll CJ. Cryptogenic cirrhosis: clinical characterization and risk factors for underlying disease. *Hepatology.* 1999;29(3):664-669.
12. Poonawala A, Nair SP, Thuluvath PJ. Prevalence of obesity and diabetes in patients with cryptogenic cirrhosis: a case control study. *Hepatology.* 2000;32(4):689-692.
13. Bugianesi E, Leone N, Vanni E, et al. Expanding the natural history of nonalcoholic steatohepatitis: from cryptogenic cirrhosis to hepatocellular carcinoma. *Gastroenterology.* 2002;123(1):134-140.
14. Marrero JA, Fontana RJ, Su GL, et al. NAFLD may be a common underlying liver disease in patients with hepatocellular carcinoma in the United States. *Hepatology.* 2002;36(6):1349-1354.
15. Lindor KD, Kowdley KV, Heathcote EJ, et al. Ursodeoxycholic acid for treatment of nonalcoholic steatohepatitis: results of a randomized trial. *Hepatology.* 2004;39(3): 770-778.
16. Adams LA, St Sauver J, Feldstein AE, Lindor KD, Brown S, Angulo P. The natural history of nonalcoholic fatty liver disease: a population based study [Abstract]. *Hepatology.* 2004;40(4):582A.
17. Pagano G, Pacini G, Musso G, et al. Nonalcoholic steatohepatitis, insulin resistance, and metabolic syndrome: Further evidence for an etiologic association. *Hepatology.* 2002;35(2):367-372.

18. Marchesini G, Brizi M, Morselli-Labate AM, et al. Association of nonalcoholic fatty liver disease with insulin resistance. *Am J Med.* 1999;107(5):450-455.
19. Marchesini G, Bugianesi E, Forlani G, et al. Nonalcoholic fatty liver, steatohepatitis, and the metabolic syndrome.[erratum appears in *Hepatology.* 2003 Aug;38(2):536]. *Hepatology.* 2003;37(4):917-923.
20. Sanyal AJ, Campbell-Sargent C, Mirshahi F, et al. Nonalcoholic steatohepatitis: Association of insulin resistance and mitochondrial abnormalities. *Gastroenterology.* 2001;120(5):1183-1192.
21. Cortez-Pinto H, Chatham J, Chacko VP, et al. Alterations in liver ATP homeostasis in human nonalcoholic steatohepatitis: A pilot study. *JAMA.* 1999;282(17):1659-1664.
22. Hui JM, Hodge A, Farrell GC, Kench JG, Kriketos A, George J. Beyond insulin resistance in NASH: TNF-alpha or adiponectin? *Hepatology.* 2004;40(1):46-54.
23. Diehl AM, Li ZP, Lin HZ, Yang SQ. Cytokines and the pathogenesis of non-alcoholic steatohepatitis. [Review] [67 refs]. *Gut.* 2005;54(2):303-306.
24. Sorbi D, Boynton J, Lindor KD. The ratio of aspartate aminotransferase to alanine aminotransferase: potential value in differentiating nonalcoholic steatohepatitis from alcoholic liver disease. *Am J Gastroenterol.* 1999;94(4):1018-1022.
25. Fletcher LM, Kwoh-Gain I, Powell EE, Powell LW, Halliday JW. Markers of chronic alcohol ingestion in patients with nonalcoholic steatohepatitis: an aid to diagnosis. *Hepatology.* 1991;13(3):455-459.
26. Caldwell SH, Hespenheide EE, Redick JA, et al. A pilot study of a thiazolidinedione, troglitazone, in nonalcoholic steatohepatitis.[see comment]. *Am J Gastroenterol.* 2001; 96(2):519-525.
27. Neuschwander-Tetri BA, Brunt E, Wehmeier KR, Oliver D, Bacon BR. Improved nonalcoholic steatohepatitis after 48 weeks of treatment with the PPAR- ligand rosiglitazone. *Hepatology.* 2003;38(4):1008-1017.
28. Marchesini G, Brizi M, Bianchi G, Tomassetti S, Zoli M, Melchionda N. Metformin in non-alcoholic steatohepatitis.[see comment]. *Lancet.* 2001;358(9285):893-894.
29. Harrison SA, Torgerson S, Hayashi P, Ward J, Schenker S. Vitamin E and vitamin C treatment improves fibrosis in patients with nonalcoholic steatohepatitis. *Am J Gastroenterol.* 2003;98(11):2485-2490.
30. Abdelmalek MF, Angulo P, Jorgensen RA, Sylvestre PB, Lindor KD. Betaine, a promising new agent for patients with nonalcoholic steatohepatitis: results of a pilot study.[see comment]. *Am J Gastroenterol.* 2001;96(9):2711-2717.

Recommended Reading

Angulo P. Nonalcoholic fatty liver disease. *N Engl J Med.* 2002;346:1221-1231.

Bacon BR, Farahvash MJ, Janney CG, et al. Nonalcoholic steatohepatitis: an expanded clinical entity. *Gastroenterology.* 1994;107:1103-1109.

Diehl AM, Li ZP, Lin HZ, Yang SQ. Cytokines and the pathogenesis of non-alcoholic steatohepatitis. [Review] [67 refs]. *Gut.* 2005;54(2):303-306.Ludwig J, Viggiano TR. Non-alcoholic steatohepatitis: Mayo Clinic experiences with a hitherto unnamed disease. *Mayo Clin Proc.* 1980;55:434-438.

Neushwander-Tetri BA, Caldwell SH. Nonalcoholic steatohepatitis: Summary of an AASLD single topic conference. *Hepatology.* 2003;37:1202-1219.

Powell EE, Cooksley WG, Hanson R, et al. The natural history of nonalcoholic steatohepatitis: a follow-up study of forty-two patients for up to 21 years. *Hepatology.* 1990; 11:74-80.

Sheth SG, Gordon FD, Chopra S, et al. Nonalcoholic steatohepatitis. *Ann Int Med.* 1997; 126:137-145.

chapter 7

Metabolic Liver Disease

Kirti Shetty, MD

Introduction

The metabolic liver diseases comprise a varied group of disorders, with differing modes of onset and clinical presentations. Most of these disorders are seen primarily in children. However, improved management has led to a greater longevity in those affected, and these individuals then transition to the care of the adult gastroenterologist. Table 7-1 provides an outline of some of the more common inherited diseases of the liver, although it is by no means a comprehensive list. This discussion will focus on some of the more important disorders encountered in adult clinical practice, namely derangements of metal metabolism and the relatively uncommon, but important, disorder of α-1 antitrypsin deficiency.

Disorders of Metal Metabolism

These include the iron overload syndromes, such as hereditary hemochromatosis, as well as those involving copper dysmetabolism, exemplified by Wilson's disease (WD).

Iron Overload Syndromes

Disorders of iron overload may be either primary, due to a genetic defect such as in hereditary hemochromatosis (HH), or may occur secondarily as a result of increased turnover of red blood cells (due to frequent transfusions or hemolysis) (see Table 7-1). The following discussion will deal with hereditary hemochromatosis.

Hereditary Hemochromatosis

Prevalence and Mode of Inheritance

Hereditary hemochromatosis (HH) is the most common identifiable genetic disease in Whites.[1] The defect within the newly discovered HFE gene (localized to the

Table 7-1

OTHER TERMS PREVIOUSLY USED TO DESCRIBE NONALCOHOLIC FATTY LIVER DISEASE

- Alcohol-like hepatitis
- Fatty liver hepatitis
- Steatonecrosis
- Diabetic hepatitis
- Pseudoalcoholic hepatitis
- Nonalcoholic Laennec's disease

short arm of chromosome 6) has been well-characterized.[2] This is a missense mutation leading to the substitution of tyrosine for cysteine at the 282 amino acid position (*C282Y*). Another mutation (*H63D*), in which aspartate is substituted for histidine at position 63, has also been identified. There are two predominant genetic abnormalities that accompany the phenotypic expression of HH: the homozygous state wherein both alleles of chromosome 6 have the *C282Y* mutation, or the compound heterozygous state with the *C282Y* mutation on one allele and the *H63D* mutation on the other. In most studies, more than 90% of those with HH are homozygous for the *C282Y* mutation, while 3% to 5% are compound heterozygotes. The remainder are believed to have other genetic aberrations that remain to be fully characterized.

The prevalence of HH in a given population reflects the frequency of the specific genetic mutation. The gene frequency in populations of European descent is as high as 1:10. It is much more rare in Asian and African populations.[3]

The phenotypic expression of the genetic abnormality is a subject of debate. In studies examining populations with iron overload, a wide variability in the incidence of the *C282Y* mutation has been noted depending on the area of the world. In the United States and Australia, 85% and 100% respectively of those with iron overload were noted to have this gene mutation. However, only 65% of a similar population from Italy tested positive for the mutation, suggesting that other genetic influences may be at play.[4]

Pathophysiology of Iron Overload

In order to appreciate the abnormalities in iron handling that occur in HH, it is important to first understand normal iron metabolism. The physiologic regulatory mechanism for iron homeostasis operates by modulation of iron absorption from the gastrointestinal tract. Normally, 1 to 2 mg/day of iron is absorbed in the duodenum. In states of iron deficiency, increased intestinal iron uptake (up to 10 mg/day) is seen.

Iron absorption is regulated by three important mediators: transferrin (Tf), the major transporter of iron; the transferrin receptor (TfR); and ferritin, the intracellular storage form of iron. TfR is a key protein in iron transport, and modulation of its expression controls iron uptake. Production of TfR is regulated by iron regulatory proteins (IRPs) that directly sense the intracellular iron level. When iron levels are low,

IRPs bind to RNA stem-loops known as iron-responsive elements (IREs). This results in an increase in the amount of TfR on the cell membrane, stimulating iron uptake. The amount of intracellular ferritin decreases simultaneously, decreasing iron storage. The converse happens in conditions of iron excess.

Cellular uptake and transport of iron also occurs by mechanisms independent of transferrin and TfR. These mechanisms have recently been elucidated and involve the divalent metal transporter (DMT1). It is believed that DMT1 plays a critical role in the process of iron uptake at the cellular level.[5]

In HH, the basic defect appears to be an impairment in TfR-mediated iron uptake. This sends the false signal that iron stores are low. As a result, the alternative pathway involving DMT1 becomes dominant. Differentiating enterocytes migrating up to the villus tip increase DMT1 production, and hence enhance iron uptake. The intestinal absorption of iron therefore proceeds at rates comparable to iron deficient patients, that is, at 10 to 20 times the basal levels. This persists despite the continual accumulation of iron within the reticuloendothelial system, and later in other body sites. Iron accumulation is toxic to the liver due to the generation of hydroxyl radicals with resultant membrane lipid peroxidation and disruption of cellular function. Other effects include the induction of collagen synthesis, contributing to hepatic fibrosis, and cirrhosis. Direct DNA damage may also occur, leading to an increased risk for development of hepatocellular carcinoma (HCC).[6]

Pathology

The major pathologic findings in the advanced stages of hemochromatosis relate to the massive amounts of iron deposited in the parenchymal cells of various organs, in particular the liver, pancreas, heart, and endocrine glands. Macroscopically, the liver is enlarged and nodular. Histological examination shows large amounts of iron in the parenchymal cells, and in the late stage, in Kupffer cells, macrophages, and biliary epithelial cells. At a critical level of hepatic iron, fibrosis develops, starting in a periportal distribution, and ultimately bridging portal tract-to-tract. A mixed macro-micronodular cirrhosis eventually develops.[7]

Cardiac deposition of hemosiderin occurs both in the heart muscle fibers and in the conducting fibers of the atrioventricular node. Other organs with hemosiderin deposition are the pancreas, endocrine glands such as the pituitary and the adrenals, as well as the skin. The characteristic "bronzed" hue of the skin is imparted by the increased melanin (with or without iron) in the dermis, in association with an atrophic epidermis.

Clinical Manifestations

The classical presentation of HH patients with the triad of diabetes mellitus, skin pigmentation ("bronze diabetes"), and hepatomegaly, is becoming increasingly uncommon in this era of increased awareness of the disease. Individuals are usually detected at an asymptomatic stage on the basis of either abnormal iron studies or screening of family members.[8]

If untreated, this condition is thought to evolve in a series of stages, the first of which consists of clinically insignificant iron accumulation (0 to 20 years of age, 0 to 5 g parenchymal iron), advancing to a stage of iron overload without disease (20 to 40 years of age, 10 to 20 g parenchymal iron), and culminating in iron overload with organ damage (over 40 years of age, over 20 g of parenchymal iron).

Symptomatic Stage

Patients usually present with one or more of the following symptoms: fatigue, skin pigmentation, loss of libido, joint pain, or features of diabetes. The most prominent physical signs include skin pigmentation, hepatomegaly, testicular atrophy, and arthropathy. Symptoms occur approximately 10 times more frequently in men than in women because of physiological blood loss in the latter group.

Hepatomegaly is the most frequently encountered abnormality and is present in more than 95% of symptomatic patients. Diabetes mellitus develops in 30% to 60% of those with advanced disease. Loss of libido is common and may be related to hypothalamic or pituitary failure, with selective impairment of gonadotrophin or gonadotrophin-releasing hormone.

Arthropathy is noted in 30% to 70% of symptomatic patients and is characterized by the deposition of calcium pyrophosphate (chondrocalcinosis). Its course occurs independent of the degree of iron overload, and is not often impacted by therapeutic phlebotomy.

Cardiac symptoms may be the initial manifestation in 5% to 15% of patients, although electrocardiographic abnormalities are present in about 30%. The most prevalent cardiac complications are those of biventricular failure and cardiac arrhythmias.

Hepatocellular carcinoma (HCC) is the most common cause of death in HH. Those individuals with HH-related cirrhosis are at 200-fold higher risk of developing HCC than the general population. This risk is related to the degree of iron-overload and is especially marked in men, aged over 40, with concomitant alcohol and tobacco abuse. The lifetime risk of developing HCC in a man with HH cirrhosis is approximately 30%. Rare cases of HCC have been described in noncirrhotic patients. However, for practical and screening purposes, we may assume that underlying cirrhosis is essential for HCC development in HH

Diagnosis of Heritary Hemochromatosis

The fundamental objective in the management of HH is to detect the disease and initiate treatment before irreversible organ damage occurs. Studies have demonstrated that the prognosis of HH and the development of complications such as decompensated cirrhosis, HCC, and cardiac disease, are dependent on the amount and duration of iron excess. Intervention at the precirrhotic stage will therefore impact favorably on overall survival.

The diagnosis of HH is based on demonstrating increased iron stores, namely increased hepatic iron concentration, associated with elevated serum ferritin levels.

Diagnostic Tests

1. *Iron Studies.* The two iron studies of most value in the diagnosis of iron overload are the transferrin saturation (TS) and the serum ferritin.[9-11] An elevated TS is the earliest abnormality in HH. It is usually measured as a ratio of the fasting serum iron and the total iron binding capacity (TIBC). TS is most accurate when measured in the fasting state. If a cutoff of 45% is used, 98% to 100% of *C282Y* homozygotes are correctly identified. However, the false positive rate has been reported to range between 22% and 44%. Hence, other groups with secondary iron overload may be identified and will need further careful clinical evaluation.

Serum ferritin when used alone lacks specificity in the diagnosis of HH, because ferritin is an acute phase reactant, and is often elevated in other disease states. However, the addition of the serum ferritin to the TS confers a negative predictive value of 97% and exceeds the accuracy of any single test. In confirmed HH, a level of serum ferritin >1000ng/mL accurately predicts the presence of hepatic fibrosis or cirrhosis.

2. *Genotypic Testing.* Testing for the HFE mutations (*C282Y* and *H63D*) can now be done by polymerase chain reaction using whole blood samples. Fasting transferrin saturation less than 45% and a normal serum ferritin require no further evaluation. Genotype testing is indicated in those individuals with abnormal studies and those who are first-degree relatives of identified homozygotes.[12]
3. *Liver Biopsy.* The utility of histologic analysis of the liver is in documenting the presence of cirrhosis, to exclude iron overload in the presence of equivocal serum markers, and to detect other possible etiologies of liver disease. The importance of age in determining the progression of HH to fibrosis and cirrhosis has been confirmed in several studies. Cirrhosis is rarely, if ever, seen in any patient less than 40 years of age. Hence, liver biopsy is indicated in those *C282Y* homozygotes over the age of 40, those with serum ferritin levels greater than 1000 ng/mL, and in those with clinical evidence of liver disease (abnormal hepatic biochemical tests or hepatomegaly) or with other risk factors for hepatic involvement such as alcohol abuse. Iron stores may be assessed by liver biopsy.[7] Qualitative iron determination may be done using a Perls' Prussian blue stain. If increased iron stores are suggested, quantitative determinations are indicated. The hepatic iron index (HII) may be calculated from such a determination (HII=hepatic iron concentration in micromoles (micmol) per gram (g) dry weight divided by age in years). A level in excess of 1.9 micmol/g/year is strong evidence of homozygous hemochromatosis. However, up to 15% of *C282Y* homozygotes lack this characteristic feature, and it is no longer considered essential for diagnosis. Liver biopsy is also useful in compound or *C282Y* heterozygotes with elevated TS, in order to determine the etiology of the abnormal iron studies.

Figure 7-1 summarizes a suggested approach to the diagnosis and management of HH.

Treatment

Indisputable evidence supports the fact that prevention of iron deposition in target organs significantly reduces the morbidity and mortality attributable to HH. Once the diagnosis is made, a course of iron depletion and monitoring should be initiated.[9-11,13] Initially, patients should undergo therapeutic phlebotomy once or twice weekly with regular monitoring of hemoglobin and hematocrit values. Each unit of blood is equal to 250 mg of iron, and in some patients with total iron stores greater than 30 g, adequate reduction of iron stores may take up to 3 years to achieve. The target ferritin level should be below 50 ng/mL and transferrin saturation under 30%. At the point when these criteria are reached, a maintenance schedule may be initiated.

One caution to be kept in mind is the recognition that the risk of cardiac dysrhythmias is particularly high during periods of rapid iron mobilization. Pharmacologic doses of vitamin C accelerate mobilization of iron and should be avoided during this period.

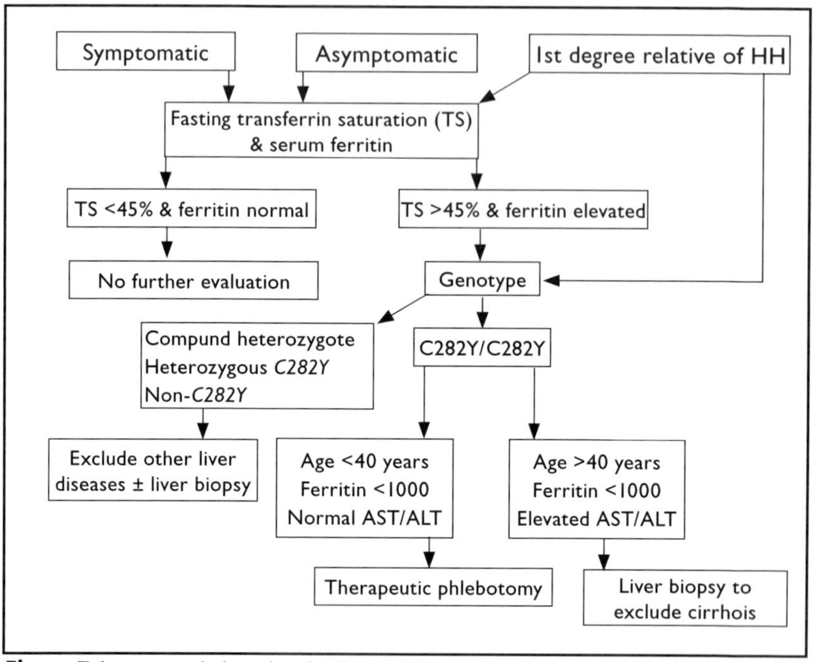

Figure 7-1. Proposed algorithm for the diagnosis and management of hereditary hemochromatosis (HH)

While phlebotomy improves or reverses some of the manifestations of HH such as fatigue, skin pigmentation, or insulin requirements, other manifestations such as cirrhosis, arthopathy or hypogonadism are rarely improved. Most studies report that the risk of developing HCC does not decrease after adequate iron removal. Thus, cirrhotic patients should continue careful surveillance for HCC, although the optimal method or frequency of surveillance remain unclear. At the present time, annual or 6-monthly alphafetoprotein with abdominal ultrasound is an accepted screening modality.

Liver transplantation is indicated for those with advanced disease.[14] Some evidence suggests that these individuals have significantly diminished post-transplant survival rates, although more recent studies dispute this finding.

Other Iron Overload States

Hematological Disorders

Chronic hemolytic anemias, such as thalassemia major, and conditions characterized by ineffective erythropoiesis, such as sideroblastic anemia, are both characterized by excessive iron stores.[15] This occurs due to increased gut absorption, as well as the parenteral iron load delivered by multiple blood transfusions. Iron loading can be controlled by the use of chelating drugs. Desferroxamine (DFO) is the most effective practical chelating agent. However, it is poorly absorbed orally and, for best results, must be administered as a subcutaneous pump. Prospective studies have demonstrated the utility of DFO in reducing iron stores, and hence the risk of diabetes, cardiac disease, and early death in those with hemolytic anemia.[16] Its utility is greatly limited by its mode of administration and difficulties encountered in achieving adequate compliance amongst its users. Research efforts are underway in the development of oral iron chelators.

Iron Overload in Chronic Liver Disease

It is thought that cirrhosis alone may cause iron accumulation in the liver, although the pathophysiology behind this is unclear. Explant studies have demonstrated increased hepatic iron concentrations in approximately 20% of those with cirrhosis.[17] Serum and hepatic iron stores have also been found to increase in those with chronic HCV. It is believed that iron overload may interfere with response to antiviral therapy in HCV, and that repeated phlebotomy may be of therapeutic benefit, although that premise remains unproven.

Iron Overload Associated with Metabolic Disorders

It is believed that conditions such as obesity, hyperlipidemia, abnormal glucose metabolism, or hypertension may be associated with a non-HLA linked iron-overload syndrome. Studies have demonstrated that these individuals have evidence of hepatic iron overload with elevated serum ferritin levels and normal transferrin saturation.[18] The overall significance and long-term prognosis of this condition remains to be elucidated.

Wilson's Disease

This is a genetic disorder characterized by accumulation of copper in the liver and brain, secondary to an inherited defect in the biliary excretion of copper.

Genetics And Pathophysiology

WD is inherited in an autosomal recessive fashion. The isolation and identification of its gene, designated *ATP7B*, has led to a greater understanding of the aberrations in copper metabolism caused by mutations in this gene.[19,20] Copper is an essential cofactor for many enzymes. Approximately 50% of ingested copper (1.5 to 3 mg/day) is absorbed in the upper small intestine. This absorbed copper is extracted from the portal circulation by hepatocytes. Intracellular copper is subsequently utilized for metabolic needs, incorporated into the secretory glycoprotein ceruloplasmin, or excreted into bile. This last route is the most crucial in the excretion of copper, as it undergoes minimal enterohepatic recirculation.

The transport of hepatocellular copper into bile is thought to involve a pathway that is dependent on *ATP7B* function. The absence or reduced function of *ATP7B* results in a decrease of biliary copper excretion, and the hepatic accumulation of this metal. The latter feature is pathognomic of WD.

The synthesis of ceruloplasmin is also believed to be dependent on *ATP7B*, which mediates copper incorporation into the ceruloplasmin molecule. Defective *ATP7B* function results in production of a noncopper containing apoprotein that is less stable, and, therefore, manifests as reduced circulating levels of ceruloplasmin.[21]

Copper is known to be hepatotoxic at excess levels. The toxic effects of copper include the generation of free radicals, lipid peroxidation of membranes and DNA, inhibition of protein synthesis, and altered levels of cellular antioxidants.

When the storage capacity of the liver for copper is exceeded or when hepatocellular damage results in the release of cellular copper into the circulation, levels of nonceruloplasmin-bound copper in the circulation become elevated. It is from this pool of copper that the extrahepatic deposition of this metal is thought to occur. The brain is the most important site for the extrahepatic accumulation of copper. Copper-induced neuronal injury is responsible for many of the neurologic and psychiatric manifestations of WD.

Pathology

The main organ systems involved are the liver, brain, kidneys, eyes, and joints.[22]

Hepatic Pathology

In the early stages, the liver may be only mildly enlarged. Light microscopic changes at this stage are nonspecific and consist of macro- and microsteatosis, with glycogenated nuclei. On electron microscopy, distinctive mitochondrial changes may be identified. These consist of enlargement and widening of intercristal spaces, and increased matrix granularity. With progression of the disease, copper-protein is sequestered in lysosomes, and may be detected as granules on copper immunohistochemistry.

The intermediate stage of WD is characterized by the features of chronic active hepatitis consisting of periportal inflammation, interface hepatitis, and bridging fibrosis. In its final stages, cirrhosis in either a micronodular or a mixed macro-micronodular histologic pattern is noted. Mallory bodies may be present in up to half of all biopsies. In patients with fulminant hepatic failure, parenchymal necrosis may overshadow other histological features. Histochemical confirmation of copper deposition may be helpful when positive, but its absence does not exclude copper overload.

Neuropathology

Macroscopically, most of the overt changes within the brain occur in the lenticular nuclei that show atrophy, discoloration, and cystic degeneration. Microscopic changes occur most commonly in the thalamus, followed by the putamen and cerebral cortex. Characteristic neuroglial changes occur with an increase in astrocytes distinctive for WD, known as Opalski cells. The swollen glia are subject to liquefaction, creating small cavities.

Miscellaneous Pathological Changes

Functional changes in the kidneys are disproportionate to any microscopic changes. Proximal or distal tubular dysfunction is common and leads to tubular proteinuria, metabolic acidosis, aminoaciduria, glycosuria, hyperphosphaturia, uricosuria, and hypercalciuria.

Bone pathology is observed, with the spine and knee joints being most commonly involved. Osteoporosis, osteomalacia, adult rickets, chondrocalcinosis, and subchondral cyst formation can be noted.

Ophthalmologic changes include the Kayser-Fleischer (K-F) rings, which are due to granular deposition of elemental copper on the inner surface of the cornea in Descemet's membrane. The sunflower cataract, another manifestation of WD, is due to copper deposition in the anterior and posterior lens capsule. Both these manifestations are reversible with effective therapy.

CLINICAL MANIFESTATIONS

Many of the early symptoms of WD are subtle and nonspecific, accounting for the frequency of delayed diagnoses. Symptoms are rare in the first 5 years of life, but about half of all affected individuals become symptomatic by their teens. Early symptoms are usually hepatic, with the full-blown syndrome becoming apparent after deposition of copper in other organs, primarily the central nervous system and the cornea. Most individuals manifest the disease by the age of 40 years, and delayed diagnosis beyond this age is rare.

The major clinical syndromes associated with WD may be summarized as follows:[23]

- *Asymptomatic stage*: This is of variable duration. It is usually identified in those with a family history of Wilson's, or in the course of the work-up of abnormal hepatic biochemistries. Physical examination usually discloses hepatomegaly, splenomegaly, or corneal Kayser-Fleischer rings.
- *Acute Wilsonian Hepatitis*: This is characterized by the sudden onset of hemolytic anemia and gastrointestinal symptoms, subsiding within 1 to 2 weeks. Even though a moderate indirect hyperbilirubinemia is often noted at this stage, liver biopsy is rarely performed, and the diagnosis is often overlooked.
- *Fulminant Hepatic Failure*: A dramatic manifestation of WD is that of acute liver failure. If timely liver transplantation is not performed, this condition is uniformly fatal. There are several unique features of this form of fulminant hepatitis: these include an associated nonimmune hemolytic anemia, markedly elevated serum copper levels, modest transaminitis given the severity of the decompensation, hypoalbuminemia, and low alkaline phosphatase.
- *Chronic Active Wilsonian Hepatitis/Cirrhosis*: Some young individuals present with chronic liver disease indistinguishable from other types of chronic hepatitis, often associated with fever, polyarthralgias, amenorrhea, and delayed puberty. If unrecognized, this progresses to cirrhosis, characterized by the many manifestations of decompensated liver disease. The development of hepatocellular carcinoma, once considered a rarity, has now been described in at least 15 patients in the worldwide literature.
- *Neurologic Wilson's*: This is almost invariably associated with cirrhosis. Patients with neurologic involvement are often older than those who present with hepatic symptoms. Neurologic manifestations are varied and include Parkinsonian characteristics of dystonia, hypertonia, and rigidity, along with chorea, tremors, and dysarthria. A variety of psychologic disturbances may be noted, ranging from mild memory impairment to overt psychosis.

Diagnostic Approach

The criteria for the confirmation of WD vary according to the patient's age and mode of presentation.

The following tests have been found to be most useful in either confirming or excluding Wilson's as the etiology for liver disease.[24]

Ophthalmic Evaluation

A slit-lamp examination of the cornea may detect golden-greenish granular deposition within Descemet's membrane, designated as the K-F ring (Figure 7-2). In association with characteristic neurologic symptoms, the K-F ring is diagnostic of WD. Conversely, its absence in a patient with neurologic manifestations, virtually excludes the disease. However, the K-F ring is not specific for WD, and may also be present in individuals with cholestatic syndromes leading to copper retention. Therefore, in the asymptomatic patient, additional tests would be necessary to confirm WD.

Serum Ceruloplasmin

Two types of assays are available for the measurement of serum ceruloplasmin. The immunologic assay tends to give higher readings, caused by the antibody reaction with not only circulating apoceruloplasmin, but also holoceruloplasmin. The enzymatic assay, which measures ceruloplasmin by its oxidase activity toward various substrates, is more accurate, and is preferred in clinical practice. A concentration lower than 20 mg/dL is found in 96% of those with WD. However, such a result alone is not diagnostic, as 10% of heterozygous carriers who never manifest the disease, also have values under 20 mg/dL. Levels of ceruloplasmin are also decreased in states of severe copper deficiency, in patients with severe fulminant hepatitis, significant protein-losing nephropathy or enteropathy, and in the rare disorders of hereditary hypoceruloplasminemia or aceruloplasminemia.

Using the serum ceruloplasmin alone as a screening test for WD is fraught with problems. One prospective study demonstrated that a subnormal ceruloplasmin had a positive predictive value of only 6% (ie, of 2867 patients tested, 17 had subnormal ceruloplasmin and only 1 of these was found to have WD).[25] Conversely, studies on patients with well-established WD have demonstrated that between 22% and 28% of these patients have ceruloplasmin levels above 15 mg/dL. It should also be remembered that ceruloplasmin is an acute phase reactant and may be elevated in inflammatory states, pregnancy, or in response to exogenous administration of estrogens.

Serum Free-Copper Concentration

The total serum copper, which is the sum of ceruloplasmin copper (90%) and nonceruloplasmin copper (10%), may be deceptively low in WD. This is due to hypoceruloplasminemia, which leads to low measured levels of total copper, despite an elevation in free copper levels. The serum nonceruloplasmin-bound or free copper concentration has been proposed as a diagnostic test for WD.[26] This may be calculated by subtracting ceruloplasmin copper (typically three times the serum ceruloplasmin) from the total copper. Normally, the free copper level is under 10 mcg/dL. In WD, levels of free copper are typically greater than 25 mcg/dL.

The major drawback of nonceruloplasmin-bound copper as a diagnostic test for WD is that it is dependent on the adequacy of the methods for measuring both serum copper and ceruloplasmin, and may be difficult to interpret. It is of greater value

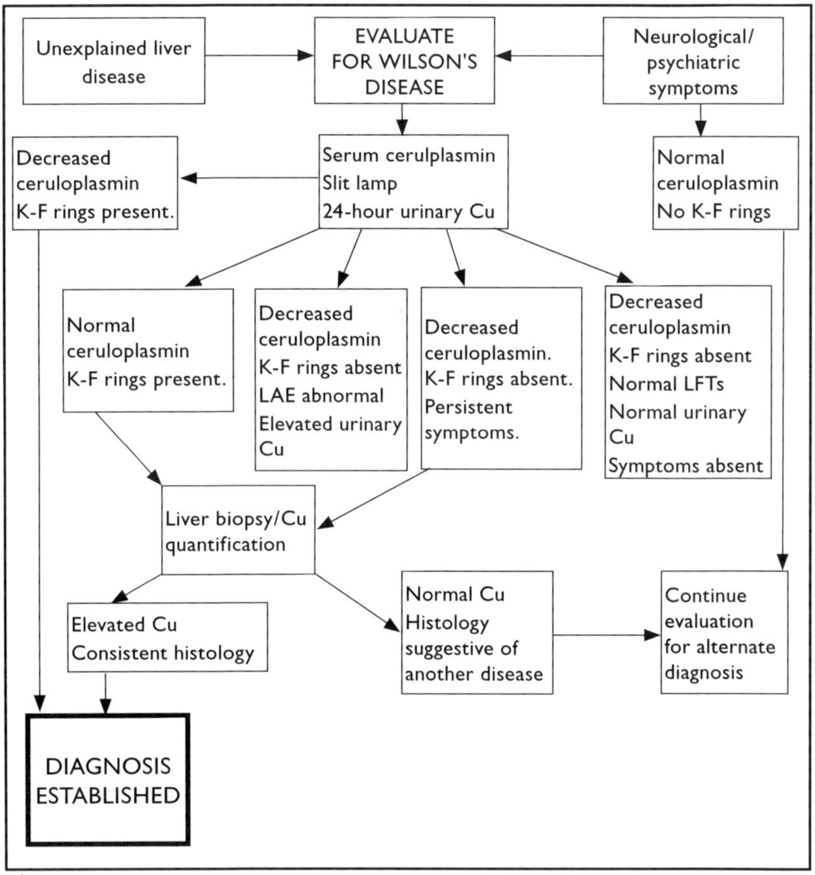

Figure 7-2. Approach to suspected Wilson's Disease.

in monitoring pharmacotherapy in known WD. Nonceruloplasmin-bound copper concentration <5mcg/dL, in combination with very low 24-hour urinary copper excretion, may signal systemic copper depletion that may occur in some patients with prolonged treatment.[24]

Urinary Copper Excretion

This is increased to more than 100 mcg/24 hrs in most symptomatic patients. Recent studies suggest that 16% to 23% of those diagnosed with WD have 24-hour excretion levels under 100 mcg.[27] Hence, using a cut-off level of 40 mcg/24 hours, which is the normal reference limit in most clinical laboratories, may be a better threshold for diagnosis. Interpretation of these results is further complicated by the overlap seen in other types of liver disease and in heterozygotes for WD, who may have intermediate levels of copper excretion. In one study of patients with chronic liver disease, 5 of 54 patients had urinary copper excretions above 100 mcg/24 hours.[28]

D-penicillamine administration prior to the urinary copper estimation may be a useful adjunctive test. This test has been standardized in a pediatric population, in which 500 mg of D-penicillamine was administered orally at the beginning and then 12 hours later during the 24-hour urine collection. When the urinary copper content is increased to above 1600 mcg/24 hours, it provides a clear distinction between WD and many other chronic liver diseases.

Hepatic Copper

Determination of hepatic parenchymal copper concentration remains the "gold-standard" for diagnosing WD. While a liver biopsy is not considered essential, most physicians prefer to have this confirmatory information available before subjecting an individual to lifetime therapy. A hepatic copper concentration of greater than 250 mcg/g dry tissue (normal: less than 50 mcg/g) is diagnostic of WD, especially in association with characteristic histologic findings.

Biopsies for quantitative copper determination should be taken with a disposable biopsy needle and placed dry in a copper-free container. This core of tissue may either be dried overnight in a vacuum oven, or preferably frozen immediately and shipped to a laboratory for quantitative copper determination. Paraffin-embedded specimens can also be analyzed for copper content. The major drawback to copper estimation is the fact that copper distribution within the liver can be inhomogenous, hence leading to an underestimation of the true copper concentration.

The hepatic parenchymal copper content provides useful diagnostic information when the diagnosis is not straightforward. In untreated patients, normal hepatic copper content (<40 µg/g dry weight) excludes a diagnosis of WD.[29]

Genetic Studies

The large number of disease-specific mutant alleles of *ATP7B* limits the practical application of genetic screening for the disease. Within a family in which a specific defective gene has been identified, such testing may replace liver biopsy in the diagnostic work-up.

Symptomatic Patients

Neurologic Presentation

The disease may be relatively easy to confirm in those who have a neurologic mode of presentation. Almost all such patients exhibit K-F rings, and 95% of them have serum ceruloplasmin concentrations below 20 mg/dL.

Hepatic Presentation

These patients are younger than those with neurologic symptoms, and corneal copper deposits are not necessarily present. The ceruloplasmin concentrations are not as reliable, as about 10% to 15% of these individuals have levels in the low-normal range (up to 30 mg/dL). A liver biopsy is often crucial in resolving the diagnostic dilemma.

Asymptomatic Patients

Screening of family members of affected individuals is mandatory. Unexplained transaminemia or an incidentally discovered K-F ring may also provide a basis for screening. Screening tests involve corneal slit-lamp examination and determination of the serum ceruloplasmin concentration. A value under 20 mg/dL is highly suspicious for WD, and one over 30 mg/dL virtually excludes the diagnosis, except in pregnant women and those taking estrogens. These conditions may cause the ceruloplasmin to rise to within the normal range in affected individuals.

Treatment

The mainstay of treatment consists of pharmacological therapy, which should be started as soon as the diagnosis is confirmed and continued for life. Significant morbidity and mortality may be prevented by the treatment of asymptomatic patients.[30,31]

Pharmacologic Therapy

D-Penicillamine

D-penicillamine (3-mercapto-D-valine) is an orally-administered chelating agent capable of markedly reducing the effects of copper toxicity. Importantly, this was the first medication that was shown to effectively prevent disease progression, and to reverse some of the neurological and hepatic manifestations of the disease. Its major effect is to promote the urinary excretion of copper. The daily dose ranges from 750 mg to 2 g in divided doses.

Side effects of penicillamine may be grouped either as early or late-occurring. Early sensitivity reactions occur in about 10% of patients and consist of fever, cutaneous eruptions, lymphadenopathy, neutropenia, or thrombocytpoenia. These reactions should prompt discontinuation of the medication. Late reactions include nephrotoxicity, a lupus-like syndrome, Goodpasture's syndrome, and dermatologic toxicities including progeric skin changes, pemphigoid lesions, and lichen planus. Very late side effects include polymyositis, myasthenia gravis, and serous retinitis.

The clinical response may often be delayed for months, and there may be an initial worsening of neurological symptoms in 10% to 50% of patients. Worsening hepatic enzymes have also been reported. However, most individuals tolerate the medication well and are able to be maintained on it for several decades. Recovery of hepatic synthetic function and improvement in clinical symptoms is typically seen in the first 2 to 6 months of treatment.

Adequacy of treatment is monitored by measuring urinary copper excretion. This should be in the range of 200 to 500 mcg/24 hours. Regular supplementation with pyridoxine is required at a dose of 25 to 50 mg daily.

In the past, patients who experienced allergic reactions underwent hyposensitization and gradual reintroduction of the medication, along with steroid administration. The emergence of safer and better-tolerated alternative therapies has made such an approach unnecessary.

Trientine Dihydrochloride

This is an alternative chelating agent, which has a more favorable side-effect profile than D-penicillamine and is considered as clinically effective. The daily dose is 1 to 2 g in divided doses. Sideroblastic anemia is a rare side effect in patients receiving more than 2 g of trientine daily, and is thought to be secondary to copper deficiency. It is easily reversible with reduction of the dose. Trientine is useful both as initial therapy in patients with severe neurological and hepatic disease, as well as in maintenance regimens.

Zinc Salts

These (acetate, gluconate, and sulphate) have been used in the treatment of WD since the 1960s. Zinc has a different mechanism of action in that it interferes with the intestinal absorption of copper by inducing metallothionein in enterocytes. Therefore, copper is chelated in enterocytes, which are later shed naturally along with the ingested copper in the feces. The rate at which copper is depleted is slow. Hence, zinc is not recommended as the sole agent for initial therapy of symptomatic patients. However, it is an effective maintenance therapy, and recent studies substantiate earlier claims of its long-term effectiveness. The average dose is 50 mg of elemental zinc 3 times daily. Common side effects include headaches and gastrointestinal upsets. Zinc acetate may be better tolerated than other formulations.

Tetrathiomolybdate

Tetrathiomolybdate is an investigational drug used primarily for initial treatment before switching to trientine or zinc; it is used to avoid the neurologic deterioration that accompanies chelation treatment in some patients. It is presently undergoing a comparison study with the combination of trientine and zinc for effectiveness in patients with neurologic WD.

British Anti-Lewisite (BAL)

British Anti-Lewisite (BAL), or 2,3-dimercapto-1-propanol, is now mainly of historic interest. It is a chelating agent that works by promoting cupriuresis. Its use is limited by its intramuscular mode of administration, and unfavorable side-effect profile.

Combination Therapy

Few published data are available on combining agents in treatment of WD. One approach is to combine two medications with different and complementary modes of action, for example using zinc with an oral chelating agent, such as trientine. This concept is now undergoing formal testing as part of a trial of initial therapy for neurologic WD. The potential role of tetrathiomolybdate as an alternative combination therapy awaits formal approval and commercial production in this country.

Dietary Measures

Certain copper-containing foods, such as shellfish, nuts, mushrooms, organ meats, and chocolate should be avoided in the first year of treatment. Well-water or water brought into the household through copper pipes should be checked for copper content. A water-purifying system is advisable if the copper content of the water is high.

Recommendations for Treatment

In clinical practice, patients may be treated differently based on their symptoms and stage of disease.[24]

1. *Symptomatic patients*: Initial treatment should include a chelating agent (penicillamine or trientine).
2. *Asymptomatic patients*: These individuals are usually identified through family screening. Treatment with chelating agents or with zinc is effective in preventing disease symptoms and progression.
3. *Maintenance therapy*: After adequate treatment with a chelator, stable patients may be converted to treatment with zinc. The usual requirements to be satisfied before making the transition to maintenance zinc therapy are as follows:
    a. Normal serum aminotransferases and hepatic synthetic function
    b. Normal nonceruloplasmin-bound copper concentration

c. 24-hour urinary copper excretion in the 200 to 500 mcg range. Maintenance therapy should be continued indefinitely to avoid the risk of hepatic decompensation

4. *Therapy in pregnancy*: Therapy should be maintained during pregnancy, although the doses of D-penicillamine or trientine should be reduced during the last trimester, as the fetus sequesters some of the excess copper. There have been reports of more than 100 successful pregnancies in women on these therapies.
5. *Role of liver transplantation*: This is indicated in patients with Wilsonian fulminant hepatitis, whether occurring as the first manifestation of the disease as a result of therapeutic noncompliance. It may also be indicated for severe hepatic insufficiency that is not responsive to several months of intensive chelation treatment. Transplant recipients have an excellent long-term prognosis, with 1-year survival rates reported in the 80% range.

MONITORING OF THERAPY

Compliance with the therapeutic regimen is crucial in the management of this condition. Several methods of monitoring compliance have been described.[24]

1. Measurement of nonceruloplasmin (free) copper: This is the most reliable indicator of copper depletion, as described in an earlier section. In appropriately treated individuals, the nonceruloplasmin copper should be 10 mcg/dL or less. In untreated or inadequately treated individuals, this value is often elevated above 25 mcg/dL.
2. Measurement of urinary copper, if properly implemented, also provides an important clue to compliance. During the early phase of treatment with chelating agents, the urinary copper excretion is often greater than 1000 mcg/dL. This declines to about 250 to 500 mcg/24 hours over time. Values under 250 mcg/24 hours suggest noncompliance with therapy or an erroneous diagnosis.

   With zinc therapy, copper absorption is retarded, and the parameters used to monitor compliance vary accordingly. A rise in the urinary copper to over 150 mcg/24 hours, rather than a decline, would indicate noncompliance. Plasma and urinary zinc levels may also be directly measured. With adequate therapy, urinary zinc levels should exceed 1000 mcg/24 hours.

In those who are compliant with pharmacotherapy, the long-term outcome of WD is excellent. Neurologic or psychiatric symptoms show a gradual recovery over months or years. Those with established cirrhosis or chronic hepatitis often stabilize their liver disease, with little or no progression.

MENKE'S DISEASE

This is a rare x-linked disorder of copper metabolism resulting from mutations within a gene encoding a copper transporting ATPase, ATP7A, homologous to the gene defect in WD. It is characterized by neurological degeneration, connective tissue and vascular involvement, depigmented and brittle hair, and death in infancy and early childhood. Copper absorption from the gut is reduced with low serum copper and ceruloplasmin levels. The liver is not affected in this disorder, but it has provided us with some valuable insights into the pathophysiology of abnormal copper metabolism, and hence a greater understanding of WD.

α-1 Antitrypsin Deficiency

α-1 antitrypsin (A1AT) deficiency is a relatively common autosomal recessive disorder characterized by hepatic involvement, pulmonary emphysema, panniculitis, and arterial aneurysms.

α-1 Antitrypsin and Its Gene

The A1AT gene is located on the q arm of chromosome 14.[32] The final protein product of the gene (A1AT) is a 52-kD serum glycoprotein predominantly derived from the liver. A1AT belongs to a class of protease inhibitors known as serpins, which function mainly as serine protease inhibitors. The plasma concentration of A1AT increases 3- to 5-fold during the host response to tissue injury and inflammation. Its principal physiologic function is to inhibit the destructive neutrophil proteases: elastase, cathepsin G, and proteinase 3.

Variants of α-1 Antitrypsin

A variety of mutations within the A1AT gene can result in a deficiency or absence of the protease inhibitor in serum. More than 75 allelic variations for A1AT have been identified. In humans, these variants are classified according to the protease inhibitor (PI) phenotype system, as defined by agarose electrophoresis. The PI classification system assigns a letter of the alphabet from A-Z to each group of allelic variants with the same electrophoretic properties. The most common normal variant migrates to an intermediate isoelectric point, designated PiM. The PiM variant is found in 65% to 70% of Whites in the United States. It is not associated with clinical disease, as serum concentration and functional activity for A1AT is within the normal range.

Individuals with the most common severe deficiency have an A1AT allelic variant that migrates to a high isoelectric point, designated PiZ. The mutation responsible for the PiZ type migration of A1AT is a single amino acid substitution (glu 342 to lys 342). In clinical practice, more than 90% of cases are caused by the PiZ mutation.

Mechanism of Hepatic Disease in α-1 Antitrypsin Deficiency

Hepatic disease has been described most commonly in association with the PiZ allele.[33] Several theories exist as to the mechanism for liver injury. The most widely accepted of these is the so-called "accumulation theory." It is believed that the PiZ mutation affects the uniquely flexible conformation of the active site loop region of A1AT. This results in abnormalities of its folding at the time of synthesis. The abnormal forms of the protein undergo polymerization and intracellular degradation with accumulation. The resultant intracellular inclusions are thought to have hepatotoxic effects. The mechanism whereby the retention of mutant A1AT leads to progressive hepatic injury is still to be elucidated. In transgenic mice expressing the human A1AT gene, nodular clusters of altered hepatocytes are seen. These progress to fibrotic dysplastic nodules, and eventually to foci of hepatocellular carcinoma.

However, difficult to reconcile with the accumulation theory is the observation that only a subset of homozygous (PiZZ) A1AT deficient individuals (approximately

10% to 15%) develop significant liver damage. It is believed that additional inherited traits or environmental factors exist that exaggerate the cellular pathophysiological consequences of mutant A1AT accumulation.

INCIDENCE AND MODE OF INHERITANCE

The incidence of homozygous (PiZZ) A1AT deficiency is highest in people of Scandinavian and Northern European ancestry, affecting approximately 1 in 1600 to 1800 live births.[34] Recent studies suggest that the incidence in the United States is almost identical to that in Scandinavian populations. There are estimated to be more than 100,000 persons with A1AT deficiency in the United States. Its main manifestation is the development of pulmonary emphysema by the third or fourth decade of life. It is also associated with a lesser risk of hepatic disease. It is the most common genetic indication for liver transplantation in the pediatric population and is an important cause of chronic liver disease and hepatocellular carcinoma in adults.

Clinical Manifestations of Liver Disease

Liver involvement is usually noted in the first 2 months of life and is characterized by persistent jaundice, and abnormal hepatic biochemical tests.[35] Approximately 10% of affected individuals may present with manifestations of cirrhosis and portal hypertension in early infancy, and an even smaller proportion with fulminant hepatic failure.

In later life, the presentation of this disease may be nonspecific. It should be suspected in any adult presenting with chronic hepatitis, cirrhosis, evidence of portal hypertension, or hepatocellular carcinoma.[36]

The heterozygous A1AT MZ phenotype is not thought to cause liver disease in children by itself. Some studies in adults suggest a relationship between heterozygosity and the development of liver disease, but no convincing evidence exists to link liver injury to the heterozygous state alone.

Liver disease has been described for several other allelic variants of A1AT. Compound heterozygotes of the type PiSZ are affected by liver injury similar to PiZZ. Liver disease has also been reported with the variant PiMmalton.

Pulmonary Manifestations of α-1 Antitrypsin Deficiency

Chronic obstructive airway disease (COAD) is seen in approximately 75% to 80% of individuals over their lifetime. Affected individuals are invariably smokers and typically develop pulmonary emphysema in the third to fourth decade of life. Smoking has been estimated to shorten the life of these patients by approximately 20 years.

The characteristic pulmonary pathological abnormality is diffuse panacinar emphysema. In deficiency states, the lack of A1AT in the pulmonary interstitium results in the unopposed action of proteases, the gradual destruction of pulmonary connective tissue, and the loss of alveolar units. It is thought that the oxidants associated with cigarette smoke promote lung disease by oxidatively inactivating the active site residue of the A1AT molecule, thereby resulting in a 1000-fold diminution in antiprotease activity.

Other Clinical Manifestations of α-1 Antitrypsin Deficiency

An ulcerative neutrophilic cutaneous panniculitis associated with fever is seen in a minority of affected individuals. These lesions typically occur on the trunk, and are often precipitated by minor trauma. A clinical response to exogenously administered A1AT and dapsone has been described.

An association between A1AT deficiency and renal disease in infancy has been described, although not well characterized. Also suggested is an association between A1AT deficiency and immune complex diseases such as rheumatoid arthritis, and Wegener's granulomatosis. Certain malignancies are also reported to occur more commonly in those with this disorder. Whether this represents primary protease-antiprotease imbalance or a linkage phenomenon remains to be determined.

Natural History of α-1 Antitrypsin Deficiency

Several registries of these patients have attempted to study their long-term outcome, but these data are still incomplete. The National Institutes of Health study suggests that the actuarial survival of PiZZ individuals to the age of 60 is only 16%, compared to 85% in the normal population. The Danish registry reports that the life expectancy in PiZZ individuals is 52 years in smokers, compared to 68 years in nonsmokers.

The natural history of liver disease in A1AT deficiency has been studied prospectively by Sveger, in a Swedish nationwide screening study.[37] Of the 127 PiZZ individuals identified by screening all newborn infants, more than 85% had persistently normal transaminases at 18 years of age. However, it is unclear as to whether occult liver disease exists in these individuals and whether they will progress to overt liver disease in adulthood. The prognosis of hepatic disease in A1AT deficiency is difficult to predict. One study suggested that persistence of hyperbilirubinemia, hard hepatomegaly, early development of splenomegaly, and prolongation of prothrombin time were all indicators of poor prognosis. In another study, elevated transaminase levels, prolonged prothrombin time, and a lower trypsin inhibitor capacity correlated with a worse prognosis.

Diagnosis

The serum A1AT phenotype may be determined by isoelectric focusing or by agarose electrophoresis at acid pH. The serum concentrations of A1AT may be helpful when used with phenotype to distinguish individuals who are homozygous for the Z allele from SZ compound heterozygotes. This is important in genetic counseling. It should be remembered that serum A1AT levels may be misleading, as they increase in response to inflammatory states and may be falsely elevated even in affected individuals.

The pathognomic histological feature of homozygous PiZZ A1AT deficiency is the appearance of periodic acid-Schiff-positive, diastase-resistant globules in the endoplasmic reticulum of hepatocytes. However, these are not specific for this condition and may be seen in PiMM individuals with other liver diseases. Other histological features include variable degrees of hepatocellular necrosis, inflammatory cell infiltration, periportal fibrosis, and cirrhosis.

Treatment

Avoidance of cigarette smoking, even in those with no definitely documented pulmonary disease, is of paramount importance. Smoking has been shown to accelerate the progression of lung involvement and significantly truncate life expectancy in affected individuals.[37]

No specific therapy is available for liver disease, apart from supportive care. In the decompensated cirrhotic, liver transplantation is the only corrective therapy. This has been shown to be associated with good survival rates in both children and adults: 90% at 1 year and 80% at 5 years. A number of PiZZ individuals have relatively preserved hepatic function, and may never need liver transplantation. The etiology of hepatic involvement in A1AT deficiency is not thought to be related to deficient levels of the protein, and so replacement therapy is not indicated.

For those with pulmonary disease, replacement therapy with recombinant plasma A1AT is available, either by intravenous or intratracheal administration. It is indicated in those with established and progressive emphysema. Lung transplantation is also an option for those with severe emphysema. Data from the Lung Transplant registry show actuarial survival in this group to be similar to that in other groups.

In summary, the inherited metabolic disorders of the liver offer an intriguing glimpse into the many complex pathophysiological mechanisms mediated by the liver. Exciting new advances in molecular medicine have exponentially increased our understanding of these disorders. It is hoped that with these greater insights come the hope of new and more effective therapies.

References

1. Bomford A. Genetics of haemochromatosis. *Lancet.* 2002;360:1673-1681.
2. Feder JN, Gnirke A, Thomas W, et al. A novel MHC class I-like gene is mutated in patients with hereditary haemochromatosis. *Nat Genet.* 1996;13:399-408.
3. Merryweather-Clarke AT, Pointon JJ, Sherman JD, Robson KJH. Global prevalence of putative haemochromatosis mutations. *J Med Genet.* 1997;34:275-278.
4. Imperatore G, Pinsky LE, Motulsky A, Reyes M, Bradley LA, Burke W. Hereditary hemochromatosis : perspectives of public health, medical genetics, and primary care. *Genet Med.* 2003;5:1-8.
5. Pietrangelo A. Physiology of iron transport and the hemochromatosis gene. *Am J Physiol.* 2002;282:G403-414.
6. Britton RS. Metal-induced hepatotoxicity. *Semin Liver Dis.* 1996;16:3-12.
7. Nash S, Marconi S, Sikorska K, Naeem R, Nash G. Role of liver biopsy in the diagnosis of hepatic iron overload in the era of genetic testing. *Am J Clin Pathol.* 2002; 118:73-81.
8. Brissot P, Moirand R, Jouanolle AM, Guyader Le Gall JY, Deugnier Y, David V. A genotypic study of 217 unrelated probands diagnosed as "genetic hemochromatosis" on "classical" phenotypic criteria. *J Hepatol.* 1999;30:588-593.
9. Tavill AS. Diagnosis and management of hemochromatosis. AASLD Practice Guidelines. *Hepatology.* 2001;33:1321-1328.
10. Bacon BR, Powell LW, Adams PC, et al. Molecular medicine and hemochromatosis: at the crossroads. *Gastroenterology.* 1999;116:193-207.
11. Pietrangelo A. Hereditary hemochromatosis—a new look at an old disease. *N Engl J Med.* 2004;350:2383-2397.
12. Robson KJH, Merryweather-Clarke AT, Cadet E, et al. Recent advances in understanding hemochromatosis: a transition state. *J Med Genet.* 2004;41:721-730.
13. Powell LW. Hemochromatosis. *Clin Liv Dis.* 2000;4(1)211-228.
14. Khanna A. Liver transplantation for metabolic liver diseases. *Surg Clin N Amer.* 1999; 79(1): 153-162.

15. Gabuti G, Borgna-Pignatti C. Clinical manifestations and therapy of transfusional haemosiderosis. *Bailleres Clin Haematol.* 1994;7:919-937.
16. Brittenham GM, Griffith PM, Nienhuis AW, et al. Efficacy of desferrioxamine in preventing complications of iron overload in patients with thalassemia major. *N Engl J Med.* 1994;331:567-573.
17. Ludwig J, Hashimoto E, Porayko M, Moyer T, Baldu W. Hemosiderosis in cirrhosis: a study of 447 native livers. *Gastroenterology.* 1997;112:882-888.
18. Mendler MH, Turlin B, Moirand R, et al. Insulin resistance-associated hepatic iron overload. *Gastroenterology.* 1999;117(5):1155-1163.
19. Bull PC, Thomas GR, Rommens JM, Forbes JR, Cox DW. The Wilson Disease gene is a putative copper transporting P-type ATPase similar to the Menkes gene. *Nat Genet.* 1993;5:344-350.
20. Tanzi RE, Petrukhin K, Chernov I, et al. The Wilson disease gene is a copper transporting ATPase with homology to the Menkes disease gene. *Nat Genet.* 1993; 5:338-343.
21. Holtzman NA, Gaumnitz BM. Studies on the rate of release and turnover of ceruloplasmin and apoceruloplasmin in rat plasma. *J Biol Chem.* 1970;245:2354-2358.
22. Schilsky ML. Diagnosis and treatment of Wilson's disease. *Ped Transplantation.* 2002;6:15-19.
23. Cuthbert JA. Wilson's disease. Update of a systemic disorder with protean manifestations. *Gastroenterol Clin N Am.* 1998;27:655-681.
24. Roberts EA, Schilsky ML. A practice guideline on Wilson disease. AASLD practice guidelines. *Hepatology.* 2003;37:1475-1492.
25. Cauza E, Maier-Dobersberger T, Polli C, et al. Screening for Wilson's disease in patients with liver diseases by serum ceruloplasmin. *J Hepatol.* 1997;27:358-362.
26. Roberts EA, Cox DW. Wilson disease. *Baillieres Clin Gastroenterol.* 1998;12:237-256.
27. Steindl P, Ferenci P, Dienes HP, et al. Wilson's disease in patients presenting with liver disease: a diagnostic challenge. *Gastroenterology* 1997;113;212-218.
28. LaRusso NF, Summerskill WH, McCall JT. Abnormalities of chemical tests for copper metabolism in chronic active liver disease : differentiation from Wilson's disease. Gastroenterology. 1976;70:653-655.
29. Ludwig J, Moyer TP, Rakela J. The liver biopsy diagnosis of Wilson's disease. Methods in pathology. *Am J Clin Pathol.* 1994;102:443-446.
30. Sternlieb I. Wilson's Disease. *Clin Liver Dis.* 2000;4(1):229-239.
31. Schilsky ML. Treatment for WD: What are the relative roles of penicillamine, trientine, and zinc supplementation? *Curr Gastro Reports.* 2001;3:54-59.
32. Teckman JH, Qu D, Perlmutter DH, Molecular pathogenesis of liver disease in alpha-1-antitrypsin deficiency. *Hepatology.* 1996;24:1504-1516.
33. Perlmutter DH. Liver injury in alpha-1 antitrypsin deficiency. *Clin Liv Dis.* 2000; 4(1):220-229.
34. Coakley RJ, Taggart C, O'Neill S, McElvaney NG. Alpha-1-antitrypsin deficiency: biological answers to clinical questions. *Am J Med Sci.* 2001;321(1):33-41.
35. Perlmutter DH. Alpha-1-antitrypsin deficiency : diagnosis and treatment. *Clinics in Liver Disease.* 2004;8:839-59.
36. Reid CL, Wiener GJ, Cox DW, Richter JE, Geisinger KR. Diffuse hepatocellular dysplasia and carcinoma associated with the Mmalton variant of alpha-1 antitrypsin. *Gastroenterology.* 1987;93:181-187.
37. Sveger T. Liver disease in α1-antitrypsin deficiency detected by screening of 200,000 infants. *N Engl J Med.* 1976;294:1316-22.

chapter **8**

Vascular Diseases Involving the Liver

Richard K. Gilroy, MBBS, FRACP and Michael F. Sorrell, MD

Hepatic Circulation

The vascular system of solid organs has arterial inflow and venous outflow. The liver is unusual in that it derives inflow from both an arterial and venous source. The hepatic artery (HA) contributes 25% of the liver's blood supply and 50% of the hepatic parenchyma oxygen supply. The HA is closely related anatomically to the bile ducts and is critical to these structures in that it is the exclusive supplier of blood flow to the biliary system.[1]

The portal vein (PV) contributes the majority of the liver's blood flow (75%) and accounts for the remaining 50% of the oxygen supply. There are no direct vascular connections between the PV and HA circulations. Blood from both systems enters the hepatic sinusoids at different levels and then unites to empty into central veins (CV). From the CV, the circulation enters the principal hepatic venous outflow tracts known as the hepatic veins (HV). There are three major HVs (right, middle, and left). Blood leaves the HV to enter the inferior vena cava (IVC) at a level just below the diaphragm before entering the right atrium (Figure 8-1).

The liver is divided into eight segments. The segmental division is derived from the vascular supply emanating from the major branches of the left and right portal vein. Accompanying the PV branches to the segments are equivalent first-order divisions of the left and right HAs and bile ducts. The major HVs do not correspond to the segmental division of the liver. The three superior HVs, also known as the right, middle, and left HV, lie in the fissures between the hepatic segments. Figure 8-2 provides a useful reference for understanding the segmental anatomy of the liver and illustrates common hepatic resection planes.

Histologically, Rappaport divided the liver parenchyma into acini incorporating the terminal hepatic arteriole, portal venule, and bile duct with the adjacent liver parenchyma.[2,3] The terminal vessels of the portal triad form the center of the acinus, and each acinus interdigitates with those adjacent to form the acinar agglomerates.

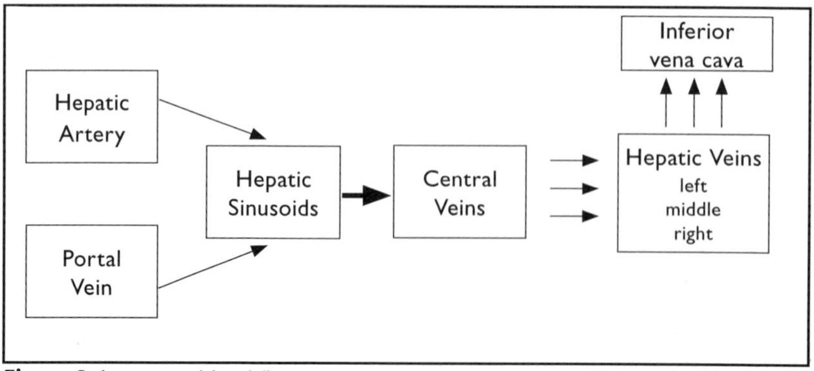

Figure 8-1. Hepatic blood flow.

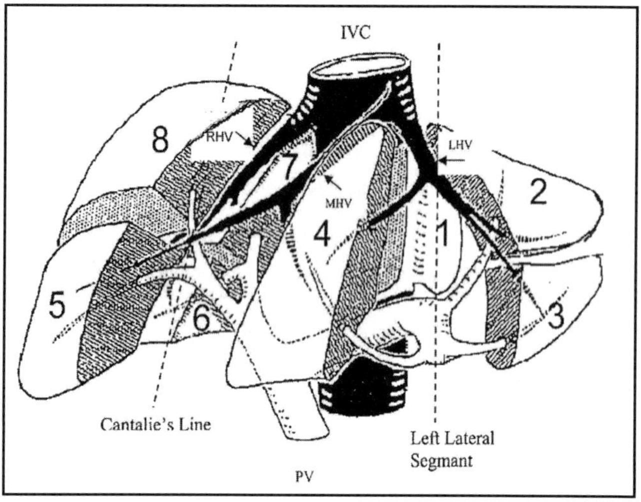

Figure 8-2. Segmental anatomy of the liver.

Physiologically, a gradient of oxygen and nutrient delivery to the surrounding parenchyma is established by the acinar structure. This gradient allows the liver parenchyma, lying between the portal triad and CV, to be separated into zones (Figure 8-3). Zone 1 contains hepatocytes in close proximity to the sinusoidal inflow and has high oxygen concentrations while zone 3 has lower oxygen tensions and is adjacent to the CV (outflow).

These anatomic gradients, by in large, explain the pattern of injury seen in hypoperfusion syndromes where zone 3 hepatocyte injury predominates. With outflow obstruction, hepatocyte loss is also seen in pericentral regions (zone 3), however, in contrast to a hypoperfusion injury, vascular congestion adjacent to the CVs is also present. Additional details on the specific patterns of injury associated with the specific vascular pathologies will be discussed later.

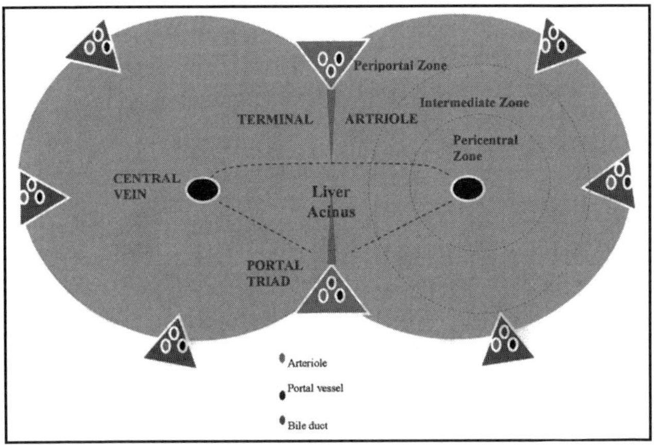

Figure 8-3. Zones of the liver parenchyma.

Vascular Diseases

Clinical characteristics of the vascular diseases of the liver are largely dependent on:

1. The nature of the pathologic process (partial or complete obstruction to the outflow or inflow tracts with accompanying inflammation).
2. The extent of hepatic involvement (segmental vs diffuse involvement).
3. The rate of evolution of the pathology.
4. The amount of the accompanying liver parenchymal necrosis.
5. Specific vasculature involvement (HA vs HV).

Insults to the liver's vasculature can be the consequence of a more generalized systemic process (eg, hypoperfusion during shock or congestion with heart failure) or can result from primary disease processes confined to the liver itself (eg, veno-occlusive disease). Table 8-1 lists the vascular diseases of the liver and site of involvement. This chapter will be limited to reviewing diffuse vascular pathologies of the liver and will not cover vascular tumors.

Budd-Chiari Syndrome (BCS)

George Budd initially described BCS in 1945.[4] The syndrome consisted of a triad of hepatomegaly, abdominal pain, and ascites.[4] Hans Chiari later contributed the characteristic histology of centrilobular injury, sinusoidal congestion, and added obliterating phlebitis of the HVs to the description.[5]

BCS results from obstruction to HV outflow. This most often follows a thrombotic event that may affect the HV at any level from the small HV to where the IVC enters the right atrium.[6] Most commonly, the medium and large hepatic veins are involved. Primary BCS is outflow obstruction originating from an endoluminal venous lesion (eg, venous thrombosis or venulitis). Secondary BCS occurs when processes outside the venous system cause HV obstruction, for example, malignant invasion of the

Table 8-1

Vascular Diseases of the Liver

Diffuse Involvement

Hepatic venous outflow obstruction:

- Budd-Chiari syndrome
- VOD
- Suprahepatic inferior vena-cava compression

Congestive hepatopathy:

- Portal vein thrombosis

Ischemic Hepatitis

Peliosis hepaticus

Systemic vascular disease:

- Polyarteritis nodosa
- Other vasculitis (SLE, GCTA)
- Atherosclerosis
- Infectious (HIV related bartonella)
- Cutaneous bacillary angiomatosis

Malignancy associated (HD, hairy cell leukemia)

Trauma/Iatrogenic

Segmental Involvement

Benign:

- Hemangioma
- Osler-weber-rendu

Malignant vascular neoplasms:

- Primary (Hemangioendothelioma, Kaposis Sarcoma, Hepatocellular carcinoma)
- Metastatic

hepatic vein by tumor. IVC membranes are another cause of BCS. These membranes may cause BCS in the absence of thrombosis.

Table 8-2 lists some of the causes of HV and IVC (large vein) thrombosis. In addition to the listed diseases, granulomatous disease and venulitis of the small HV can cause BCS in the absence of large vein occlusion. Although right heart failure and veno-occlusive disease (VOD) can present with a BCS-like picture, these are not considered part of the syndrome.[7]

The etiologies underlying BCS vary with age and ethnicity. In Western societies, myeloproliferative disorders are the most common identifiable precipitant of thrombosis, whereas, in Southern Africa and Asia, constricting IVC membranes are the most common causes.[8-11] These disorders do not necessarily occur in isolation, and more than one of the many disorders associated with BCS can coexist.

Table 8-2

CAUSES OF BUDD-CHIARI SYNDROME

Hepatic Vein Obstruction

Nonmembranous:

- Prothrombotic
    - Antithrombin III deficiency
    - Protein C or S deficiency
    - Paroxysmal nocturnal hemoglobinuria
    - Factor V Leiden mutation
    - Factor II G20210A mutation
    - Lupus anticoagulant
    - Antiphospholipid antibodies
- Malignancy associated
    - Myeloproliferative disorders
    - Hepatocellular carcinoma
    - Other neoplasms (mucin producing)
- Pregnancy
- Medications (oral contraceptive pill)
- Infections
- Systemic lupus erythematosus
- Bechet's disease
- Collagen vascular diseases
- Inflammatory bowel disease
- Cirrhosis
- Polycystic liver disease
- Idiopathic

Webs

Membranes

Iatrogenic (Complication of surgery)

The myeloproliferative condition most commonly associated with BCS is polycythemia rubra vera. Essential thrombocythemia and myelofibrosis are less commonly associated with BCS.

Membranous obstruction of the vena cava (MOVC) can cause obstruction to hepatic outflow. The etiology of the membrane is unknown. Infection is thought to account for some of the cases. There are suggestions that occult procoagulant conditions and trauma to the IVC at the level of the diaphragm predispose an injury that results in thrombosis. As a consequence of this, an obstructing membrane develops.[10,12] The greatest reported incidence of BCS from MOVC is from Nepal.[13] Some

Table 8-3

PROCOAGULANT STUDIES PERFORMED IN BUDD-CHIARI SYNDROME

Hematologic	*Procoagulant*
Prothrombin time	Lupus anticoagulant
Partial thromboplastin time	Anticardiolipin antibody
Hemoglobin and hematocrit	Protein C level
Platelet count	Protein S level
Total red cell mass	Factor II mutation
Bone marrow aspirate	Factor V Leiden
Flow cytometry CD55 and CD59	Antithrombin level
Erythroid colony cultures	Fasting homocysteine level
MTHFR polymorphism	

believe MOVC is a clinical disorder that should be separately considered when BCS is reviewed. These authors believe there are features unique to MOVC, in contrast to simple BCS, to warrant this.[9,10] An alternative name created for this MOVC is obliterative hepatocavopathy.[10]

Identified procoagulant conditions appear less common in MOVC.[10] When BCS occurs with MOVC, thrombosis is typically present in the IVC. This thrombosis may extend to involve the HV.

It is important to note coexisting procoagulant disorders are common in BCS.[14-18] Identification of one defect or disorder does not preclude the diagnostic existence of another concurrent procoagulant disorder. In addition, the complexity of the procoagulant screen (Table 8-3) will expand as additional procoagulant disorders are identified.

Clinical Presentation

The most common age at presentation is 35 years. The incidence in women is approximately twice that of men.[9,19] Up to 25% of BCS in women occurs in the context of pregnancy or the postpartum period. Table 8-4 outlines some of the clinical and biochemical features of BCS and their relative frequency.

The clinical manifestations are unpredictable and depend upon the extent and rate of evolution of the thrombotic process. This creates a highly variable spectrum of clinical presentation ranging from no symptoms to acute fulminant hepatic failure. The cardinal triad is abdominal pain, hepatomegaly, and ascites. Patients may present with acute symptoms but commonly are found to have underlying chronic disease.[8,20-22] Up to 15% of patients with BCS have cirrhosis at initial presentation.[22]

In pediatric populations, the first manifestation may be splenomegaly detected on routine health maintenance examination. On occasion, these children have a history of umbilical vein catheterization, although there appears to be no association between catheterization and BCS.

Table 8-4

THE CLINICAL AND LABORATORY FINDINGS IN BUDD-CHIARI SYNDROME AND THEIR RELATIVE FREQUENCY ON PRESENTATION

Clinical	*Frequency*	*Laboratory*	*Frequency*
Abdominal pain	2.5% to 72%	Albumin >30g/L	65%
Ascites	70% to 90%	Bilirubin >2.0 mg/dL	10% to 50%
Hepatomegaly	60% to 90%	PT secs	Median 14
Leg edema	50% to 70%	AST or ALT <100	30% to 50%
Jaundice	6% to 33%	Established cirrhosis	6% to 15%
Fever	Uncommon		
Splenomegaly	Rare		
Fulminant failure	Rare		

The diagnosis of BCS should also be considered in patients with chronic liver disease suffering from intractable ascites. In addition, patients with a known prothrombotic tendency and liver disease, or those with fulminant hepatic failure and hepatomegaly, should be evaluated for BCS.

In countries where MOVC is a common cause of BCS, symptoms of a complicating hepatocellular carcinoma can be the presenting complaint.[39,40] The incidence of hepatocellular carcinoma in BCS with MOVC ranges considerably.[9,23] Hepatocellular carcinoma is uncommon in BCS resulting from procoagulant disorders.[23-28] Presently, there is no recommendation for screening for hepatocellular cancer in patients with chronic BCS in the absence of MOVC.

Pathophysiology

Obstruction to the hepatic venous outflow tract results in increased sinusoidal pressure and congestion. Reductions in portal perfusion occur as a consequence of the obstruction. Subsequently, stasis and congestion leads to hypoxic hepatocyte damage.[29] Clinically, acute phlebitis and capsule distension produce abdominal pain and fever.

The injury is most prominent in zone 3 where congestion and cell drop out is most marked.[7] Fibrosis develops as early as 14 days after the acute insult. Fibrosis may lead to bridging, nodular regenerative hyperplasia, and ultimately cirrhosis.

PV thrombosis occurs in 20% of cases of BCS.[30] This appears as a consequence of reduced PV flow, PV congestion, and (commonly) an underlying procoagulant pathology. In most patients with BCS, hepatic venous outflow obstruction is incomplete due to a variety of accessory HVs that drain into the IVC above or below the site of obstruction. The most common accessory veins are the accessory inferior hepatic and caudate veins, which drain into the IVC inferior to the major HVs. These segments of the liver that have preserved venous drainage often undergo hypertrophy.[31] In chronic

BCS, caudate lobe hypertrophy is common and can be so large as to compress the infrahepatic IVC.

Investigations

The diagnosis of BCS requires demonstration of an obstructed venous outflow. Doppler-ultrasound is the most easily accessed noninvasive method and has a sensitivity of over 85% in expert hands.[32,33] This procedure provides information on the perihepatic vascular anatomy and the level and extent of obstruction.[34] Doppler-ultrasound identifies PV thrombosis if present.[30] Magnetic resonance (MR) venography can provide additional anatomic information and is a noninvasive alternative when sonographic studies are incomplete.[34] MR scanning is helpful in differentiating benign macroregenerative nodules from hepatocellular carcinomas in patients with long-standing BCS.[35] Dual-phase CT scanning has no increased diagnostic value in BCS.

Venography, by retrograde cannulation of the hepatic veins, provides the most accurate evaluation of BCS. During venography, the amount of contrast media administered must be carefully monitored. This is particularly important in individuals with acute severe liver disease or those with underlying renal dysfunction.

After confirmation of BCS, a comprehensive procoagulant screen is mandatory (see Table 8-4). This should be obtained before initiation of anticoagulation. More than one procoagulant condition may be present. Identifying the existence of a procoagulant disorder(s) allows appropriate management for the patient and directs family counseling where indicated.

Deficiencies in Protein C, Protein S, and antithrombin III predispose to HV thrombosis; however, low circulating levels also develop in liver disease. It is uncommon for patients with inherited deficiencies to have values greater than 10% to 20% of normal.[29] Diagnosis, however, may be difficult in the setting of pre-existing or extensive liver disease. In these circumstances, family pedigrees may assist in establishing a diagnosis. Formulas that adjust these parameters for the degree of liver injury have been created, however, these have not been validated.[16]

Liver biopsy may help in establishing the diagnosis of BCS in difficult situations and provides information on chronicity.[23] Liver biopsy does not provide independent prognostic information for individuals with BCS in either the acute or the chronic setting.[7]

Management

Figure 8-4 provides an algorithm for BCS. Management mandates assessment of disease duration and severity before selecting any therapeutic path.

Generally, anticoagulation is advocated in BCS. It targets control of the underlying prothrombotic state, prevents thrombus propagation, and avoids portal vein thrombosis, which if present can limit therapeutic options.

Evidence supporting the use and efficacy of anticoagulation in BCS is, however, circumstantial, as there are no randomized trials. It should be initiated in the asymptomatic individuals with underlying procoagulant states. No data exist to recommend long-term anticoagulation in asymptomatic patients without an established procoagulant disorder, although, in the absence of a major contraindication, it is generally utilized. In symptomatic patients, anticoagulation is often combined with diuretics and endoscopic therapy.[6] Initial anticoagulation is achieved with heparin followed by a vitamin K antagonist.

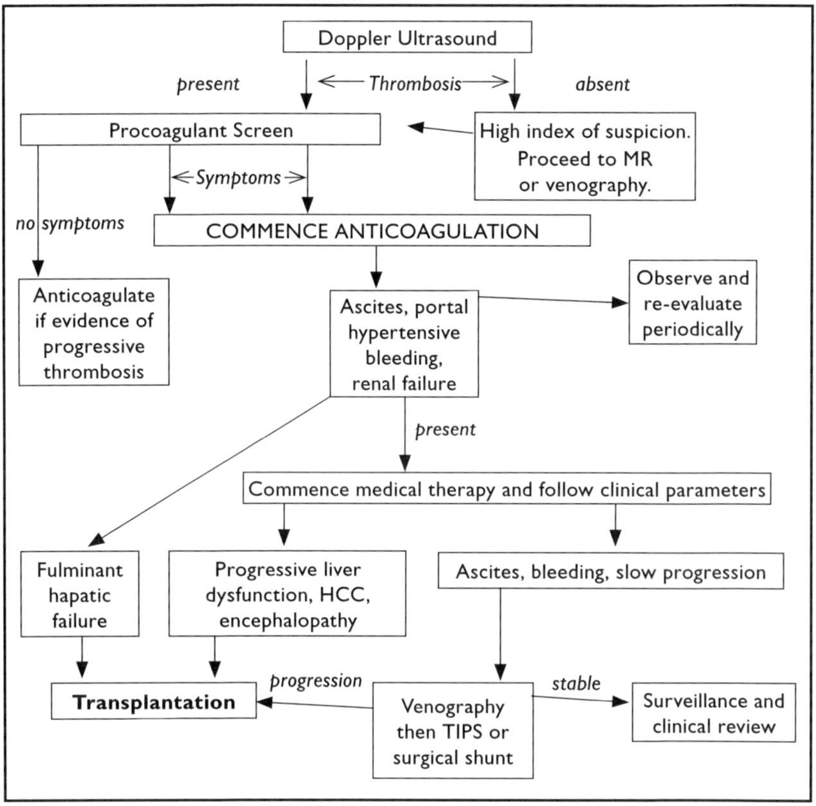

Figure 8-4. Approach to suspected Budd-Chiari Syndrome.

There are no data comparing the safety and efficacy of low molecular weight heparin versus unfractionated heparin in BCS. Data on the use of heparin in other thrombotic disorders favor low molecular weight heparin for both efficacy and safety reasons.[36] The incomplete ability to reverse the anticoagulant effect of low molecular weight heparin warrants caution in patients with a history of recent bleeding. Unlike unfractionated heparin, low molecular weight heparin is not reversed completely with protamine sulfate.[37] It is important to recognize that anticoagulation may complicate the management of BCS complications, in particular variceal hemorrhage and ascites.

Those who do not improve or develop severe complications are considered for more invasive management including thrombolysis (usually catheter directed), TIPS, surgical shunting and liver transplantation.

Experience with the use of thrombolysis is limited to case reports and small series.[38,39] It appears more effective in acute thrombosis, particularly when catheter directed and combined with stenting.[38-40] HV stenosis and rethrombosis can occur despite postprocedure anticoagulation.[24]

Percutaneous angioplasty with stenting has achieved excellent patency rates for HV and IVC obstruction.[7,8,21,41] This procedure is suited to those with short segment stenosis or occlusion. It is also employed in those with MOVC. Unfortunately, revisions may be required to retain patency in up to 70% of patients.[42-44] The risk/benefit ratio for this modality of treatment is unknown.[7]

In the presence of favorable anatomy (at least partially patent PV and terminal IVC), TIPS can be performed.[42-43,45-46] In the presence of complete HV obstruction, the procedure may be performed by utilizing the caudate lobe's venous supply. However, even with what appears to be complete obstruction, cannulation of a remnant hepatic vein stump may be possible.[43] A recent report suggests a survival advantage for TIPS in acute BCS.[30] No randomized multicenter trials, however, exist, comparing TIPS to other treatment modalities. Limitations of the current literature include ill-defined selection criteria for the cohorts studied, failure to present procedure failure rates, lack of randomization or control populations, and the heterogeneous nature of the disease BCS.[6]

Surgical shunts have traditionally been the standard alternative to liver transplantation. Surgical options include portocaval, mesocaval, and mesoatrial shunts. There is no data confirming the superiority of any particular procedure on survival. Mesocaval shunting appears more desirable when liver transplantation is required later while side-to-side portocaval shunting may have superior patency rates. In patients where the suprahepatic IVC is occluded, mesoatrial shunts may be used, in the uncommon circumstance of alternatives not being technically possible.

Surgical shunt dysfunction occurs in approximate 30% of cases; however, it is less common than shunt dysfunction following TIPS. Anticoagulation is initiated during the early postoperative period. With surgical shunts, patency appears to predict survival.[47] However, in a recent multivariate analysis, there appeared to be no survival benefit for surgical shunts when compared to no intervention.[48] Independent factors that predict clinical success after surgical correction include response of ascites to diuretics, age, low Child-Pugh score, absence of significant hepatic fibrosis and normal serum creatinine.[48,49] There are, as yet, no trials comparing the efficacy of TIPS and surgical shunts.

Liver transplantation is used for fulminant hepatic failure and where severe symptoms continue (eg, refractory ascites) despite treatment.[50] This is the only intervention that is associated with a survival advantage when compared to no intervention.[7] Post-transplant, 1-year survival is 88% and is comparable to that for transplantation for other diseases.[51-53] There appears to be an increased thrombosis risk after transplantation and recurrent BCS has been reported.[51,54] Anticoagulation is, therefore, recommended in all patients following transplantation. Liver transplantation potentially corrects some prothrombotic disorders (eg, Protein C deficiency). No consensus exists for discontinuing anticoagulation after transplantation in patients with disorders potentially corrected by liver grafting.[16]

Outcomes

The natural history of BCS is poorly understood.[7] Patient age, severity of liver disease, and refractory ascites appear to be the best predictors of long-term outcome.[48] The risk of death is greatest during the first year after diagnosis.[48]

After liver transplantation, patients require life-long immunosuppression. This is associated with many side effects—one being an increased risk of malignancy. Unknown is the long-term effect that immunosuppression may have in patients with

Table 8-5

FACTORS THAT INCREASE THE RISK FOR DEVELOPING VENO-OCCLUSIVE DISEASE

- Female gender
- Older patient age
- Irradiation (concurrent or previous)
- Karnofsky score less than 90
- Chemotherapy use
- Subsequent course of high dose chemotherapy
- Past history of VOD
- Abnormal liver enzymes before treatment
- Chronic hepatitis (both viral and nonviral)

myeloproliferative disorders. Acute leukaemic transformation has been reported.[51] The progression of any underlying blood dyscrasia, which has resulted in BCS, likely will influence patient survival well beyond transplantation.[51] Hepatocellular carcinoma is rarely associated with BCS in the absence of MOVC. The degree of risk of hepatocellular carcinoma is undefined.[28]

VENO-OCCLUSIVE DISEASE

VOD is a nonthrombotic obstruction of the sinusoids and central veins as a consequence of injury to the sinusoidal wall.[55,56] The histologic features are sinusoidal fibrosis, necrosis of pericentral hepatocytes, and, late in the course, fibrosis, and obliteration of the CVs.[57-60] This results in intrahepatic obstruction to the venous outflow of the liver.[56] Another descriptive name for this disorder is sinusoidal obstruction syndrome.[56,61]

VOD in general develops rapidly. In the United States and Europe, it most commonly follows high-dose chemotherapy, particularly bone marrow transplantation.[56,62-63] The reported incidence approaches 50% in some studies, and mortality for severe VOD approximates 70% in this setting.[64-66] In the nononcology setting, VOD has also been associated with the use of Azathioprine in solid organ transplantation, rheumatologic, and inflammatory bowel disease.[59,67-68]

Risk factors for developing VOD are outlined in Table 8-5.[64,69] Previous radiotherapy and bone marrow transplantation appear to increase the risk.[70] The use of cyclosporine after bone marrow transplantation is not an independent predictor of VOD.

Traditional medicines and natural therapies containing pyrrolizidine alkaloids like heliotrine have caused VOD.[71] These alkaloids are the common causes of VOD in under-developed countries.[72] Ironically, these herbs, on occasion, are prescribed as traditional medicines for the management of liver disease. With the increasing use of natural therapies in the United States, the incidence of VOD attributed to these agents is likely to increase.[73]

Table 8-6

CAUSES OF VENO-OCCLUSIVE DISEASE

Chemotherapies	*Herbal Medications*
Actinomycin-D	Senecio
Gemtuzumab	Crotalaria
Dacarbazine (DTIC)	Heliotropium
Cytosine arabinoside (Ara-C)	Gordolobo yerba
6-thioguanine (6-TG)	Skullcap
Azathioprine	Comfrey
Busulphan	
Cyclophosphamide	
Total Body Irradiation	

Table 8-6 lists agents associated with VOD. Toxicities from many of these agents appear dose-dependent. The use of multiple agents is not uncommon in the oncology setting, and while VOD is common after high-dose chemotherapy, it should be remembered that other forms of hepatotoxicity (eg, graft vs host disease or drug-induced hepatitis) also occur and can have features similar to VOD.

Clinical Presentation

A combination of signs and symptoms are used to diagnose VOD in the clinical setting. In many instances, a liver biopsy cannot be safely performed due to thrombocytopenia. A biopsy is not prerequisite for the diagnosis of VOD. Outlined in Table 8-7 are the criteria utilized in establishing VOD in the postchemotherapy setting.[64,74-75] Unfortunately, these criteria are neither highly sensitive nor specific for VOD. Therefore, the clinician must always consider other important post-bone marrow transplant liver diseases while evaluating for VOD.[76]

Clinically, VOD is characterized by jaundice, weight gain, ascites, painful hepatomegaly, and refractory thrombocytopenia. These features all develop early on in the post-bone marrow transplant period.[77] The earliest sign is weight gain follow by edema, ascites, and then painful hepatomegaly. Jaundice although common is often the last to appear. In bone marrow transplantation, VOD generally occurs within 20 days although, the rate of evolution may vary. With total body irradiation, there may be a delay of up to 3 months in the development of VOD.

Mild VOD is a self-limiting disease requiring no intervention while moderate VOD is defined by the need for specific interventions to manage the complications of VOD. Severe GVHD is time dependent and requires either the symptoms of VOD to persist for more than 100 days or to be present at the time of death.[64,78-79] Severe VOD has a mortality rate greater than 70%.

The differential diagnosis of VOD is extensive (Table 8-8). Certain clinical features provide clues leading to a diagnosis of VOD. Hepatomegaly is a critical feature of VOD when compared to drug toxicity or viral hepatitis. When hepatomegaly is identi-

Table 8-7

Clinical Criteria for Veno-Occlusive Disease[64,74,75]

Baltimore

Any two of the following occurring before 21 days:

1. Hepatomegaly and/or upper abdominal pain
2. Jaundice
3. Ascites and/or unexplained weight gain exceeding 2.5%

Seattle

Any two of the following features present before 20 days:*

1. Bilirubin >2mg/dL
2. Hepatomegaly and abdominal pain
3. Ascites
4. Weight gain >5%

*Original criteria modified in 1993[78]

fied, the differential diagnosis includes acute fatty liver and hepatic vein thrombosis. These conditions are generally differentiated by ultrasound evaluation. An important clinical feature is the timing of onset of symptoms and signs. The diagnosis of VOD is unlikely when the onset of signs occurs more than 4 weeks after high-dose chemotherapy. Hepatic graft-vs-host disease and acute viral hepatitis are more likely at this time. Clues to a diagnosis of graft-vs-host disease include the presence of skin rash and diarrhea, both of which are uncommon with VOD.

Investigation

The degree of transaminase elevation is not helpful in establishing a diagnosis of VOD. The AST and ALT may be normal, although generally mildly elevated. Elevations probably represent hepatocellular ischemia.[56] Before cancer therapy, the presence of an abnormal aspartate aminotransferase (AST) greater than 1.5 times the upper limit of normal is a predictor for the development of VOD. AST levels greater than four times the upper limit of normal before initiation of cancer chemotherapy appear to predict VOD severity.[64] Modest increases in alkaline phosphatase are also observed.[80]

Serum bilirubin is elevated in established VOD. The degree of rise in bilirubin appears to correlate with severity. Prothrombin time (PT) prolongation uncommonly exceeds 16 seconds, and elevations above this indicate severe disease. Serum albumin levels may be depressed and have no prognostic value in this disease.

Levels of factor VII and protein C are depressed early in the course of the evolution of VOD and predict the development of VOD.[81] Low levels of antithrombin III also occurs but have no predictive value for subsequent VOD while increases in thrombin-antithrombin complexes and fibrinogen are nonspecific. Levels of propeptide for type III procollagen, plasminogen activator inhibitor 1, and hyaluronic acid in the early postchemotherapy also appear to correlate with the onset of VOD.[81-82]

Table 8-8

Differential Diagnosis of Veno-Occlusive Disease

- Cholestasis of sepsis
- Drug induced hepatotoxicity
- Graft versus host disease
- Acute viral hepatitis (Herpes group, Hepatitis B or C)
- Budd-Chiari syndrome
- Right heart failure
- Hemolysis and Disseminated intravascular coagulation
- Ischemic hepatitis
- Malignancy
- Acalculous cholecystitis
- Fungal infection (aspergillus, candida)
- Parenteral nutrition

Doppler ultrasound is used to eliminate other causes of liver injury, such as HV thrombosis. Nonspecific findings that suggest VOD on ultrasound include gall bladder wall thickness greater than 4 mm, altered flow in segmental branches of the PV, and ascites.[83] Flow recorded in the paraumbilical vein appears to be the only ultrasound criterion associated with severity.[84]

PV thrombosis is associated with VOD.[85] Predisposing factors include reduced portal flow and reduced levels of the anticoagulant factors (protein C and antithrombin III). In the postchemotherapy setting, HV and PV thrombosis do not exclude concurrent VOD.

Liver biopsies are uncommonly performed. However, if necessary the transjugular approach is generally utilized. In early disease, the histology shows widening of the subendothelial zone of the CV. The terminal central venule demonstrates luminal narrowing and dilated and congested hepatic sinusoids. Red cell fragmentation and extravasation are not uncommon. Hepatocyte injury and necrosis are most marked around the CVs. Hepatic stellate cell hypertrophy and sinusoidal fibrosis with collagen deposition occurs to varying degrees and predominates in zone 3.[86] Asymptomatic cases of VOD with abnormal histology are common.[64] The severity of histologic abnormality appears to correlate with the grade of VOD.[87]

Hepatic venous pressure measurement has a low sensitivity (60%) for VOD, but are highly specific (>90%) when gradients exceed 10 mmHg. Pressure gradients correlate with the severity of disease and predict survival.[88]

Differential Diagnosis

The differential diagnosis of VOD is outlined in Table 8-8 and includes many of the hepatic complications of high-dose chemotherapy. These conditions must be excluded when VOD is considered. In established VOD, concurrent diseases may be present.

Prevention

No pharmacologic approaches have demonstrated a beneficial effect in preventing VOD. Unfractionated heparin has been extensively studied, and no convincing evidence to support this practice exists.[63,78,89] Trials with low molecular weight heparin are ongoing.[79] Other strategies include the use of N-acetylcysteine, prostaglandin-E1 (PGE-1), pentoxyfylline, glutamine, and ursodeoxycholic acid. Their efficacy in prevention of VOD is unproven.[77-79,89-92]

Management

Management principals are much the same as for the management of cirrhosis. Sodium restriction and diuretics provide the cornerstone for ascites control. Therapeutic paracentesis may be required. When renal failure occurs in VOD, elimination of other potential causes is essential. Encephalopathy and gastrointestinal bleeding are managed similarly to that for cirrhotic patients.

Specific therapies aiming to reduce venous occlusion after the onset of VOD include PGE-1, defibrotide, tissue plasminogen activator, and heparin. Defibrotide appears to be the most promising agent. Defibrotide is a single-stranded polydeoxyribonucleotide with fibrinolytic, antithrombotic, and anti-ischemic properties. It binds selectively to the vascular endothelium of small blood vessels and has a profibinolytic effect (93). Defibrotide does not affect the systemic coagulation system and is not associated with significant bleeding or toxicity.[94,95] In patients with severe VOD, promising response rates have occurred in non-randomized studies.[94,95] Ursodeoxycholic acid has been used in VOD, and although it may reduce hyperbilirubinemia, it does not alter outcome. The use of tissue plasminogen activator is associated with severe bleeding and does not improve outcome.[66,96]

Liver transplantation has been selectively used in patients with severe VOD who have a low likelihood of recurrent malignancy.[97] Post-transplant survival is similar to transplantation for other diseases. Interestingly, some authors have described VOD as a complication of liver transplantation in the absence of a pre-existing history of risk factors for VOD.[98,99]

A role for TIPS is not established for the management of complications associated with severe VOD.[100] The mortality in patients who have received a TIPS in VOD is greater than 70%. There appears to be no survival advantage to TIPS intervention in severe VOD. A management algorithm is outlined in Figure 8-5.

Outcome

Mild to moderate grades of VOD are associated with increased morbidity but not increased mortality when compared to matched patients in an oncology setting. Overall, VOD improves in 70% to 85% of cases within 25 days of the onset of symptoms.[77] Mortality rates exceed 70% in patients with severe VOD.[94,101] Death is due to multiorgan failure rather than simply hepatic failure. The degree of hyperbilirubinemia and fluid retention appears to be the best predictor of outcome. The development of encephalopathy is an ominous prognostic sign.

The Liver in Heart Failure

Cardiac hepatopathy, also known as congestive hepatopathy, is relatively common but often unrecognized.[102] In patients with liver dysfunction associated with cardiac failure, the failing heart dominates the clinical picture.

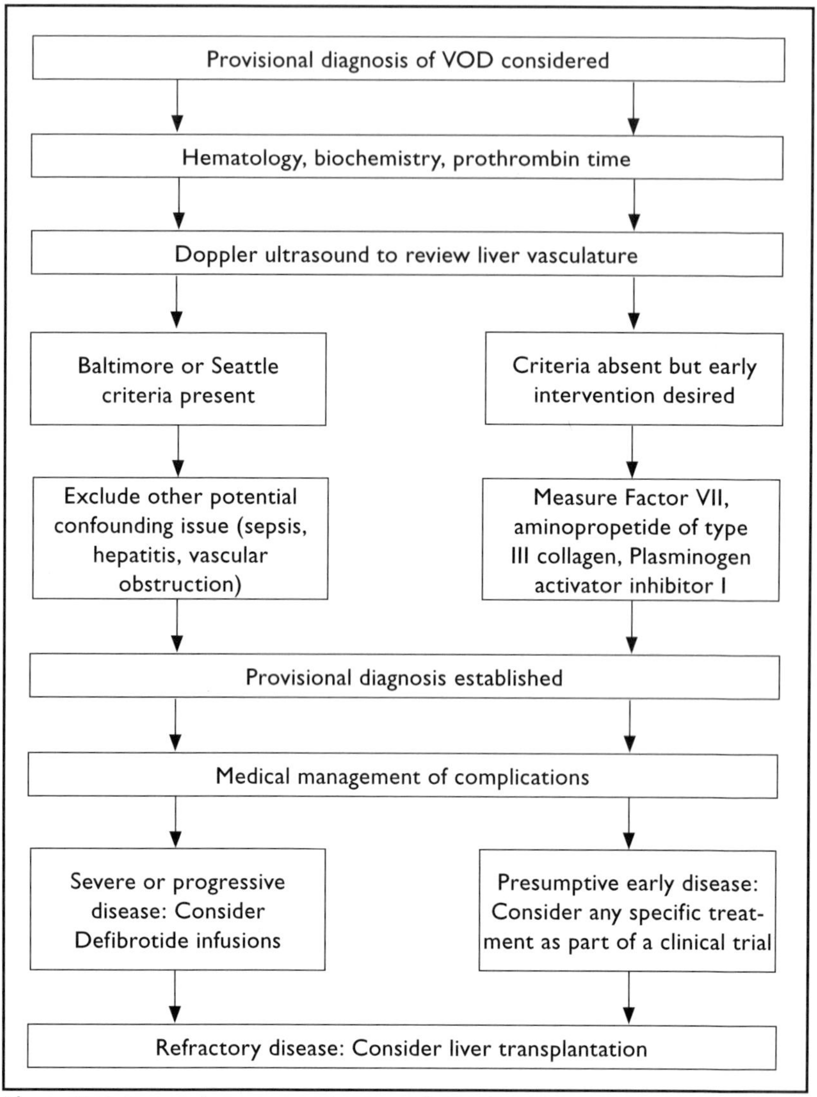

Figure 8-5. Approach to suspected veno-occlusive disease.

Clinical Presentation

The patient infrequently complains of symptoms specifically related to the liver, jaundice is uncommon, and ascites, when present, occur in the context of severe peripheral edema. The ascites may be present in the absence of peripheral edema when diuretic therapy has been initiated. The symptoms and signs of right heart failure predominate; symptoms related to the liver are generally mild with right upper-quadrant discomfort the most common complaint. Patients with tricuspid incompetence may present with a pulsatile liver. When cirrhosis is present, ascites may remain despite diuretic therapy. Typically, before presentation, the patient has a protracted history of heart failure.[103]

The majority of patients have abnormalities in gammaglutamyltransferase (GGT) and alkaline phosphatase (AP) with mild elevations in AST and ALT. Prominant elevations of these enzymes strongly suggest an alternate diagnosis. In severe heart failure, ischemic hepatitis is one such pathology.[102]

Hyperbilirubinemia does occur in a third of patients presenting with heart failure; however, persistent jaundice is uncommon and suggests the presence of coexisting hemolysis. With the exception of ascites, other manifestations of hepatic decompensation are rare. Serum ascites albumin gradients are greater than 1.1 g/dL, and the ascitic protein content is usually greater than 2.5 g/dL. The red cell count in the ascites is often more elevated than in other forms of ascites.[103,104]

Ultrasound imaging of the liver may demonstrate dilated HVs with preserved blood flow. Cirrhosis from chronic heart failure is rare, and hepatocellular carcinoma has not been reported in Western literature as a consequence of chronic heart failure.

Liver biopsy is infrequently performed in the acute setting. Most data on the histology are derived from biopsies taken upon resolution of severe heart failure or autopsy series.[102,105,106] Histology shows centrilobular congestion, sinusoidal dilation, pericentral cell drop out, and fibrosis. Cirrhosis is uncommon.[105]

Outcome

Treatment is directed toward the underlying condition and response to therapy dictates outcome. No data shows coexistent cirrhosis a contraindication to transplantation of other organs, in instances where this is being considered.

Portal Vein Thrombosis (PVT)

The etiology of PVT is divided into three categories:

1. Thrombosis resulting from direct portal vein injury leading to obstruction.
2. Thrombosis resulting from developmental anomalies of the portal vein.
3. Thrombosis as a result of an associated disease process.

Group 3 is the predominant category and contains the majority of identifiable causes of PVT in both adults and children. In adults, approximately 25% of PVT is associated with cirrhosis. In cirrhotic patients referred for liver transplantation, 16% have existing PVT.[107] There is an association between PVT and the presence of hepatocellular carcinoma.

The etiology of PVT is uncertain in approximately half the cases, although factors associated with thrombosis are identified in as many as 85% of individuals.[108,109] In children, umbilical sepsis, rather than umbilical vein catheterization, appears the main risk factor. In children with umbilical vein catheters, 100% develop thrombi within 3 days, but when followed, thrombi resolve in nearly all instances.[108] In the absence of infection or a prothrombotic disorder, umbilical catheterization does not appear a cause of chronic PVT.[110-111] Table 8-9 lists the more common identifiable causes of PVT.

Table 8-9

ETIOLOGY OF PORTAL VEIN THROMBOSIS

Children	*Adults*
Umbilical sepsis (omphalitis)	Cirrhosis
Intra-abdominal sepsis	Intraabdominal sepsis
Umbilical catheterization	Myeloproliferative disorders*
Malignancy	Procoagulant conditions*
Idiopathic	Pancreatitis
	Trauma
	Idiopathic

For elaboration of these disorders refer to Table 8-2.

Adapted from Sarin SK, Agarwal SR. Extrahepatic portal vein obstruction. *Semin Liver Dis.* 2002; 22(1):43-58.

Clinical Presentation

The acute event often goes unnoticed in childhood. Variceal bleeding in the context of splenomegaly occurs months or years after PVT. In the absence of liver disease, the variceal hemorrhage is well tolerated. Esophageal varices, which are present in 85% with chronic PVT, are the most common bleeding site.

In adults, the natural history of PVT is unknown. The most common presentation is melena from variceal bleeding. Jaundice is uncommon in the absence of sepsis or underlying liver disease. Ascites present in 10% to 35% of individuals.[110-115] The risk of bleeding for noncirrhotic PVT in adults is 17 events per 100 patient-years.[112] Mortality among patients with PVT is related to concurrent medical conditions. Although more common in the past, death from variceal hemorrhage is now rare. The prognosis in the absence of malignancy, cirrhosis, and mesenteric vein thrombosis is excellent.[108,112-113]

Liver enzymes are normal or mildly elevated in the absence of an underlying liver disease. Serum albumin, PT, and bilirubin are usually normal.

In the acute setting of PVT, ultrasound and Doppler of the PV confirms the absence of PV flow. Ascites, evidence of portal venous collaterals, and splenomegaly are absent except when the thrombosis extends to involve the splenic vein. In this situation, splenomegaly may develop rapidly. In chronic PVT, splenomegaly is present and is massive in 50% of cases. Cavernous transformation of the PV indicates chronicity.

Management

The rarity of presentations with acute PVT has prevented controlled therapeutic trials to be conducted in this condition.[116] When a procoagulant disorder is identified, auticoagulant therapy is recommended unless a major contraindication exists. In patients without cirrhosis and a recent PVT, anticoagulation therapy may facilitate recanalization in more than 80% of cases.[116] In the setting of established cavernous transformation of the PV, no data exist to support anticoagulation in the absence of a thrombophilic disorder.[116]

When bleeding is the presenting complaint in patients with chronic PVT, initial management is variceal obliteration. This is successful in 70% to 95% of cases.[106,109,112] Nonselective β-blockers are administered after control of the acute episode of bleeding and appear to reduce the risk of rebleeding.[116]

Surgical procedures to reduce portal hypertension (portosystemic shunting, portal thrombectomy, or portal reconstruction) are indicated in approximately 10% of cases.[109] Anticoagulation may be used after these procedures, especially if there is a coagulation disorder. TIPS is often technically difficult and has no advantage over other measures.

Prognosis

The outcome of PVT is dictated by the concomitant diseases leading to thrombosis rather than the consequences of PVT.[109]

Peliosis Hepatis

Peliosis hepatis is characterized by multiple, small, dilated blood-filled cavities in the hepatic parenchyma. These cysts generally lack endothelial linings and communicate directly with the hepatic sinusoids, which are usually dilated. It is most commonly associated with hepatic tumors or with cholestatic jaundice, but can be caused by several drugs including anabolic steroids, arsenic, azathioprine, oral contraceptives, danazole, thorotrast, vinyl chloride monomers, diethylstilbestrol, tamoxifen, vitamin A, hydroxyurea, and azathioprine.[117-119] *Bartonella henselae* is the most common cause of peliosis in human immunodeficiency virus; however, it may also cause this in immunocompetent individuals.[119]

With the exception of removing the causative agent, there is no specific management for this condition.

References

1. Deshpande RR, Heaton ND, Rela M. Surgical anatomy of segmental liver transplantation. *Br J Surg.* 2002;89(9):1078-1088.
2. Rappaport AM. Hepatic blood flow: morphologic aspects and physiologic regulation. *Int Rev Physiol.* 1980;21:1-63
3. Rappaport AM. The microcirculatory and acinar concept of normal and pathological hepatic structure. *Bietr Path.* 1976;157:215.
4. Budd G. *On Diseases of the Liver.* 3rd ed. Philadelphia: Blanchard & Lea; 1857.
5. Chiari H. Ueber die selbstandige phlebitis obliterans der hauptstamme der venae hepaticae als todesursache. *Beitr Z Pathol Anat.* 1899;26:1-18.
6. Janssen HL, Garcia-Pagan JC, Elias E, et al. Budd-Chiari syndrome: a review by an expert panel. *J Hepatol.* 2003;38(3):364-371.
7. Valla DC. The diagnosis and management of Budd-Chiari Syndrome: consensus and controversies. *Hepatology.* 2003;38(4):793-803.
8. Singh V, Sinha SK, Nain CK, et al. Budd-Chiari syndrome: our experience of 71 patients. *J Gastroenterol Hepatol.* 2000;15(5):550-554.
9. Okuda K, Kage M, Shrestha SM. Proposal of a new nomenclature for Budd-Chiari Syndrome: hepatic vein thrombosis versus thrombosis of the inferior vena cava at its hepatic portion. *Hepatology.* 1998;28(5):1191-1198.

10. Okuda K. Membranous obstruction of the inferior vena cava (obliterative hepatocavopathy, Okuda). *J Gastroenterol Hepatol.* 2001;16(11):1179-1183.
11. De BK, De KK, Sen S, et al. Etiology based prevalence of Budd-Chiari syndrome in eastern India. *J Assoc Physicians India.* 2000;48(8):800-803.
12. Balian A, Valla D, Naveau S, et al. Post-traumatic membranous obstruction of the inferior vena cava associated with a hypercoagulable state. *J Hepatol.* 1998;28(4):723-726.
13. Shrestha SM, Okuda K, Uchida T, et al. Endemicity and clinical picture of liver disease due to obstruction of the hepatic portion of the inferior vena cava in Nepal. *J Gastroenterol Hepatol.* 1996;11(2):170-179.
14. Deltenre P, Denninger MH, Hilliare S, et al. Factor V Leiden related Budd-Chiari syndrome. *Gut.* 2001;48(2):264-268.
15. Praderio L, Dagna L, Longhi P, et al. Budd-Chiari syndrome in a patient with ulcerative colitis: association with anticardiolipin antibodies. *J Clin Gastroenterol.* 2000; 30(2):203-204.
16. Janssen HL, Meinardi JR, Vleggaar FP, et al. Factor V Leiden mutation, prothrombin gene mutation, and deficiencies in coagulation inhibitors associated with Budd-Chiari syndrome and portal vein thrombosis: results of a case-control study. *Blood.* 2000;96(7):2364-2368.
17. Denninger MH, Chait Y, Casadevall N, et al. Cause of portal or hepatic venous thrombosis in adults: the role of multiple concurrent factors. *Hepatology.* 2000;31(3):587-591.
18. Minnema MC, Janssen HL, Niermeijer P, de Man RA. Budd-Chiari syndrome: combination of genetic defects and the use of oral contraceptives leading to hypercoagulability. *J Hepatol.* 2000;33(3):509-512.
19. Mahmoud AE, Mendoza A, Meshikhes AN, et al. Clinical spectrum, investigations and treatment of Budd-Chiari syndrome. *QJM.* 1996;89(1):37-43.
20. Langlet P, Escolano S, Valla D, et al. Clinicopathological forms and prognostic index in Budd-Chiari syndrome. *J Hepatol.* 2003;39(4):496-501.
21. Wang ZG, Jones RS. Budd-Chiari syndrome. *Curr Probl Surg.* 1996;33(2):83-211.
22. Iwai M, Kitagawa Y, Nakajima T. et al. Clinical features, image analysis, and laparoscopic and histological liver findings in Budd-Chiari syndrome. *Hepatogastroenterology.* 1998;45(24):2359-2368.
23. Dilawari JB, Bambery P, Chawla Y, et al. Hepatic outflow obstruction (Budd-Chiari syndrome). Experience with 177 patients and a review of the literature. *Medicine* (Baltimore). 1994;73(1):21-36.
24. Havlioglu N, Brunt EM, Bacon BR. Thrombocytosis and recurrent hepatic outflow obstruction (Budd-Chiari syndrome) after successful thrombolysis: case report and literature review. *Clin Appl Thromb Hemost.* 2002;8(4):369-374.
25. Simson IW. The causes and consequences of chronic hepatic venous outflow obstruction. *S Afr Med J.* 1987;72(1):11-14.
26. Matsui S, Ichida T, Watanabe M, et al. Clinical features and etiology of hepatocellular carcinoma arising in patients with membranous obstruction of the inferior vena cava: in reference to hepatitis viral infection. *J Gastroenterol Hepatol.* 2000;15(10):1205-1211.
27. Okuda H, Yamagata H, Obata H, et al. Epidemiological and clinical features of Budd-Chiari syndrome in Japan. *J Hepatol.* 1995;22(1):1-9.
28. Havlioglu N, Brunt EM, Bacon BR. Budd-Chiari syndrome and hepatocellular carcinoma: a case report and review of the literature. *Am J Gastroenterol.* 2003;98(1):201-204.

29. Menon KV, Shah V, Kamath PS. The Budd-Chiari syndrome. *N Engl J Med.* 2004; 350(6):578-585.
30. Mahmoud AE, Helmy AS, Billingham L, Elias E. Poor prognosis and limited therapeutic options in patients with Budd-Chiari syndrome and portal venous system thrombosis. *Eur J Gastroenterol Hepatol.* 1997;9(5):485-489.
31. Kahn AN, Chandramohan M, Macdonald S. Budd-Chiari Syndrome. Available at http://www.emedicine.com/RADIO/topic121.htm.
32. Bolondi L, Gaiani S, Li Bassi S, et al. Diagnosis of Budd-Chiari syndrome by pulsed Doppler ultrasound. *Gastroenterology.* 1991;100:1324-1331.
33. Chawla Y, Kumar S, Dhiman RK, et al. Duplex Doppler sonography in patients with Budd-Chiari syndrome. *J Gastroenterol Hepatol.* 1999;14(9):904-907.
34. Al-Damegh S. Budd-Chiari syndrome: a short radiological review. *J Gastroenterol Hepatol.* 1999;14(11):1057-1061.
35. Brancatelli G, Federle MP, Grazioli L, et al. Benign regenerative nodules in Budd-Chiari syndrome and other vascular disorders of the liver: radiologic-pathologic and clinical correlation. *Radiographics.* 2002;22(4):847-862.
36. Schafer AI, Levine MN, Konkle BA, Kearon C. Thrombotic disorders: diagnosis and treatment. *Hematology.* 2003:520-539.
37. Warkentin TE, Crowther MA. Reversing anticoagulants both old and new. *Can J Anaesth.* 2002;49(6):S11-25.
38. Sharma S, Texeira A, Texeira P, et al. Pharmacological thrombolysis in Budd Chiari syndrome: a single centre experience and review of the literature. *J Hepatol.* 2004;40(1):172-180.
39. Raju GS, Felver M, Olin JW, Satti SD. Thrombolysis for acute Budd-Chiari syndrome: case report and literature review. *Am J Gastroenterol.* 1996;91(6):1262-1263.
40. Sharma S, Texeira A, Texeira P, et al. Pharmacological thrombolysis in Budd Chiari syndrome: a single centre experience and review of the literature. *J Hepatol.* 2004;40(1):172-180.
41. Kaul U, Agarwal R. Management of hepatic venous outflow obstruction (Budd Chiari syndrome): balloon angioplasty with or without the use of a stent. *Cathet Cardiovasc Diagn.* 1997;42(2):240.
42. Cejna M, Peck-Radosavljevic M, Schoder M, et al. Repeat interventions for maintenance of transjugular intrahepatic portosystemic shunt function in patients with Budd-Chiari syndrome. *J Vasc Interv Radiol.* 2002;13:193-199.
43. Perello A, Garcia-Pagan JC, Gilabert R, et al. TIPS is a useful long-term derivative therapy for patients with Budd-Chiari syndrome uncontrolled by medical therapy. *Hepatology.* 2002;35(1):132-139.
44. Blum U, Rossle M, Haag K, et al. Budd-Chiari syndrome: technical, hemodynamic, and clinical results of treatment with transjugular intrahepatic portosystemic shunt. *Radiology.* 1995;197(3):805-811.
45. Ganger DR, Klapman JB, McDonald V, et al. Transjugular intrahepatic portosystemic shunt (TIPS) for Budd-Chiari syndrome or portal vein thrombosis: review of indications and problems. *Am J Gastroenterol.* 1999;94(3):603-608.
46. Gasparini D, Del Forno M, Sponza M, et al. Transjugular intrahepatic portosystemic shunt by direct transcaval approach in patients with acute and hyperacute Budd-Chiari syndrome. *Eur J Gastroenterol Hepatol.* 2002;14(5):567-571.
47. Panis Y, Belghiti J, Valla D, et al. Portosystemic shunt in Budd-Chiari syndrome: long-term survival and factors affecting shunt patency in 25 patients in Western countries. *Surgery.* 1994;115(3):276-281.

48. Zeitoun G, Escolano S, Hadengue A, et al. Outcome of Budd-Chiari syndrome: a multivariate analysis of factors related to survival including surgical portosystemic shunting. *Hepatology.* 1999;30(1):84-89.
49. Panis Y, Belghiti J, Valla D, et al. Portosystemic shunt in Budd-Chiari syndrome: long-term survival and factors affecting shunt patency in 25 patients in Western countries. *Surgery.* 1994;115(3):276-281.
50. Putnam CW, Porter KA, Weil R 3rd. Liver transplantation of Budd-Chiari syndrome. *JAMA.* 1976;236(10):1142-1143.
51. Srinivasan P, Rela M, Prachalias A, et al. Liver transplantation for Budd-Chiari syndrome. *Transplantation.* 2002;73(6):973-977.
52. Shaked A, Goldstein RM, Klintmalm GB, et al. Portosystemic shunt versus orthotopic liver transplantation for the Budd-Chiari syndrome. *Surg Gynecol Obstet.* 1992; 174(6):453-459.
53. United Network for Organ Sharing. *Homepage.* Available at http://www.unos.org. Accessed June 6, 2005.
54. Ruckert JC, Ruckert RI, Rudolph B, Muller JM. Recurrence of the Budd-Chiari syndrome after orthotopic liver transplantation. *Hepatogastroenterology.* 1999;46(26):867-871.
55. Griner PF, Elbadawi A, Packman CH. Veno-occlusive disease of the liver after chemotherapy of acute leukemia. Report of two cases. *Ann Intern Med.* 1976;85(5):578-582.
56. DeLeve LD, Shulman HM, McDonald GB. Toxic injury to hepatic sinusoids: sinusoidal obstruction syndrome (veno-occlusive disease). *Semin Liver Dis.* 2002;22(1):27-42.
57. Stillman AS, Huxtable R, Consroe P, et al. Hepatic veno-occlusive disease due to pyrrolizidine (Senecio) poisoning in Arizona. *Gastroenterology.* 1977;73(2):349-352.
58. McGee J, Patrick RS, Wood CB, et al. A case of veno-occlusive disease of the liver in Britain associated with herbal tea consumption. *J Clin Pathol.* 1976;29(9):788-794.
59. Marubbio AT, Danielson B. Hepatic veno-occlusive disease in a renal transplant patient receiving azathioprine. *Gastroenterology.* 1975;69(3):739-743.
60. Richardson PG, Elias AD, Krishnan A, et al. Treatment of severe veno-occlusive disease with defibrotide: compassionate use results in response without significant toxicity in a high-risk population. *Blood.* 1998;92(3):737-744.
61. Chojkier M. Hepatic sinusoidal-obstruction syndrome: toxicity of pyrrolizidine alkaloids. *J Hepatol.* 2003;39(3):437-446.
62. Asbury RF, Rosenthal SN, Descalzi ME, et al. Hepatic veno-occlusive disease due to DTIC. *Cancer.* 1980;45(10):2670-2674.
63. Pegram AA, Kennedy LD. Prevention and treatment of veno-occlusive disease. *Ann Pharmacother.* 2001;35(7-8):935-942.
64. McDonald GB, Hinds MS, Fisher LD, et al. Veno-occlusive disease of the liver and multiorgan failure after bone marrow transplantation: a cohort study of 355 patients. *Ann Intern Med.* 1993;118(4):255-267.
65. Barker CC, Butzner JD, Anderson RA, et al. Incidence, survival and risk factors for the development of veno-occlusive disease in pediatric hematopoietic stem cell transplant recipients. *Bone Marrow Transplant.* 2003;32(1):79-87.
66. Litzow MR, Repoussis PD, Schroeder G, et al. Veno-occlusive disease of the liver after blood and marrow transplantation: analysis of pre- and post-transplant risk factors associated with severity and results of therapy with tissue plasminogen activator. *Leuk Lymphoma.* 2002;43(11):2099-2107.

67. Vallet-Pichard A, Rerolle JP, Fontaine H, et al. Veno-occlusive disease of the liver in renal transplant patients. *Nephrol Dial Transplant.* 2003;18(8):1663-1666.

68. Holtmann M, Schreiner O, Kohler H, et al. Veno-occlusive disease (VOD) in Crohn's disease (CD) treated with azathioprine. *Dig Dis Sci.* 2003;48(8):1503-1505.

69. Strasser SI, Myerson D, Spurgeon CL, et al. Hepatitis C virus infection and bone marrow transplantation: a cohort study with 10-year follow-up. *Hepatology.* 1999; 29(6):1893-1899.

70. Radich JP, Sanders JE, Buckner CD, et al. Second allogeneic marrow transplantation for patients with recurrent leukemia after initial transplant with total-body irradiation-containing regimens. *J Clin Oncol.* 1993;11(2):304-313.

71. Stillman AS, Huxtable R, Consroe P, et al. Hepatic veno-occlusive disease due to pyrrolizidine (Senecio) poisoning in Arizona. *Gastroenterology.* 1977;73(2):349-352.

72. Datta DV, Khuroo MS, Mattocks AR, et al. Herbal medicines and veno-occlusive disease in India. *Postgrad Med J.* 1978;54(634):511-515.

73. Stewart MJ, Steenkamp V. Pyrrolizidine poisoning: a neglected area in human toxicology. *Ther Drug Monit.* 2001;23(6):698-708.

74. McDonald GB, Sharma P, Matthews DE, et al. Venocclusive disease of the liver after bone marrow transplantation: diagnosis, incidence, and predisposing factors. *Hepatology.* 1984;4(1):116-122.

75. Jones RJ, Lee KS, Beschorner WE, et al. Venoocclusive disease of the liver following bone marrow transplantation. *Transplantation.* 1987;44(6):778-783.

76. Carreras E, Granena A, Navasa M, et al. On the reliability of clinical criteria for the diagnosis of hepatic veno-occlusive disease. *Ann Hematol.* 1993;66(2):77-80.

77. Carreras E. Veno-occlusive disease of the liver after hemopoietic cell transplantation. *Eur J Haematol.* 2000;64(5):281-291.

78. Carreras E, Bertz H, Arcese W, et al. Incidence and outcome of hepatic veno-occlusive disease after blood or marrow transplantation: a prospective cohort study of the European Group for Blood and Marrow Transplantation. European Group for Blood and Marrow Transplantation Chronic Leukemia Working Party. *Blood.* 1998;92(10):3599-3604.

79. Forrest DL, Thompson K, Dorcas VG, et al. Low molecular weight heparin for the prevention of hepatic veno-occlusive disease (VOD) after hematopoietic stem cell transplantation: a prospective phase II study. *Bone Marrow Transplant.* 2003; 31(12):1143-1149.

80. Styler MJ, Crilley P, Biggs J, et al. Hepatic dysfunction following busulfan and cyclophosphamide myeloablation: a retrospective, multicenter analysis. *Bone Marrow Transplant.* 1996;18(1):171-176.

81. Tanikawa S, Mori S, Ohhashi K, et al. Predictive markers for hepatic veno-occlusive disease after hematopoietic stem cell transplantation in adults: a prospective single center study. *Bone Marrow Transplant.* 2000;26(8):881-886.

82. Salat C, Holler E, Kolb HJ, et al. Plasminogen activator inhibitor-1 confirms the diagnosis of hepatic veno-occlusive disease in patients with hyperbilirubinemia after bone marrow transplantation. *Blood.* 1997;89(6):2184-2188.

83. Hommeyer SC, Teefey SA, Jacobson AF, et al. Venocclusive disease of the liver: prospective study of US evaluation. *Radiology.* 1992;184(3):683-686.

84. Lassau N, Auperin A, Leclere J, et al. Prognostic value of doppler-ultrasonography in hepatic veno-occlusive disease. *Transplantation.* 2002;74(1):60-66.

85. Kikuchi K, Rudolph R, Murakami C, et al. Portal vein thrombosis after hematopoietic cell transplantation: frequency, treatment and outcome. *Bone Marrow Transplant.* 2002;29(4):329-333.

86. Sato Y, Asada Y, Hara S, et al. Hepatic stellate cells (Ito cells) in veno-occlusive disease of the liver after allogeneic bone marrow transplantation. *Histopathology.* 1999;34(1): 66-70.

87. Shulman HM, Fisher LB, Schoch HG, et al. Veno-occlusive disease of the liver after marrow transplantation: histological correlates of clinical signs and symptoms. *Hepatology.* 1994;19(5):1171-1181.

88. Carreras E, Granena A, Navasa M, et al. Transjugular liver biopsy in BMT. *Bone Marrow Transplant.* 1993;11(1):21-26.

89. Park SH, Lee MH, Lee H, et al. A randomized trial of heparin plus ursodiol vs. heparin alone to prevent hepatic veno-occlusive disease after hematopoietic stem cell transplantation. *Bone Marrow Transplant.* 2002;29(2):137-143.

90. Ringden O, Remberger M, Lehmann S, et al. N-acetylcysteine for hepatic veno-occlusive disease after allogeneic stem cell transplantation. *Bone Marrow Transplant.* 2000;25(9):993-996.

91. Bearman SI, Shen DD, Hinds MS, et al. A phase I/II study of prostaglandin E1 for the prevention of hepatic venocclusive disease after bone marrow transplantation. *Br J Haematol.* 1993;84(4):724-730.

92. Savarese DM, Savy G, Vahdat L, et al. Prevention of chemotherapy and radiation toxicity with glutamine. *Cancer Treat Rev.* 2003;29(6):501-513.

93. Richardson PG, Murakami C, Jin Z, et al. Multi-institutional use of defibrotide in 88 patients after stem cell transplantation with severe veno-occlusive disease and multi-system organ failure: response without significant toxicity in a high-risk population and factors predictive of outcome. *Blood.* 2002;100(13):4337-4343.

94. Corbacioglu S, Greil J, Peters C, et al. Defibrotide in the treatment of children with veno-occlusive disease (VOD): a retrospective multicentre study demonstrates therapeutic efficacy upon early intervention. *Bone Marrow Transplant.* 2004;33(2):189-195.

95. Kaleelrahman M, Eaton JD, Leeming D, et al. Role of plasminogen activator inhibitor-1 (PAI-1) levels in the diagnosis of BMT-associated hepatic veno-occlusive disease and monitoring of subsequent therapy with defibrotide (DF). *Hematology.* 2003;8(2):91-95.

96. Bearman SI, Lee JL, Barón AE, McDonald GB. Treatment of hepatic venocclusive disease with recombinant human tissue plasminogen activator and heparin in 42 marrow transplant patients. *Blood.* 1997;89:1501-1506.

97. Rosen HR, Martin P, Schiller GJ, et al. Orthotopic liver transplantation for bone-marrow transplant-associated veno-occlusive disease and graft-versus-host disease of the liver. *Liver Transpl Surg.* 1996;2(3):225-232.

98. Mor E, Pappo O, Bar-Nathan N, et al. Defibrotide for the treatment of veno-occlusive disease after liver transplantation. *Transplantation.* 2001;72(7):1237-1240.

99. Nakazawa Y, Chisuwa H, Mita A, et al. Life-threatening veno-occlusive disease after living-related liver transplantation. *Transplantation.* 2003;75(5):727-730.

100. Azoulay D, Castaing D, Lemoine A, et al. Transjugular intrahepatic portosystemic shunt (TIPS) for severe veno-occlusive disease of the liver following bone marrow transplantation. *Bone Marrow Transplant.* 2000;25(9):987-992.

101. Reiss U, Cowan M, McMillan A, Horn B. Hepatic venoocclusive disease in blood and bone marrow transplantation in children and young adults: incidence, risk factors, and outcome in a cohort of 241 patients. *J Pediatr Hematol Oncol.* 2002;24(9):746-750.

102. Myers RP, Cerini R, Sayegh R, et al. Cardiac hepatopathy: clinical, hemodynamic, and histologic characteristics and correlations. *Hepatology.* 2003;37(2):393-400.
103. Naschitz JE, Slobodin G, Lewis RJ, et al. Heart diseases affecting the liver and liver diseases affecting the heart. *Am Heart J.* 2000;140(1):111-120.
104. Runyon BA. Cardiac ascites: a characterization. *J Clin Gastroenterol.* 1988;10(4):410-412.
105. Arcidi JM Jr, Moore GW, Hutchins GM. Hepatic morphology in cardiac dysfunction: a clinicopathologic study of 1000 subjects at autopsy. *Am J Pathol.* 1981;104(2):159-166.
106. Giallourakis CC, Rosenberg PM, Friedman LS. The liver in heart failure. *Clin Liver Dis.* 2002;6(4):947-967.
107. Schiff ER, Sorrell MF, Maddrey WC. *Schiff's Diseases of the Liver.* 9th ed. Philadelphia: Lippincott Williams and Wilkins; 2003.
108. Sarin SK, Agarwal SR. Extrahepatic portal vein obstruction. *Semin Liver Dis.* 2002; 22(1):43-58.
109. Janssen HL, Wijnhoud A, Haagsma EB, et al. Extrahepatic portal vein thrombosis: aetiology and determinants of survival. *Gut.* 2001;49(5):720-724.
110. Kim JH, Lee YS, Kim SH, et al. Does umbilical vein catheterization lead to portal venous thrombosis? Prospective US evaluation in 100 neonates. *Radiology.* 2001;219(3):645-650.
111. Schwartz DS, Gettner PA, Konstantino MM, et al. Umbilical venous catheterization and the risk of portal vein thrombosis. *J Pediatr.* 1997;131(5):760-762.
112. Valla DC, Condat B, Lebrec D. Spectrum of portal vein thrombosis in the West. *J Gastroenterol Hepatol.* 2002;17 Suppl 3:S224-S227.
113. Webb LJ, Sherlock S. The aetiology, presentation and natural history of extra-hepatic portal venous obstruction. *Q J Med.* 1979;48(192):627-639.
114. Rangari M, Gupta R, Jain M, et al. Hepatic dysfunction in patients with extrahepatic portal venous obstruction. *Liver Int.* 2003;23(6):434-439.
115. Belli L, Romani F, Riolo F, et al. Thrombosis of portal vein in absence of hepatic disease. *Surg Gynecol Obstet.* 1989;169(1):46-49.
116. Condat B, Pessione F, Hillaire S, et al. Current outcome of portal vein thrombosis in adults: risk and benefit of anticoagulant therapy. *Gastroenterology.* 2001;120(2):490-497.
117. Qin LX, Tang ZY. The prognostic significance of clinical and pathological features in hepatocellular carcinoma. *World J Gastroenterol.* 2002;8(2):193-199.
118. Romagnuolo J, Sadowski DC, Lalor E, et al. Cholestatic hepatocellular injury with azathioprine: a case report and review of the mechanisms of hepatotoxicity. *Can J Gastroenterol.* 1998;12(7):479-483.
119. Cavalcanti R, Pol S, Carnot F, et al. Impact and evolution of peliosis hepatis in renal transplant recipients. *Transplantation.* 1994;58(3):315-316.

chapter 9

Benign and Malignant Tumors of the Liver

Arie Regev, MD

Benign Solid Tumors of the Liver

Introduction

Benign focal lesions are detected with increasing frequency due to the prevalent use of imaging studies of the abdomen. Many are discovered incidentally in patients with no history and no clinical evidence of liver disease. Technical advances in imaging modalities have led to the identification of smaller lesions. Patients with benign hepatic tumors are often asymptomatic, and typically have normal hepatic biochemical tests. When symptoms do occur, it is often difficult to corroborate a causative relationship to the hepatic lesion.[1] Benign liver tumors may be difficult to differentiate from malignant ones by laboratory investigations and imaging studies. Nevertheless, in some of the benign tumors accurate diagnosis is imperative not only to exclude malignancy but also because they may have specific risks such as bleeding, in the case of hepatic adenoma, and malignant potential, in hepatic adenoma and hepatobiliary cystadenoma. Histopathological evaluation remains essential in the clinical management of some liver masses; possible exceptions include FNH, hemangioma, and focal fatty change that may be unequivocally diagnosed by imaging studies. Unfortunately, in many benign lesions (eg, hemangioma and hepatic adenoma) liver biopsy carries a high risk of bleeding, and is therefore, contraindicated.

Benign tumors of the liver may arise from hepatocytes, bile-duct epithelium, the supporting mesenchymal tissue, or a combination of two or more of these (Table 9-1).

The most common benign tumors are hemangioma, hepatic adenoma, and focal nodular hyperplasia, however, many other lesions may present as a mass in the liver.

Table 9-1

BENIGN SOLID TUMORS OF THE LIVER

Epithelial Tumors
- Hepatocellular adenoma
- Bile duct adenoma
- Biliary cystadenoma

Mesenchymal Tumors
- Hemangioma
- Infantile hemangioendothelioma
- Fibroma
- Angiomyolipoma
- Lipoma
- Lymphangioma
- Benign mesenchymoma

Mixed Tumors
- Teratoma

Tumor-Like Lesions
- Focal nodular hyperplasia
- Nodular regenerative hyperplasia
- Mesenchymal hamartoma
- Microhamartoma (von Meyenburg complex)
- Inflammatory pseudotumor
- Focal fatty change
- Pseudolipoma
- Macroregenerative nodule

HEMANGIOMA

Epidemiology

Hemangioma is the most common benign tumor of the liver. The reported prevalence at autopsy ranges from 0.4% to 7.4%. Most often, they are found incidentally and have no major clinical implications. Hemangiomas may present at all ages, but are most common between the third and fifth decades and are rare in young children. They are more prevalent in women, and in the right hepatic lobe. Sex ratio is between 4:1 and 6:1.

Clinical Manifestations

Hemangiomas are asymptomatic in the majority of patients, and are most often discovered as an incidental finding. Infrequently, they may grow to a large size, causing pressure or displacement of adjacent structures. Several authors refer to hemangiomas that are larger than 4 cm in diameter as giant hemangiomas. Large hemangiomas are uncommon, and although most are asymptomatic, they are more likely to cause symptoms than smaller ones. The most common complaints are of abdominal pain or discomfort, however, early satiety, nausea, and vomiting may also occur. Pain may be due to infarction or necrosis within the hemangioma, pressure on adjacent structures, or distention of the liver capsule. However, the relationship between the symptoms and the hemangioma may be difficult to ascertain, and in many cases other causes are discovered.

Physical examination is usually unremarkable. Uncommonly, the liver may be enlarged or a palpable mass may be detected. Rarely, a bruit may be heard over the hemangioma. Hepatic biochemical tests are usually normal and are, therefore, of little help in the diagnosis of a hemangioma. On rare occasions, serum aminotransferases may be mildly elevated.

Complications

There are rare reports of a spontaneous rupture of large hepatic hemangiomas. Rupture has also been reported following a blunt abdominal trauma and during delivery. Very rarely patients with giant hemangiomas may develop consumption coagulopathy within the hemangioma and may present with evidence of disseminated intravascular coagulopathy (DIC), the so called Kasabach-Merritt syndrome.[2] There are rare reports of rapid growth of hepatic hemangiomas during pregnancy, and following the use of estrogens, however, the vast majority of hemangiomas are not affected by estrogen.

Imaging Studies

The various methods of imaging for focal nodular hyperplasia, hemangioma and hepatic adenoma and their features are compared and costrasted in Table 9-2. *Plane abdominal radiographs* are usually unhelpful. Rarely, they may show calcification. In contrast, *Ultrasonography* is very useful for the diagnosis of hepatic hemangioma. It typically shows an echogenic, homogenous lesion with well-defined borders (Figure 9-1A). *Posterior acoustic enhancement* is a common feature. Doppler usually does not detect flow within the hemangioma, because of the slow blood flow. Dynamic, triple-phase, contrast-enhanced CT scan is the study of choice for the diagnosis of hepatic hemangioma (Figure 9-2).[3] It has sensitivity and specificity of more than 85% for lesions greater than 2 cm in size. Precontrast images typically show a hypodense lesion (see Figure 9-1B). Succeeding scans, following contrast injection, show diffusion of the contrast from the periphery to the center of the lesion, with a globular pattern, until opacification is homogenous (see Figure 9-1C). Opacification is usually completed in 3 minutes, and the lesion remains isodense or hyperdense on delayed scans up to 60 minutes after injection. The center of the lesion may remain hypodense, representing central necrosis or fibrosis. This may be encountered with increasing frequency as the size increases. A nonhomogenous filling may be seen due to previous bleeding or thrombus formation within the hemangioma. *Magnetic resonance imaging* (MRI) also shows a high degree of sensitivity and specificity in the diagnosis of hemangioma, and has special value in the diagnosis of small lesions, of less than 2 cm, and in patients with contraindications to the use of iodine based intravenous contrast material. MRI typically shows a well-circumscribed, homogenous lesion, with low

Table 9-2

IMAGING FEATURES OF FOCAL NODULAR HYPERPLASIA, HEMANGIOMA, AND HEPATIC ADENOMA

	FNH	*Hemangioma*	*Adenoma*
Ultrasonography	Usually nondiagnostic Variable echogenicity Occasionally central scar	Hyperechoic lesion with well-defined borders	Usually nondiagnostic
Doppler	Arterial flow within the lesion	No internal flow	Venous signals within the lesion (nondiagnostic)
Contrast-enhanced spiral CT scan	Precontrast: Hypo or isodense lesion Homogenous arterial enhancement with a hypodense central scar May turn isodense postcontrast	Precontrast: Hypodense lesion Centripetal globular enhancement Retained contrast on delayed venous phase	Precontrast: Hypo- or isodense lesion Irregular enhancement with peripheral arterial enhancement postcontrast
MRI Unenhanced	Low signal on TI Slightly hyperintense on T2 Central scar hyperintense on T2	Well-circumscribed homogenous lesion Low signal on TI Very high signal on T2	Low to slightly hyperintense area on TI Well-defined low intensity capsule Heterogeneous enhancement on T2
Gadolinium-enhanced MRI	Homogenous arterial enhancement Hypodense central scar Contrast accumulates in central area on delayed TI	Progressive centripetal enhancement Similar to CT	Enhancement as in CT

Table 9-2 (continued)

Imaging Features of Focal Nodular Hyperplasia, Hemangioma, and Hepatic Adenoma

	FNH	Hemangioma	Adenoma
Angiography	Dilated hepatic artery Highly vascular lesion, with a central vascular supply Spoke-wheel pattern in one third of the patients	Venous lakes with well-defined circular shape Displaced arterial branches Delayed venous phase	Hypervascular lesion: 50% Hypovascular lesion: 50% Peripheral vascular supply
Scitigraphy with ^{99m}Tc-labeled RBC	Equal or increased uptake in 50% to 70% of the patients	Increased uptake in the lesion during venous phase Retention on delayed images	Hypoconcentration of the colloid (focal defect) in most patients

signal intensity on T1-weighted images and high signal intensity on T2. Intravenous contrast enhancement with gadolinium shows a centripetal opacification similar to contrast enhanced CT.

^{99m}Technetium pertechnetate-labled red blood cells (^{99m}Tc-RBC) pool study may occasionally be helpful in controversial cases. It typically shows initial hypoperfusion during the arterial flow phase, followed by gradual increase in the isotope in the lesion, with retention of the isotope in the lesion in delayed images. ^{99m}Tc-RBC scan has a low sensitivity for lesions smaller than 2 cm. Sensitivity for lesions larger than 2 cm ranges from 69% to 82%, with specificity close to 100%.

Single photon emission CT (SPECT) with ^{99m}Tc-RBC shows persistent isotope activity within the lesion. SPECT has sensitivity and specificity close to those of MRI (90% to 95%) in lesions greater than 2 cm. It is best used to clarify doubtful CT lesions.

Angiography is rarely needed for the diagnosis of a hemangioma. It is used only when other modalities have failed to yield a definitive diagnosis. Hemangiomas are usually shown to displace large hepatic arterial branches to one side. The hepatic arteries are not enlarged, and taper normally to small vessels before filling the vascular spaces. The vascular space usually has a well-defined circular shape and typically shows a prolonged opacification.

Pathology

Biopsy is usually not necessary for diagnosis and may result in significant bleeding. On gross examination, hemangiomas appear as a spongy, purple compressible lesion.

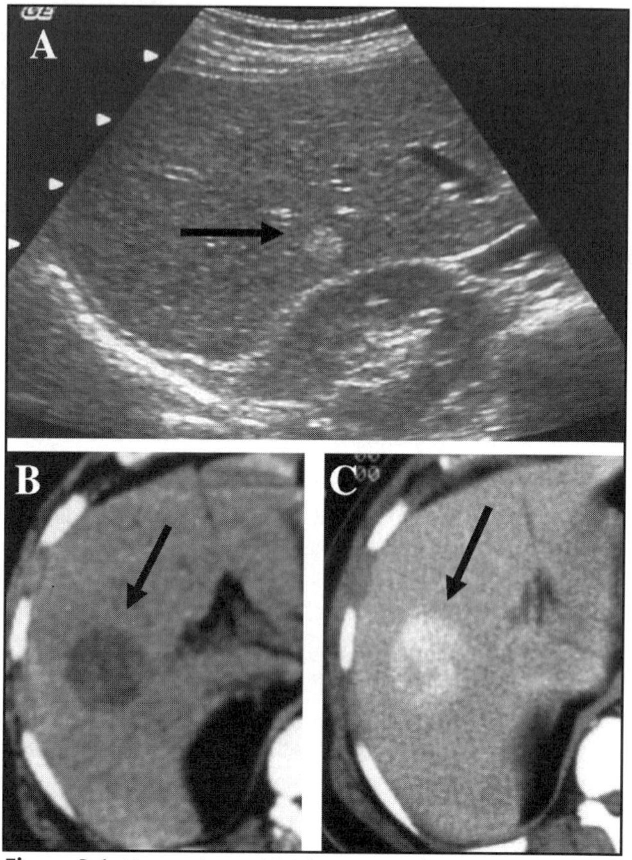

Figure 9-1. Hemangioma. (A) Ultrasonography: A transverse view of the right hepatic lobe shows a well-circumscribed echogenic mass measuring 2x2 cm, which is consistent with a hemangioma (arrow). (B) Abdominal CT scan, precontrast injection, shows a well-circumscribed mass with low attenuation in the right hepatic lobe (arrow). (C) The hemangioma demonstrated in 2B is shown in a late image (5 min), following the administration of intravenous contrast. The lesion shows a persistent enhancement in a globular pattern, typical of a hemangioma. (Courtesy of J. Casillas, MD, Department of Radiology, University of Miami, Miami, FL.)

Microscopically, they are composed of endothelial-lined vascular walls of varying thickness. Intraluminal thrombi may be present, and may organize to form fibrous septa and calcifications.

Management

Under most circumstances hemangiomas require no treatment. The rare reports of bleeding should not be considered as an indication for surgical treatment. Indications

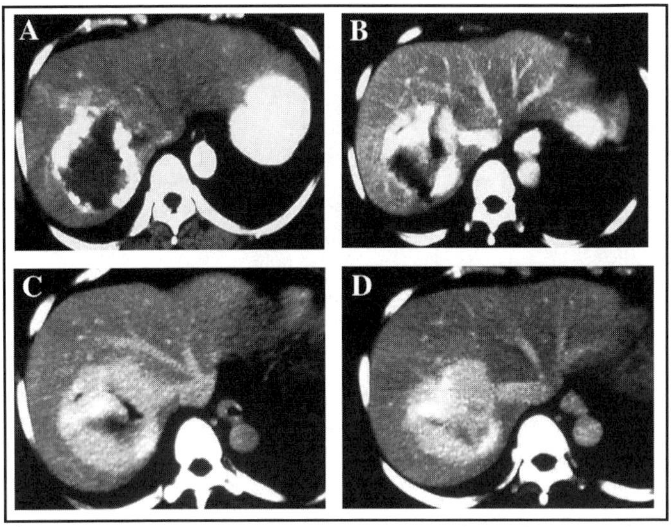

Figure 9-2. Hemangioma. Dynamic, contrast-enhanced CT scan demonstrates diffusion of the contrast from the periphery to the center of the lesion, at consecutive stages of intravenous contrast injection. (A) 40 sec; (B) 60 sec; (C) 90 sec; (D) 120 sec. (Courtesy of J. Casillas, MD, Department of Radiology, University of Miami, Miami, FL.)

for surgery include 1) a large symptomatic lesion, 2) complications such as bleeding, and 3) uncertain diagnosis, especially when malignancy cannot be excluded.

In these unusual cases, resection may be indicated. Resection or enucleation of a hemangioma may be performed safely by an experienced surgical team with a mortality rate near 0%. Other modalities of therapy, such as hepatic artery ligation or embolization and radiation therapy, although reported, are not likely to yield good long-term results.

Focal Nodular Hyperplasia

Epidemiology

Focal nodular hyperplasia (FNH) is the second most common benign solid tumor of the liver (Figure 9-3). Its prevalence at autopsy ranges from 0.3% to 0.6%. It has been reported to occur most frequently in young women, although it may occur in both genders, and the sex difference is less striking than that for hepatic adenoma. The peak incidence is between the third and fifth decades of life, but it is seen at any age. Generally, it is more common than hepatic adenoma, and its association with the use of oral contraceptives is controversial. The pathogenesis of FNH is not completely clear. It is thought to originate in a vascular malformation that leads to a local hyperplastic response of the hepatic parenchyma. FNH is sometimes associated with other vascular malformations such as hepatic hemangiomas and neoplasms of the brain.

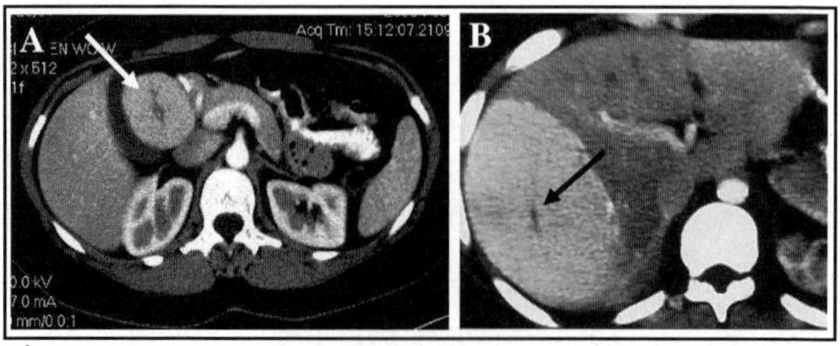

Figure 9-3. Focal nodular hyperplasia (FNH). (A) Arterial phase of a contrast-enhanced CT shows an enhanced lesion protruding from the left hepatic lobe, with a nonenhancing central scar (arrow). (B) Arterial phase of a contrast-enhanced CT shows an enhanced lesion in segments 5 and 6, with a nonenhancing central scar (arrow). (Courtesy of J. Casillas, MD, Department of Radiology, University of Miami, Miami, FL.)

Clinical Manifestations and Natural History

FNH is usually asymptomatic (in 50% to 90% of the cases). About three-fourths of the lesions are discovered incidentally on a routine ultrasonography or during abdominal surgery. FNH may present as a nontender mass in the right upper abdomen. Rarely patients may present with abdominal pain resulting from hemorrhage, rupture or necrosis in the lesion. Physical examination is normal in 80% of the patients. The remainder may present with hepatomegaly, abdominal mass or tenderness. Hepatic biochemical tests are usually normal, and are of little value in the diagnosis of FNH. The prognosis of an unresected FNH is excellent. The majority of FNH lesions will not increase in size after diagnosis, and will probably remain asymptomatic. Rupture causing hemoperitoneum and shock is exceedingly rare, and malignant transformation has not been described. Large pedunculated lesions have rarely been reported to undergo torsion or necrosis.

Imaging Studies

Imaging studies are diagnostic for FNH in the majority of patients, and usually make it possible to distinguish between FNH and hepatic adenoma (see Table 9-2). Detection of a central scar is characteristic.[4]

Ultrasonography commonly identifies a nodular mass, with variable echogenicity. It may occasionally demonstrate the central scar, but in many cases it is nondiagnostic. Doppler may show arterial flow inside the lesion. A hypoechoic rim may be demonstrated, and should raise the suspicion of malignancy.

CT scan may show a hypodense or isodense lesion that enhances homogenously during the arterial phase of contrast injection, and returns to its precontrast density within 1 minute. Central scar is demonstrated in 60% of the patients. In contrast to a hemangioma, no venous pooling is seen during late images; however, the central scar may show hyperattenuation.[5]

MRI usually shows an isointense homogenous lesion on T1-weighted images, and an isointense to slightly hyperintense mass on T2-weighted images.[6] The central scar is demonstrated in 78% of the cases. Injection of gadolinium shows early enhancement of the lesion, and may increase the intensity of the central scar, showing delayed intensity of the scar in T1 weighted images. Gadolinium injection helps to distinguish FNH from malignant vascular tumors.

^{99m}*Tc sulfur colloid liver scans* demonstrate equal or enhanced uptake in the lesion compared to the rest of the hepatic parenchyma in 50% to 70% of the patients. This is in contrast to hepatic adenoma, which usually shows hypoconcentration of the colloid (defect), and shows hyperconcentration in less than 7%. This has been attributed to the high numbers of Kupffer cells within the FNH, compared to lower numbers or decreased function in hepatic adenoma. Liver scan may assist in distinguishing FNH from hepatic adenoma, however, its reliability is poor in lesions less than 4 cm in size.

Single photon emission tomography (SPECT) may enhance the sensitivity compared to planar scitigraphy, but also shows low reliability in lesions smaller than 2 cm in size.

Although it is seldom required for the diagnosis of FNH, *angiography* may demonstrate a dilated hepatic artery with one or more highly vascular lesions. The vessels within the lesion are very torturous, and septation of the tumor mass may be visible in about half of the cases during the capillary phase. A "spoke wheel" pattern with central arterial supply and radiating vessels is seen in about one third of the cases. Nevertheless, angiographic findings frequently do not distinguish between FNH and hepatic adenoma, especially in lesions smaller than 3 cm in size.

Pathology

Macroscopically, FNH is a firm sharply demarcated light–brown nodular lesion, which is usually found in peripheral areas of the liver. It is frequently single, although multiple lesions have been described. The average size is less than 5 cm, rarely exceeding 10 cm in diameter. Typically, it has a dense central scar with radiating fibrous septa, which divide the lesion into lobule-like structures that may resemble cirrhotic nodules. Occasionally foci of hemorrhage or necrosis may be encountered. A single artery supplies the lesion and is not accompanied by a portal vein or a bile duct. Microscopically, FNH closely resembles cirrhosis. The septa typically contain numerous bile ductules, blood vessels, and inflammatory cells. The hepatocytes, between the septa, are indistinguishable from those of a normal liver. They are arranged in cords forming sinusoids, however they lack portal tracts and central veins. Kupffer cells are present.

Differential Diagnosis

The differential diagnosis of FNH includes benign lesions such as hemangioma and hepatic adenoma and malignant tumor such as hepatocellular carcinoma, fibrolamellar carcinoma, intrahepatic cholangiocarcinoma, and metastases.

Hemangiomas typically show a characteristic centripetal enhancement on contrast injection. *Hepatic adenoma* is usually larger than FNH and lacks the characteristic central scar. Nevertheless, occasionally these lesions may bleed internally or may develop a central necrosis. This may create a similar appearance to the central scar of FNH on CT. In contrast, MRI may differentiate a central scar from a central hemorrhage or necrosis, since the latter shows a low signal on T2, whereas a central scar shows a high signal. Contrary to FNH, *Hepatocellular carcinoma* (HCC) usually appears in patients with pre-existing liver disease. It may show vascular invasion and metastatic spread.

The most common malignant tumors in patients with no pre-existing liver disease are metastases. *Hepatic metastases* may be hypervascular, but usually lack a central scar. Most are hypodense, showing a ring enhancement on the vascular phase of enhanced CT scan.

In *fibrolamellar carcinoma,* a calcified central scar may be seen in up to 55%, making the differential diagnosis from FNH extremely difficult. Intrahepatic cholangiocarcinoma is less vascular than FNH, although it also may have a central scar. It may also show local invasion, which is not a feature of FNH.

Management

Since the incidence of complications is extremely low, the recommended treatment in asymptomatic FNH is observation.[7] To ensure stability of the lesion size, it is recommended to repeat abdominal imaging 3, 6, and 12 months after the diagnosis. If the lesion is highly suggestive of FNH and does not change over a period of 1 year, no further observation is indicated. If the lesion is enlarging on consecutive imaging studies, resection should be considered. There is no convincing data on increased risk in association with oral contraceptives or pregnancy, and it is probably unjustified to recommend resection of the lesion when pregnancy is contemplated. Pedunculated lesions may require local resection to prevent torsion. Resection is also recommended for severely symptomatic lesions, however, other possible causes for symptoms should be ruled out, and the association between the lesion and the symptoms needs to be clearly ascertained prior to surgery.

Hepatic Adenoma

Epidemiology

Hepatic adenoma, also called hepatocellular adenoma, is a solid tumor, seen mainly in women of childbearing age. It has a strong association with estrogens in general and oral contraceptives in particular. Hepatic adenomas were considered to be rare until the mid-1960s. However, since the 1970s there has been a marked increase in the number of reported cases, which has been attributed to the introduction of oral contraceptives in the 1960s. Association has also been described with diabetes mellitus, glycogen storage diseases, and pregnancy. There are also reported cases in men and children without known predisposing factors. Adenomas are found more commonly in women using higher doses of estrogen and for a longer duration. Women after the age of 30, who took oral contraceptives for more than 5 years, are at significantly increased risk. In women who have never used oral contraceptives, the annual incidence is 1 to 1.3 per million; however, it increases to 3 to 4 per 100,000 in long-term users of oral contraceptives. Women who use oral contraceptive agents for more than 9 years have been estimated to have 25 times the normal risk of developing hepatic adenoma. Still in 10% the exposure may be as short as 6 to 12 months. Adenomas have been shown to regress with cessation of oral contraceptive therapy, and to increase in size during pregnancy. The incidence has decreased in the last decade, compared to the 1970s and 1980s, probably as a result of lower concentrations of estrogens in oral contraceptives.

Multiple hepatic adenomas occur in association with glycogen storage diseases (GSD) types I and III. They usually occur before the third decade of life. A rare condition in which ten or more adenomas are encountered has been named liver adenomatosis. This may occur in both men and women, and may not be associated with the use of oral contraceptives.

Natural History and Complication

Hepatic adenoma does not result in significant complications in the majority of patients. Nevertheless, there are several reports of bleeding into the tumor as well as rupture with intra-abdominal hemorrhage.[7] Bleeding from an adenoma may occur spontaneously or after a blunt trauma, and may result in hemoperitoneum, hypotension and shock. The initial manifestation is typically acute abdominal pain. These complications seem to be more common during pregnancy or within 6 weeks postpartum. Patients with hepatic adenoma are also at increased risk of transformation into carcinoma within the tumor. The frequency of this uncommon complication is not well established.

Clinical Manifestations

Hepatic adenomas are often found incidentally, usually by abdominal imaging studies. Less than one-fourth present with abdominal symptoms. When symptoms do occur, they consist most commonly of pain or discomfort in the epigastrium or right upper quadrant. Abdominal symptoms occur more frequently during menstruation or shortly thereafter. Acute or severe abdominal pain may be due to hemorrhage into the tumor, rupture into the peritoneum or tumor necrosis. Rupture and bleeding may lead to hypotension, and shock. Malignant transformation of an adenoma may present with an abdominal mass in 25% to 35% of the cases and occasionally with hepatomegaly. Laboratory studies are usually normal in patients with hepatic adenomas. Alkaline phosphatase (AlkP) and gamma-glutamyl transpeptidase (GGT) may occasionally be elevated, mainly in patients with bleeding or rupture. Serum levels of alpha-fetoprotein are not elevated. Liver adenomatosis (10 or more adenomas) is more likely to be associated with elevated serum levels of AlkP and GGT.

Pathology

Hepatic adenomas are usually solitary tumors, ranging in size from 1 to 30 cm. Most range from 8 to 15 cm in diameter. Occasionally two or more lesions may be present. Macroscopically, adenomas appear as well-circumscribed, light brown tumors that may or may not be encapsulated. They arise in otherwise normal liver tissue, usually in subcapsular locations. Foci of hemorrhage or necrosis are found frequently. Microscopically, adenoma may mimic normal liver tissue. It is composed of cells closely resembling normal hepatocytes, which are arranged in plates separated by sinusoids. Consequently, liver biopsy typically lacks pathognomonic characteristics, and is commonly nondiagnostic, although it may occasionally suggest the diagnosis of hepatic adenoma. Adenoma cells may have a slightly atypical appearance and may be larger than normal liver cells. There are few or no bile ducts, portal tracts, or central veins within the adenoma. In addition, Kupffer cells may be markedly reduced in number. Since adenomas have no portal tracts, they are perfused solely by peripheral arterial feeders. The tendency to bleed may arise from the hypervascular nature of the adenoma, which contains dilated sinusoids with thin walls and poor connective tissue support under arterial pressure.

Imaging Studies

Imaging studies (see Table 9-2) are usually insufficient to make a definite diagnosis of hepatic adenoma. *Ultrasonography* shows a well-demarcated mass with variable internal echogenicity which is non diagnostic. On *CT scan,* adenoma appears as a hypo or isodense mass that enhances in an irregular pattern upon injection of contrast material. The absence of a central scar helps in differentiating adenoma from focal nodular hyperplasia; however, bleeding into an adenoma may produce a hypodense center that remains hypodense after contrast injection, and may be indistinguishable from a central scar. In the presence of multiple lesions the diagnosis of hepatic adenomas should be considered a diagnosis of exclusion, since metastatic disease, or multifocal hepatocellular carcinoma are more common causes.

MRI shows a low-to-slightly hyperintense signal on T1-weighted images and hetergenous enhancement on T2. T1 images may show a well-defined low-intensity capsule.

Hepatic arteriography may add important information since hepatic adenomas are frequently associated with enlargement of the hepatic artery. The lesion itself may appear either hypovascular or hypervascular. Blood vessels are frequently seen entering the lesion from the periphery in a parallel pattern (spoke-wheel appearance). Arteriovenous shunting and portal venous invasion suggest hepatocellular carcinoma rather than adenoma.

^{99m}*Technetium colloid scan* was frequently used in early studies. It often demonstrates decreased uptake of the colloid, especially in lesions larger than 4 cm. This finding has been attributed to decreased numbers of Kupffer cells in these lesions, however, it is an inconsistent finding which is not reliable in differentiating an adenoma from a focal nodular hyperplasia.

Management

Liver biopsy is best avoided when the diagnosis of hepatic adenoma is suspected, due to the high risk of bleeding. Even when biopsy is performed, the diagnosis remains uncertain in a significant number of patients (approximately in 25%). Due to the significant risks of bleeding, especially in larger adenomas, and the small risk of rupture and malignant transformation, the recommended approach for hepatic adenoma is segmental or lobar resection whenever possible. In cases of ruptured hepatic adenoma resection should be performed if possible. An alternative is embolization of the hepatic artery feeding the tumor. In patients with unresected adenoma, it is recommended to avoid pregnancy because of the risk of rapid increase in size, as well as increased risk of hemorrhage and rupture. Mortality from elective resection of hepatic adenoma is less than 1%; however, it may increase to 5% or 8% for emergency resection in bleeding or ruptured lesion.

Other Benign Tumors

Angiomyolipoma is a rare liver tumor diagnosed most commonly in women in the fourth to seventh decade. It is composed of fat tissue, epithelioid cells, smooth muscle cells, and thick-walled vascular channels. Its size ranges from 0.8 to 36 cm. Ultrasonography shows a homogeneous, highly echogenic, well circumscribed lesion, and CT shows a hypodense lesion with density measurement characteristic of fat tissue. It is commonly misdiagnosed as hepatic adenoma, hepatocellular carcinoma, or FNH. For symptomatic or suspicious lesions resection is the treatment of choice.

Bile duct adenoma is a rare hepatic tumor found more commonly after the fifth decade of life. It is virtually never symptomatic and is usually diagnosed incidentally at laparotomy or autopsy. Bile duct adenoma is almost always solitary, and its size is usually less than 1 cm. Microscopically, it is characterized by a local proliferation of normal-appearing small bile ducts and fibrous stroma, containing numerous lymphocytes. Its main significance is in the differential diagnosis from metastatic carcinoma, cholangiocarcinoma, or other focal hepatic lesions.

Infantile hemangioendothelioma, although a rare finding, is the most common benign hepatic tumor in children, accounting for more than 50% of the cases. It presents almost always in the first 6 months of life and is twice as common in girls. It may be associated with congestive heart failure resulting from massive arteriovenous shunting, which may lead to a high mortality rate (up to 70%) among the affected children. Spontaneous regression occurs frequently.

Pseudolipoma of the liver is a rare lesion composed of mature adipose tissue, which is found outside the liver tissue but within the Glisson's capsule. The speculated origin is from epiploicae appendices or omental fat. Fat necrosis and calcification may occur.

Tumor-Like Lesions

Inflammatory pseudotumor is a rare hepatic lesion of uncertain etiology. It affects all ages, with a men to women ration of 8:1. It typically presents with fever, pain, and weight loss, associated with a liver mass and abnormal hepatic biochemical tests. The reported size ranges from 1 to 35 cm. Macroscopically, the lesion is devoid of a capsule and has no distinct borders. Microscopically, it is composed of spindled cells mixed with mononuclear inflammatory cells, predominantly plasma cells, in a fibrous stroma. Inflammatory pseudotumor may initially be misdiagnosed as a liver abscess, Hodgkin's disease, or sarcoma. Cultures from the lesion are invariably negative. The natural history may vary from spontaneous regression to persisting severe symptoms. Resection is necessary in persisting symptomatic lesions and in cases in which a firm histologic diagnosis cannot be made preoperatively.

Macroregenerative nodules, also known as dysplastic nodules, occur in the setting of advanced chronic liver disease, usually with cirrhosis. They are found in cirrhotic livers due to any underlying liver disease, and are considered a premalignant condition. Similar lesions have been described in massive or submassive necrosis due to acute liver injury.

In gross examination, macroregenerative nodules appear distinct from the surrounding cirrhotic parenchyma because of difference in color and a tendency to protrude from the liver's surface. Central necrosis or hemorrhage within the nodule suggest hepatocellular carcinoma. Microscopically, the hepatocytes within the nodule may show low-grade and high-grade dysplastic features, but they do not meet the criteria of hepatocellular carcinoma. MRI may assist in differentiating between macroregenerative nodule and hepatocellular carcinoma. When this lesion is recognized, the patient should be followed closely by repeat imaging studies, and serum levels of alfa-feto-protein.

Focal fatty change in the liver may manifest as a focal lesion or as diffuse infiltration. It varies in size, and may be single or multiple. It may or may not be associated with diffuse fatty infiltration, obesity, diabetes mellitus, hypercholesterolemia,

Table 9-3

Classification of Malignant Tumors of the Liver

Epithelial Tumors

- Hepatocellular carcinoma
- Cholangiocarcinoma
- Biliary cystadenocarcinoma
- Squamous cell carcinoma
- Mucoepidermoid carcinoma

Mesenchymal Tumors

- Angiosarcoma
- Epethelioid hemangioendothelioma
- Undifferentiated (embryonal) sarcoma
- Fibrosarcoma
- Leiomyosarcoma
- Epithelioid leiomyoma (leiomyoblastoma)
- Malignant mesenchymoma
- Malignant rhabdoid tumor

Mixed Tumors

- Hepatoblastoma
- Carcinosarcoma

corticosteroid therapy, malnutrition, total parenteral nutrition, and alcoholism. Hepatic biochemical tests may be normal or mildly elevated. Imaging studies, such as ultrasonography, CT scan, and MRI, may usually delineate this lesion, but it may be difficult to differentiate from other processes. Ultrasonography shows a hyperechoic lesion with ill-defined borders. CT scan shows a hypodense, sharply demarcated area, with no mass effect on hepatic and portal veins. Helical contrast enhanced CT scan typically demonstrates normal vessels coursing through the hypodense lesion. MRI shows increased intensity in T1, which is a typical finding for fatty infiltration and may appear only rarely in other conditions such as malignant melanoma and iron overload. When the diagnosis is uncertain, a liver biopsy should be performed, and is usually diagnostic.

Biliary microhamartoma (von Meyenburg complex) is a relatively common lesion, which is usually detected as an incidental finding at surgery or autopsy. It is commonly solitary or may appear as multiple lesions. It usually measures a few millimeters, but may be as large as 0.5 cm in diameter. Biliary microhamartoma is typically asymptomatic and is associated with normal hepatic biochemical tests. Histologically, it appears as an abnormal proliferation of ductules or small bile ducts of various sizes, which are surrounded by fibrous stroma. It is a frequent finding (more than 90%) in patients with adult polycystic kidney disease, and is also associated with solitary hepatic cysts.

Table 9-4

PREDISPOSING CONDITIONS AND RISK FACTORS FOR HEPATOCELLULAR CARCINOMA

Chronic hepatitis B
Chronic hepatitis C with cirrhosis
Cirrhosis of any cause
Metabolic disorders:
- Hemochromatosis
- α-1 antitrypsin deficiency
- Wilson's disease
- Tyrosinemia
- Glycogenosis type I and III

Carcinogens:
- Aflatoxin
- Anabolic steroids
- Thorium dioxide

Others:
- Membranous obstruction of inferior vena-cava

MALIGNANT TUMORS OF THE LIVER

INTRODUCTION

Malignant tumors of the liver are either primary or metastatic. Metastases are by far the most common form of hepatic malignancy in adults. In contrast, in children primary malignant tumors of the liver, although rare, are more common than benign or metastatic tumors. Liver metastases arise primarily from malignant tumors of the gastrointestinal tract, lung, and breast. Primary malignant liver tumors may arise from hepatocytes, bile duct epithelium or supporting mesenchymal tissue (Table 9-3). The most common primary malignant tumor of the liver in adults is hepatocellular carcinoma (HCC), which accounts for up to 85% of the primary hepatic cancers.

HEPATOCELLULAR CARCINOMA

Epidemiology

Hepatocellular carcinoma (HCC) is currently the fifth most common cancer worldwide. Although it is still uncommon in the United States, its incidence is clearly on the rise.[8] The age-adjusted incidence in the US in 1998 was 3.0 per 100,000 of the population per year. The incidence is significantly higher (>15 per 100,000) in sub-Saharan Africa and Southeast Asia. It increases progressively with increasing age, except for the fibrolamellar variant of HCC that typically affects young adults. The median age at diagnosis is in the fourth decade in high incidence areas; however, it presents at a significantly older age in other region. In most populations, there is male predominance ranging from 2:1 to 5:1. The major risk factors for HCC are chronic hepatitis B and chronic hepatitis C with cirrhosis. Other risk factors are metabolic disorders such as hemochromatosis and α-1 antitrypsin deficiency and environmental carcinogens such as aflatoxin and cirrhosis of any etiology.

Etiology

The exact mechanism for the development of HCC is unknown, but several predisposing conditions and risk factors have been identified (Table 9-4). Chronic hepatitis B virus (HBV) infection is the most common etiologic factor in high incidence areas, whereas cirrhosis due to hepatitis C virus (HCV) is the major predisposing factor in other areas. HBV may lead to HCC through chronic hepatic inflammation and regeneration leading to proliferation of hepatocytes. In addition, HBV may cause malignant transformation through integration of the HBV DNA into the DNA of the host cells and interaction of HBV-specific proteins with hepatic genes. The X protein of HBV has been shown to act as a transactivator for some cellular promoters and oncogenes which may lead to accelerated proliferation of hepatocytes. HCV-related cirrhosis appears to be the dominant predisposing factor to HCC in many developed countries. The role of HCV in the pathogenesis of HCC is still unclear. The RNA of HCV does not become integrated into the host genome and nearly all cases of HCV-related HCC are associated with cirrhosis. Concomitant excessive alcohol drinking increases the risk of HCC in HCV patients. Alcoholic cirrhosis is also an independent risk factor for HCC. Hemochromatosis is strongly associated with HCC, with a relative risk exceeding 200. Although cirrhosis almost invariably precedes the development of HCC in patients with hemochromatosis, there are several reports of HCC occurring without cirrhosis.

HCC may also occur with α-1 antitrypsin deficiency, Wilson's disease and other metabolic diseases (see Table 9-4); however, the risk with these disorders is substantially lower.

Clinical Manifestations

In the vast majority of patients, the tumor arises on a background of cirrhosis. Nevertheless, many patients in China and Africa, and some in Western countries are not aware of their liver disease prior to the diagnosis of HCC. In many patients the tumor is clinically indolent during early phases, whereas in advanced stages it often becomes symptomatic. In patients with known cirrhosis, a sudden and unexplained deterioration in their condition should prompt an evaluation for HCC. The most common symptoms are of abdominal discomfort and weight loss. The discomfort is usually in the epigastric and right upper quadrant area. It may progress gradually to a constant pain. A sudden increase in the pain intensity may result from bleeding into the tumor, or portal vein thrombosis. Rarely, severe abdominal pain may result from rupture of the tumor and intraperitoneal hemorrhage. Other common symptoms are fatigue, weakness and decreased appetite. Increased abdominal girth and jaundice may occur in patients with advanced decompensated liver disease. Uncommonly, the patient may present with symptoms of metastatic disease such as cough and exertional dyspnea caused by pulmonary metastases, or bone pain, due to skeletal metastases.

Physical examination may be unremarkable in early stages of the disease, or may show hepatomegaly and progressive wasting in later stages. Most patients have a hard, nodular and occasionally tender liver. An arterial bruit may be heard over the tumor in 7% to 29% of the patients, and 20% to 50% will have ascites or splenomegaly at the time of diagnosis. Low or moderate-grade fever may occur in up to 40% of the patients, and blood tinged ascites may occur in up to 20%. Rarely cutaneous metastases, metastases to the umbilicus (Sister Joseph's node) or metastases to Virchow's nodes may be found. A variety of nonmetastatic paraneoplastic manifestations have been described in association with HCC. These manifestations have been attributed to production of biologically active peptide by the tumor cells. They include hypoglycemia, erythrocytosis, hypercalcemia, hypertension, hypercholesterolemia, watery diarrhea syndrome, neuropathy, and sexual changes such as feminization. The majority of HCCs produce alpha fetoprotein (AFP), an α_1-globulin, which can be easily detected in the patient's blood, and is used for screening in patients with cirrhosis or chronic HBV infection. Abnormal levels may be detected in 70% to 80% of HCC patients and may range from slightly above the normal adult level, which is 6 to 8 ng/mL, to over 10 millions ng/mL. Generally, there is no clear correlation between the serum level of AFP and the size or prognosis of the tumor. However, in an individual patient AFP level is usually lower when the tumor is small and may increase rapidly as the tumor grows in size. Levels of more than 400 ng/mL are considered diagnostic in a cirrhotic patient with a typical focal lesion. An abnormal type of prothrombin, des-γ-carboxy prothrombin may be elevated in 60% to 90% of patients with HCC. Serum levels of carcinoembryonic antigen (CEA) may also be raised in HCC patients, although usually to a slight degree.

Natural History

Several factors determine the natural history of HCC, including: number and size of tumors on diagnosis, degree of differentiation and presence of macroscopic or microscopic vascular invasion. In addition, the liver function and Child-Pugh score are important predictors of the patient's prognosis. The rate of tumor growth is extremely variable. Doubling time may vary from less than 1 month to more than 20 months. Moreover, the tumor growth pattern may vary from a constant growth rate in some tumors to a gradual decline in growth rate in others. Other tumors may exhibit an initial slow-growth phase followed by a rapid increase in tumor growth rate. Rapidly growing HCC may present with increasing pain, abdominal distension, weight loss, and jaundice, whereas slow growing tumor may be asymptomatic for a long time. Symptomatic HCCs usually have worse prognosis than asymptomatic ones. In almost half the patients, HCC may be detected as a multinodular disease, which may represent a second primary tumor or a metastatic tumor. Second primary tumors appear to be less aggressive compared to metastatic tumors; however, differentiation between the two is extremely difficult on the basis of clinical data, and may be possible only after the tumor is resected. Distant metastases are typically found in the lungs, bones, brain, and adrenals.

Staging

Several staging systems have been proposed for HCC. The commonly used TNM (tumor, node, metastasis) system does not accurately predict patient survival. The Okuda system has been used for years and is based on tumor size, presence of ascites, and serum levels of bilirubin and albumin. It has been shown to accurately predict the natural history of untreated HCC. The recently proposed Barcelona Clinic Liver Cancer (BCLC) staging system uses the patient's performance stage, Child-Pugh class, and tumor stage. This staging system was shown to be a relatively accurate predictor of survival.[9]

Pathology

Macroscopically, HCC may appear in 3 different forms: nodular, diffuse, or massive. The nodular type appears as a distinct lesion, which is sharply delineated from the surrounding liver tissue, whereas the diffuse type is characterized by diffuse involvement of the liver. The massive type typically occupies a large area and infiltrates the neighboring liver tissue with satellite nodules. Microscopically, the World Health Organization classified HCC as trabecular, acinar, compact, or scirrhous. The tumor cells may be arranged in cords separated by sinusoids (trabecular) in gland-like structures (glandular), or in a compact solid mass devoid of sinusoid (compact). In the scirrhous- type cords, tumor cells are separated by fibrous tissue. Each histologic type is further classified as well, moderate, and poorly differentiated. This classification has been shown to be an independent predictor of prognosis.

Imaging

Ultrasonography is a highly sensitive technique that is commonly used for screening of asymptomatic cirrhotic patients. It typically shows HCC as a solid tumor with irregular or ill-defined margins, and occasionally nonhomogenous echogenicity. It may detect tumors as small as 1 to 2 cm, but it usually cannot distinguish with certainty HCC from other solid lesions such as adenoma or FNA. Doppler ultrasound is useful for detecting thrombosis in the portal or hepatic veins, which raise suspicion for vascular invasion. Contrast enhanced CT is a sensitive and specific technique for the detection of HCCs of 2 cm or larger. The use of spiral triple-phase CT increases the sensitivity considerably and this should be the technique of choice when CT is used in cirrhotic patients.[10] It typically shows early arterial phase contrast enhancement, which is often heterogeneous ("mosaic sign"), and commonly associated with a tumor capsule. Small HCCs, in contrast, are often characterized by a homogenous arterial phase enhancement, which may also be seen in benign lesions such as regenerative nodules, dysplastic nodules, small hemangiomas, and arterial-to-portal shunts. This may make the differentiation from a small HCC difficult. In as many as 27% of the HCCs, the tumor may be detected only on arterial phase images and is not seen on unenhanced or portal venous phase images. Large centrally located tumors are commonly associated with peripheral intrahepatic biliary dilatation. This dilatation usually results from a duct compression rather than biliary invasion, which is uncommon in HCC. Intraarterial infusion of lipiodol followed by a CT scan 10 to 14 days later increases the sensitivity, as the HCC tissue retains the lipiodol. Although rarely used in most centers, Lipiodol injection may be beneficial when HCC is highly suspected (eg, high serum levels of AFP) but has not been demonstrated by other techniques. CT angiography (CT with contrast injection into the hepatic artery) is not used routinely due to its invasiveness, however, it has increased sensitivity and may provide important information regarding the size and location of the tumor in problematic cases.

MRI may occasionally be helpful in distinguishing HCC from a large dysplastic nodule. The latter will show a characteristic pattern of high signal intensity (bright appearance) on T1-weighted images and low signal intensity (dark appearance) on T2-weighted images.

Diagnosis

The diagnosis of HCC may be based on histopathologic criteria when a tissue sample is available, or on a combination of imaging studies and serum level of alpha fetoprotein.[11] Needle biopsy should be performed cautiously due to the vascular nature of this tumor. Another possible risk of a needle biopsy is seeding the needle track with tumor cells. The likelihood of seeding has been estimated to range from 0.006% to 1%. A focal hepatic lesion in a patient with cirrhosis should be suspected as HCC until proven otherwise. According to the Barcelona criteria of the European Association for the Study of Liver Disease (EASL), demonstration of a focal lesion larger than 2 cm with arterial hypervascularization on two imaging techniques (eg, ultrasonography, spiral CT, MRI, or angiography) is diagnostic for HCC in a cirrhotic patient.[9,12] Furthermore, a combination of one imaging technique showing a foal lesion larger than 2 cm with arterial hypervascularization, in association with alfa fetoprotein level of 400 ng/mL or higher is also considered diagnostic for HCC.[9] Cytologic examination of ascetic fluid is invariably negative for tumor cells.

Screening and Surveillance

Surveillance programs using periodical abdominal ultrasonography and serum levels of AFP have become the standard of care in most centers in the United States. Based on the risk for HCC, these programs are targeted at patients with cirrhosis as well as patients with chronic HBV infection who are not cirrhotic. For patients with cirrhosis, 6-month interval for ultrasonography and AFP is considered cost effective; however, no randomized study has shown a survival benefit for screening patients at high risk of HCC.

Treatment

Currently, the only chance for cure in patients with HCC is with a surgical resection or liver transplantation.[11,13] Liver transplantation, when possible, is the treatment of choice in the majority of HCC patients. Based on the Milan Criteria,[14] transplantation should be limited to patients with a solitary lesion less than 5 cm in diameter or for patients with fewer than three tumors, each smaller than 3 cm. It has been shown that larger tumors are associated with an increased frequency of vascular invasion and higher risk of recurrence post-transplant. The 5-year post-transplant survival of patient fulfilling the Milan criteria is approximately 70%. Although recently challenged by several authors, these criteria are used by most transplant centers in the United States and Europe. In contrast to liver transplantation, resection can be performed only in patients with compensated liver disease, and is possible in a minority of the patients. It can be performed by segmentectomy, partial hepatectomy, or hemihepatectomy. Generally, surgical resection is feasible in tumors that are confined to one hepatic lobe with no vascular invasion. Resection may be a preferred option in centers with limited access to transplantation or a long waiting-time (exceeding 6 to 10 months). The risk of tumor recurrence is approximately 50% in 2 years.[15] Other approaches are based on local ablation of the tumor and are considered primarily palliative. These include percutaneous ethanol injection, radiofrequency ablation, cryoablation, or microwave coagulation. Local ablative therapies may be used as a bridge to transplantation during the waiting period. Larger tumors can be treated by embolization of the supplying branch of the hepatic artery, or by direct hepatic artery injection of chemotherapy followed by local embolization. Chemoembolization has recently been shown to provide survival benefit in HCC patients.[16] The procedure may be complicated by postembolization syndrome (abdominal pain, fever, chills, nausea, vomiting, and leukocytosis) and transient, but occasionally irreversible hepatic decompensation. Cytotoxic therapy administered via the intra-arterial route is believed to be superior to systemic chemotherapy in HCC. Hepatic artery ligation has also been shown to be effective in reducing tumor size. In contrast, systemic chemotherapy with various cytotoxic agents has not been found to be effective. Similarly, there is no strong evidence suggesting benefit from treatment options such as tamoxifen, octreotide, proton beam radiation, or antiandrogens. Hepatitis B vaccination has been shown to decrease the incidence of HCC.[11,17,18]

Fibrolamellar Hepatocellular Carcinoma

Fibrolamellar hepatocellular carcinoma is a subtype of HCC exhibiting distinct features both clinically and histopathologically. As apposed to the typical HCC, it occurs primarily in noncirrhotic livers of young adults. Its incidence is approximately 1% of all HCCs, and is equal for male and female patients. The serum levels of AFP are elevated in less than 20% of the patients. About half the patients may exhibit a central scar, which commonly contains small calcifications. Calcifications are uncommon both in HCC and in FNH which may help differentiating between the lesions. Histologically, it is composed of large eosinophilic cells arranged in trabecules, which are surrounded by fibrous bands with lamellar stranding. Since fibrolamellar carcinomas are usually localized and sharply demarcated, and usually arise in noncirrhotic livers, they are more often suitable for resection than the usual forms of HCC. In addition, the outcome of liver transplantation far exceeds that observed in the nonfibrolamellar type of HCC.

Cholangiocarcinoma

Cholangicarcinoma is a malignant tumor of bile duct epithelium that accounts for approximately 10% of all primary liver cancers. It is uncommon in Western countries; however, its prevalence is higher in parts of Southeastern and Eastern Asia. Less than 10% of the cholangiocarcinomas are intrahepatic, most of them in elderly patients. The rest are located in the extraheptic biliary tree, 50% to 60% in the bifurcation of the common bile duct (Klatskin tumor), and the rest in other areas of the bile duct. Several predisposing factors have been recognized including 1) sclerosing cholangitis, 2) inflammatory bowel diseases, 3) chronic hepatobiliary parasitic infections (eg, Clonorchis sinensis; Opisthorchis viverrini), 4) choledochal cyst, 5) biliary atresia, and 6) exposure to biliary tract carcinogens (eg, thorium dioxide). Patients with distal cholangiocarcinoma usually present with painless jaundice, pruritus, weight loss, and acholic stools. In patients with distal lesions, the gallbladder may be distended, and easily palpable. Intrahepatic lesion may be indistinguishable from HCC. The diagnosis is made by demonstrating the lesion on magnetic resonance cholangiography (MRC), endoscopic retrograde cholangiogrphy (ERC), or percutaneous transhepatic cholangiogrphy (PTC). Cholangiography allows obtaining specimens for cytological examination by brushing or biopsy, but the yield of this test is low, and its sensitivity is less than 60%. Cholangiography also allows insertion of stents for biliary drainage. Cholangiocarcinoma carries poor prognosis and is typically advanced by the time it presents clinically. Chemotherapy and irradiation have not been shown to have a beneficial effect. Less than 20% of the tumors are respectable, and in these cases, complete resection is the treatment of choice. However, even when a lesion is deemed resectable the 5-year survival ranges from 10% to 30%. Treatment with liver transplantation is controversial, and 5-year survival probably does not exceed 25%.

Other Malignant Tumor

Hepatoblastoma is a malignant tumor of fetal hepatocytes, which is the most frequent malignant hepatic tumor in children. Its peak incidence is in the first 2 years of life, and it is rare beyond the second decade. It is usually a solitary lesion that ranges in size from a few centimeters to 15 cm or more. It is typically associated with very high serum levels of AFP, which is elevated in 90% of the cases. It may be resectable in almost 40% of the patients, and the outcome of resection in these patients is excellent. The survival rate declines progressively, as the stage of the tumor increases.

Angiosarcoma is a rare mesenchymal neoplasm of the liver. It consists of vascular spaces lined by malignant endothelial cells. It has been associated with exposure to the radioactive contrast agent thorium dioxide, vinyl chloride polymer, arsenic, and androgenic anabolic steroids. Its peak incidence is in men in their sixth to seventh decade of life.

Most patients present late in the course of the disease and distant metastases are already present in more than 60%, mostly in the lungs and spleen. Most patients die within 6 months. Chemotherapy and radiotherapy are of limited value, and liver transplantation is contraindicated due to the high risk of recurrence.

Epithelioid hemangioendothelioma is a rare hepatic tumor of vascular origin. It may present from the second to the eighth decade, and its prognosis is extremely variable. It is typically a slow growing tumor and may be associated with long survival even in the presence of metastatic disease. The diagnosis can be made with a fine-needle aspiration, and immunohistochemical staining reveals expression of factor VIII antigen. A 5-year survival rate of 43% has been achieved with liver transplantation. Due to its slow growth rate, extrahepatic involvement is not considered an absolute contraindication to liver transplantation.

Clinical Approach to a Solid Liver Lesion

The evaluation and management of solid hepatic lesions is a cooperative venture that requires a multidisciplinary approach. Detailed history, physical examination, hepatic biochemical tests, imaging studies, and histopathological assessment are all of major importance in making the diagnosis.[19] The appropriate selection of imaging techniques depends on the clinical context. The specific approach may vary with the presentation of the lesion, the demographic details of the patients, and the medical history.

The diagnostic approach in a solid tumor found in a young, previously healthy women, should focus on the differential diagnosis of hemangioma, FNH, and adenoma. In contrast, in a middle-aged man with a recent history of colon cancer and no previous history of liver disease, the most likely diagnosis would be a metastatic lesion.

A different diagnosis should be suggested in a patient with pre-existing cirrhosis or chronic HBV, where the likely diagnosis would be HCC or a macroregenerative nodule. The diagnostic approach should, therefore, include a detailed history and physical examination to assess whether an underlying liver disease or a comorbid illness is present. In addition, hepatic biochemical tests, tumor markers, serological markers for viral hepatitis, and contrast-enhanced dynamic CT scan should be obtained. Ultrasonography is a useful screening test; however, in most instances, it is not sufficient for a final diagnosis. Triphasic contrast-enhanced CT scan is usually necessary for an accurate diagnosis. It also assists in detecting additional small hepatic masses and evaluating for other intra-abdominal lesions. In the absence of a history or clinical evidence suggestive of malignancy or pre-existing liver disease, a solid liver lesion is most likely benign. The most common solid benign hepatic lesions are hemangioma (approximately 4%), FNH (0.4%), and adenoma (less than 0.004%). FNH and hemangioma typically have characteristic features on imaging studies, and are diagnosed with a high degree of accuracy with no histological examination. When a hemangioma is suspected, delayed venous phase images should be requested. In questionable lesions, contrast-enhanced MRI may add important information. Occasionally, a diagnostic laparoscopy in a specialized Medical Center may help in establishing the diagnosis. Angiography may also add important information and should be considered prior to surgery. When the likely diagnosis is FNH in an asymptomatic patient, this patient may be followed by ultrasonography or CT scans every 3 to 6 months for 1 year. Liver biopsy is usually not recommended and is better avoided when adenoma is suspected, because of the risk of bleeding and low diagnostic yield.

References

1. Charny CK, Jarnagin WR, Schwartz LH, et al. Management of 155 patients with benign liver tumours. *Br J Surg.* 2001;88(6):808-813.
2. Vilgrain V, Boulos L, Vullierme MP, et al. Imaging of atypical hemangiomas of the liver with pathologic correlation. *Radiographics.* 2000;20(2):379-397.
3. Kim T, Federle MP, Baron RL, Peterson MS, Kawamori Y. Discrimination of small hepatic hemangiomas from hypervascular malignant tumors smaller than 3 cm with three-phase helical CT. *Radiology.* 2001;219(3):699-706.
4. Kehagias D, Moulopoulos L, Antoniou A, et al. Focal nodular hyperplasia: imaging findings. *Eur Radiol.* 2001;11(2):202-212.
5. Brancatelli G, Federle MP, Grazioli L, Blachar A, Peterson MS, Thaete L. Focal nodular hyperplasia: CT findings with emphasis on multiphasic helical CT in 78 patients. *Radiology.* 2001;219(1):61-68.
6. Mortele KJ, Praet M, Van VH, Kunnen M, Ros PR. CT and MR imaging findings in focal nodular hyperplasia of the liver: radiologic-pathologic correlation. *Am J Roentgenol.* 2000;175(3):687-692.
7. Reddy KR, Kligerman S, Levi J, et al. Benign and solid tumors of the liver: relationship to sex, age, size of tumors, and outcome. *Am Surg.* 2001;67(2):173-178.
8. El-Serag H, Davila J, Petersen N, McGlynn K. The continuing increase in the incidence of hepatocellular carcinoma in the United States: an update. *Ann Intern Med.* 2003;139(10):817-823.
9. Bruix J, Sherman M, Llovet JM, et al. Clinical management of hepatocellular carcinoma. Conclusions of the Barcelona-2000 EASL conference. European Association for the Study of the Liver. *J Hepatol.* 2001;35(3):421-430.

10. Peterson MS, Baron RL. Radiologic diagnosis of hepatocellular carcinoma. *Clin Liver Dis.* 2001;5(1):123-144.
11. Befeler AS, Di Bisceglie AM. Hepatocellular carcinoma: diagnosis and treatment. *Gastroenterology.* 2002;122(6):1609-1619.
12. Llovet JM, Fuster J, Bruix J. The Barcelona approach: diagnosis, staging, and treatment of hepatocellular carcinoma. *Liver Transpl.* 2004;10(2 Suppl 1):S115-S120.
13. Omata M, Yoshida H. Prevention and treatment of hepatocellular carcinoma *Liver Transpl.* 2004;10(2 Suppl 1):S111-S114.
14. Mazzaferro V, Regalia E, Doci R, et al. Liver transplantation for the treatment of small hepatocellular carcinomas in patients with cirrhosis. *N Engl J Med.* 1996;334(11): 693-699.
15. Poon RT, Fan ST, Lo CM, Liu CL, Wong J. Intrahepatic recurrence after curative resection of hepatocellular carcinoma: long-term results of treatment and prognostic factors. *Ann Surg.* 1999;229(2):216-222.
16. Llovet JM, Bruix J. Systematic review of randomized trials for unresectable hepatocellular carcinoma: Chemoembolization improves survival. *Hepatology.* 2003;37(2):429-442.
17. Chang MH, Chen CJ, Lai MS, et al. Universal hepatitis B vaccination in Taiwan and the incidence of hepatocellular carcinoma in children. Taiwan Childhood Hepatoma Study Group. *N Engl J Med.* 1997;336(26):1855-1859.
18. Chang MH. Decreasing incidence of hepatocellular carcinoma among children following universal hepatitis B immunization. *Liver Int.* 2003;23(5):309-314.
19. Rubin RA, Mitchell DG. Evaluation of the solid hepatic mass. M*ed Clin North Am.* 1996;80(5):907-928.

chapter 10

Liver Disease in Pregnancy

Rena Desai Callahan, MD and K. Rajender Reddy, MD

Introduction

Liver disease during pregnancy is an entity with unique considerations as the health of both the mother and her fetus is involved. Early diagnosis and timely intervention can reduce perinatal and maternal morbity and mortality, so it is important to have a high index of suspicion for potential conditions affecting the liver. The wide spectrum of liver disease in the pregnant female can be categorized as 1) liver disease unique to pregnancy, 2) intercurrent liver disease in pregnancy, and 3) chronic liver disease in pregnancy. This chapter will explore the epidemiology, etiology, diagnosis, and management of the myriad liver diseases that occur in the pregnant female.

There are several overlapping symptoms, signs, and laboratory parameters associated with these entities. Therefore, gestational age should be used to guide the differential diagnosis for hepatic biochemical test abnormalities during pregnancy. For example, hyperemesis gravidarum is a first trimester condition, whereas intrahepatic cholestasis of pregnancy (ICP) may present in the second trimester. Pre-eclampsia and the HELLP syndrome (Hemolysis, Elevated Liver tests, Low Platelets) predominantly occur in the third trimester. While they may occur at any time, conditions such as acute viral hepatitis may be more severe during the third trimester and portal hypertension during the second trimester or labor.

Liver in Normal Pregnancy

Pregnancy is associated with several expected physical and physiologic changes. In order to recognize the pathologic changes that result from liver disease, it is first necessary to understand the normal physiology of the liver during pregnancy (Table 10-1).

History and physical exam may reveal a variety of nonpathologic features. For instance, fatigue from increased energy demands and frequent urination due to bladder compression from the enlarged uterus are commonly noted. Heart rate is increased, whereas blood pressure is decreased. Palmar erythema may be seen which

Table 10-1

Normal Changes in Laboratory Parameters During Pregnancy

	Decreased	*Unchanged*	*Increased*
Hepatic	Albumin Bile salts	ALT AST Bilirubin LDH	Alkalinephosphatase Gamma globulins Lipids
Hematologic	Hematocrit Hemoglobin	MCV Platelets PT PTT	Clotting factors ESR Fibrinogen White blood cells
Endocrine and metabolism	Fasting glucose	Free T3 Free T4 TSH	α-1 and 2 globulins Ceruloplasmin Cholesterol Estrogen hCG hPL Plasma insulin Progesterone TBG Total T3 Total T4 Transferrin
Renal	BUN Creatinine Uric acid	Urine protein	Creatinine clearance GFR Urine glucose

ALT = Alanine Aminotransferase; AST = Aspartate aminotransferase; BUN = Blood urea nitrogen; ESR = Erythrocyte sedimentation rate; GFR = Glomerular filtration rate; hCG = Human chorionic gonadotropin; hPL = Human placental lactogen; LDH = Lactate dehydrogenase; MCV = Mean corpuscular volume; PT = Prothrombin time; PTT = Partial Thromboplastin Time; TBG = Thyroid binding globulin; TSH = Thyroid stimulating hormone

Adapted from Bacq Y, Zarka O, Brechot J-F, et al. Liver function tests in normal pregnancy: a prospective study of 103 pregnant women and 103 matched controls. *Hepatology.* 1996;23:1030-1034.

is due to the hyperestrogenic state of pregnancy. Additionally, varicose veins over the lower extremities may be noted. Minute ventilation increases resulting in a mild respiratory alkalosis.

Pregnancy routinely results in significant hemodynamic shifts. During pregnancy, plasma volume is known to increase by approximately 40%. The rise begins in the sixth week and continues through the 32nd week of gestation. Red blood cell mass also increases, albeit proportionally less than plasma volume. Therefore, the hematocrit decreases, resulting in dilutional anemia. The anticipated increase in cardiac output and heart rate peak at 32 weeks. However, net blood flow to the liver remains the same or is slightly decreased. Blood pressure initially decreases due to systemic vasodilation. However, starting at 24 weeks, blood pressure should begin to rise, reaching prepregnant levels by term. Despite compression of the vena cava by the gravid uterus, there should be a net increase in venous return.. Laboratory values of platelet count, prothrombin, prothromboplastin time, antithrombin III, or protein C do not change. However, pregnancy is a hypercoagulable state in which levels of fibrinogen and other clotting factors may be elevated.

Measurements of proteins and lipids are affected by pregnancy. Triglycerides, cholesterol, ceruloplasmin, transferrin, and α-1 and 2 globulins may all increase. Cholesterol and triglycerides both steadily increase up to term and return to prepregnant levels at about 20 weeks postpartum. The increase in triglycerides is related to overproduction of very low-density lipoproteins, which are needed to serve as a fetal energy source. A concomitant decrease in high-density lipoprotein cholesterol may be seen. Greater hepatic production of immunoglobulins may produce a false-positive rapid plasma reagin (RPR) test due to cross reactivity.

Hepatic biochemical tests display pregnancy-related variation as well. Alkaline phosphatase may rise three to four times higher than nonpregnant values due to the contribution of placental alkaline phosphatase that begins at 20 weeks gestation. In the second trimester, the bile salt pool decreases. Additionally, biliary cholesterol may increase. There is also a decrease in albumin, urea, and uric acid in the third trimester. The decrease in albumin is dilutional, whereas the change in urea and uric acid occurs secondary to increased renal clearance.

Imaging During Pregnancy

Imaging studies play a significant role in the evaluation of liver disease during pregnancy. However, the use of diagnostic imaging in pregnancy raises concerns for the safety of the fetus, but it must be remembered that a delayed diagnosis due to avoidance of imaging also poses risk of substantial fetal harm. Imaging modalities may be divided into those that use ionizing radiation, such as plain x-ray films, angiography, computed tomography (CT), and nuclear scans, and those that do not, including magnetic resonance imaging (MRI) and ultrasound. Use of ionizing radiation and higher radiation dose increases potential for harm. The risk also increases at a gestational age of 3 to 10 weeks that corresponds to the period of organogenesis. In general, MRI and ultrasound are considered safe for the fetus. However, the use of MRI during the first trimester should be avoided due to limited data on its effect on organogenesis. Other imaging modalities should be used with caution and only after a complete discussion of potential risks with the patient has taken place.

Liver Disease Unique to Pregnancy

The diseases involving the liver that are exclusive to pregnancy include intrahepatic cholestasis of pregnancy (ICP), acute fatty liver of pregnancy (AFLP), hyperemesis gravidarum, preeclampsia, and HELLP.

Intrahepatic Cholestasis of Pregnancy

Definition and Epidemiology

ICP is an idiopathic cholestatic condition that is characterized by pruritus that is intense at times. Pruritus may markedly impair the quality of life of the mother but more significantly, can result in fetal morbidity or mortality. ICP occurs in only 0.01% of pregnancies in the United States. Higher rates are reported in Sweden where 1% to 2% of pregnancies are affected. In Chile, rates are as high as 6.5% among the general population and 24% among Auracian Indians.[2] ICP generally presents in the third trimester, but has been known to begin at any time between 6 weeks gestation to immediately postpartum. Risk factors include a positive family history and a history of oral contraceptive related cholestasis. The recurrence rate in subsequent pregnancies is high and is approximately 60% (Table 10-2).

Etiology

While the cause of ICP is unknown, a genetic and environmental etiology is suggested by the increased prevalence within certain ethnic communities (Swedish, Chilean, and Auracian Indians). Studies have been undertaken to associate specific HLA haplotypes with development of disease. However, there is no definitive evidence for a specific genetic defect. ICP may be precipitated by pregnancy-related hormonal effects on metabolism. For example, estrogen may impair sulfation, leading to an increase in glucoronide metabolites that are known to promote cholestasis. There may be a familial predisposition to this hormonal sensitivity.

Diagnosis

Symptoms of ICP include progressive pruritus that is prominent in the arms, legs, and trunk. During history and exam, the patient is often noted to be very uncomfortable and scratching oneself. Excoriations are usually observed on the extremities. Jaundice occurs in 20% of ICP cases and may follow the pruritus by approximately 2 weeks. These findings generally disappear a few days postpartum. Another symptom of ICP may be steatorrhea.

In ICP, there is an increase in fasting serum bile acids, especially conjugated primary bile acids such as cholic acid. The rise in gamma glutamyl transferase (GGT), expected with other cholestatic conditions, may be absent in ICP, lending measurement of bile acids of greater importance in formulating the diagnosis. Bilirubin is often elevated, but usually remains less than 5 mg/dL. It consists primarily of the conjugated fraction. Alanine aminotransferase (ALT) and aspartate aminotransferase (AST) are usually 2 to 10 times the upper limit of normal, but can be as high as 50 times that of the normal value. A modest increase in triglycerides and cholesterol may also be observed.

Imaging with ultrasound may be useful in excluding other causes of pruritus and jaundice including cholelithiasis and biliary tract disease. An enlarged gallbladder is

Table 10-2

Recurrence of Liver Disease in Subsequent Pregnancies

Liver Disease	*Recurrence Rate*
Acute Fatty Liver of Pregnancy	Rare
Intrahepatic Cholestasis of Pregnancy	45% to 70%
Hyperemesis Gravidarum	48%
Pre-eclampsia	20% to 42%
HELLP	3% to 19%

Adapted from Martin JN J, Rinehart BK, May WL, et al. The spectrum of severe preeclampsia: comparative analysis by HELLP syndrome classification. *Am J Obstet Gynecol.* 1999;180:1373-1384; Eliakim R, Abulafia O, Sherer DM. Hyperemesis gravidarum: a current review. *Am J Perinatol.* 2000;17:207-218; Sandhu BS, Sanyal AJ. Pregnancy and liver disease. *Gastroenterol Clin N Am.* 2003;32:407-436; Sibai BM, Ramadan MK, Chari RS, Friedman SA. Pregnancies complicated by HELLP syndrome (hemolysis, elevated liver enzymes, and low platelets): subsequent pregnancy outcome and long-term prognosis. *Am J Obstet Gynecol.* 1995;172(1 Pt 1):125-9; Sullivan CA, Magann EF, Perry KG Jr, Roberts WE, Blake PG, Martin JN Jr. The recurrence risk of the syndrome of hemolysis, elevated liver enzymes, and low platelets (HELLP) in subsequent gestations. *Am J Obstet Gynecol.* 1994;171:940-943.

sometimes noted in patients with ICP. Liver biopsy, which is generally not indicated, shows nonspecific findings of cholestasis such as centrilobular bile stasis.

Treatment/Management

The serum bile acids, albumin, and alkaline phosphatase should be followed closely as changes in these parameters may indicate worsening disease. Therapy with ursodeoxycholic acid (UDCA) has been demonstrated to improve both pruritus and abnormalities of hepatic biochemical tests. UDCA is a tertiary bile acid that replaces lithocholic acid, a potential hepatotoxic agent that is commonly increased in ICP. UDCA may also decrease absorption of cholic and chenodeoxycholic acid. The dosage is usually 15 mg/kg/day, divided twice a day. In some animal studies, therapy with UDCA had displayed teratogenic potential. However, it is considered to be safe for the fetus when administered late in pregnancy, which is the time ICP manifests.

Cholestyramine, a bile acid binding resin has been shown to improve pruritus, but neither hepatic biochemical tests nor fetal prognosis. Additionally, use of cholestyramine must proceed with caution as it may lead to decreased absorption of fat-soluble vitamins, notably vitamin K, which may result in greater risk of hemorrhagic complications. S-adenosyl methionine (SAMe) may decrease both pruritus and hepatic biochemical test abnormalities. However, results with SAMe therapy in ICP have varied across studies. Other medications used to decrease pruritus include phenobarbital and dexamathasone. Potential complications associated with ICP include an increased risk of preterm delivery, meconium, and fetal distress, which result in a perinatal mortality of approximately 3%. Due to this risk, delivery of the fetus by 38 weeks is considered with earlier delivery when jaundice and bile acids >1.8 mg/dL are present. There is a higher incidence of postpartum cholelithiasis in pregnancies complicated by ICP. Both fetal and maternal outcomes have been improving with close monitoring which includes fetal non stress tests, amniocentesis, and induction of labor following demonstration of fetal lung maturity.

Acute Fatty Liver of Pregnancy

Definition and Epidemiology

Acute fatty liver of pregnancy is a rare condition occurring in approximately 1 in 10,000 pregnancies. This entity was first described in 1940 by Sheehan and termed, "acute yellow atrophy of pregnancy." Although relatively rare, when AFLP occurs, it has serious implications. Both maternal and fetal mortality approach 20%. Much lower mortality rates were described in a recent study by Ch'ng et al, and may be attributed to greater vigilance and recognition of the condition at early stages. The risk of AFLP appears to be increased with multiple gestation pregnancies, male births, and primiparous females.

Etiology

Mitochondrial dysfunction, specifically long chain 3 hydroxyl coA dehydrogenase (LCHAD) deficiency (a failure of beta oxidation), may contribute to the development of AFLP. Recent research has demonstrated an increased risk of AFLP when there exists a homozygous LCHAD deficiency in the fetus combined with heterozygous LCHAD deficiency in the mother. Females with a history of AFLP should consider genetic testing for specific LCHAD mutations.[3] Short chain deficiency has also emerged as a potential contributor to the development of AFLP.

Diagnosis

Symptoms of AFLP include sudden anorexia, nausea, vomiting, abdominal pain, polydipsia, fever, and malaise. Jaundice is observed in the majority of cases, which occurs one to two weeks after the onset of other symptoms. Headache and other CNS disturbances are sometimes present. The onset of symptoms of AFLP usually occurs between 30 and 38 weeks gestation, but may occur as early as 26 weeks or even postpartum.

The differential diagnosis of AFLP includes HELLP and other causes of fulminant hepatic failure including hepatitis E and HSV hepatitis (Table 10-3). Laboratory data and imaging studies can be used to distinguish between these causes. The diagnosis is primarily clinical and may need to be confirmed by a liver biopsy. Laboratory abnormalities are common and include moderately increased transaminases, usually less than 1000. Prolonged prothrombin time (PT), partial thromboplastin time (PTT), thrombocytopenia, and decreased fibrinogen are often found and warn of disseminated intravascular coagulation (DIC). Bilirubin may also be increased with values generally between one and 10 mg/dL. Leukocytosis is often present. Hypoglycemia is a common finding in AFLP and is related to decreased liver synthetic function. Hyperammonemia and increased creatinine are also seen.[11]

Ultrasound imaging of AFLP displays increased echogenicity consistent with fatty infiltration and CT demonstrates low attenuation. The overall liver architecture is generally intact, and, therefore, false-negative imaging studies are common. Biopsy is recommended in cases when hepatic biochemical tests and coagulation studies do not

Table 10-3

Signs of AFLP vs HELLP Syndrome

	Decreased	*Unchanged*	*Increased*
AFLP Early	Fibrogen Glucose Platelets	LDH	ALT AST Ammonia Bilirubin PT PTT
AFLP Late	Fibrogen Glucose Platelets	LDH	ALT AST Ammonia Bilirubin PT PTT
HELLP Early	Haptoglobin Platelets<150K	Ammonia Bilirubin Fibrinogen Glucose LDH PT PTT	ALT AST LDH
HELLP Late	Haptoglobin Platelets <50K	Ammonia Fibrinogen Glucose PTT	ALT AST Bilirubin LDH PT

Adapted from Martin JN J, Rinehart BK, May WL, et al. The spectrum of severe preeclampsia: comparative analysis by HELLP syndrome classification. *Am J Obstet Gynecol.* 1999;180:1373-1384.

normalize after delivery or when diagnosis is uncertain, particularly in the early stages, so that early delivery can be initiated. Liver biopsy may be contraindicated in cases of severe underlying coagulopathy due to the bleeding risk. Centrilobular microvesicular fatty infiltration of hepatocytes is the most common microscopic finding in AFLP.

Treatment/Management

Delivery of the fetus and monitoring in the intensive care unit is the cornerstone of treatment of AFLP. Postponing delivery, especially in severe cases, may have dire consequences. Patients may require supportive care, fluid resuscitation, glycemic control, correction of coagulopathies, platelet transfusions, antihypertensive therapy, and antiseizure medication. There have been a few cases in which liver transplant was performed. Complications of AFLP are severe and may include maternal cerebral edema, gastrointestinal hemorrhage, renal failure, DIC, and sepsis. Up to half of the patients develop preeclampsia, which complicates both diagnosis and management. Acute renal failure and DIC develop in more than 70% of patients with AFLP. Children with homozygous LCHAD deficiency may manifest nonketotic fasting hypoglycemia and hepatic encephalopathy several months after birth to a mother with AFLP. Recurrence of AFLP is uncommon partly due to the unwillingness or inability for the patient to become pregnant again.

Acute Fatty Liver of Pregnancy and Intrahepatic Cholestasis of Pregnancy

An association between acute fatty liver (AFLP) and intrahepatic cholestasis of pregnancy (ICP) has been reported.[4] This patient appeared to experience both clinical entities during pregnancy, and exhibited pruritus as the first symptom. ICP was diagnosed first, during a timeframe considered too early for manifestation of AFLP. After delivery, aminotransferase levels did not normalize as expected, and, therefore, AFLP was suspected and diagnosed. It is unclear if patients with a similar progression have a less severe form of AFLP with an earlier presentation or true, concomitant ICP and AFLP. It is thought that in these patients ICP may protect against complications of AFLP since it may induce premature or earlier delivery.

Hyperemesis Gravidarum

Definition and Epidemiology

Liver involvement is common in hyperemesis gravidarum (HG), a condition of protracted emesis during pregnancy resulting in electrolyte derangements. While nausea and vomiting are very common in pregnancy with reported rates as high as 80%, hyperemesis gravidarum only occurs in 0.5% of pregnancies. An increased incidence has been noted in nulliparous females, multiple gestation pregnancies, and gestational trophoblastic disease. Since liver dysfunction only occurs in 50% of HG, and usually with more severe course of HG and with laboratory abnormalities resolving concurrently with the disease, the dysfunction is thought to be a secondary event in HG.

Etiology

The cause of HG is unknown. Hormonal variations in pregnancy may play a role in the etiology. Specifically, elevated thyroxine levels may be involved. The mechanism of hormonal involvement may occur via beta human chorionic gonadotropin (HCG), which is known to elevate thyroid hormone levels by cross activating the thyroid stimulating hormone (TSH) receptor. Some studies have shown higher beta HCG levels in patients with HG. The HCG induced elevated thyroid hormone level may predispose a pregnant female to develop HG. However, a direct causal relationship has not yet been established. Recently, an association between HG and *Helicobacter pylori* (*H. pylori*) seropositivity has been demonstrated. In one study, 90.5% of females with HG were *H. pylori* positive in comparison to 46.5% of controls.[5] Antibiotic treatment of *H. pylori* resulted in improvement of HG in several patients.

Diagnosis

Symptoms and signs of HG include weight loss, electrolyte abnormalities, ketonemia, ketonuria, dehydration, and renal damage. Many patients have also noted ptyalism. When liver involvement is marked, jaundice may be present. HG starts in the first trimester during the fourth to tenth week, peaks at the eighth to twelfth week, and resolves by 20 weeks gestation.

The differential diagnosis of liver disease and nausea during pregnancy is broad and includes drug toxicity, viral hepatitis, AFLP, HELLP, cholelithiasis, and peptic ulcer disease. In diagnosing HG, liver biopsy is not recommended and would only be expected to show minor, nonspecific changes. Similarly, imaging is not necessary and is only used to evaluate the complications of this condition. Laboratory values and clinical findings assist in making the diagnosis of HG.

This condition may be accompanied by transient hyperthyroidism as discussed previously. Abnormalities in transaminases are seen in half, with values generally less than 1000 IU/L. A mild conjugated and unconjugated hyperbilirubinemia also occurs in half. Other laboratory values may reflect dehydration (eg, increased urine specific gravity, increased blood urea nitrogen and hematocrit, hypokalemia, hypochloremia, hyponatremia).

Treatment/Management

Inpatient admission is usually required to manage HG. Bowel rest and maintaining hydration with intravenous fluids are essential. In severe cases, enteral feeding may restore nutrition. Lab monitoring should include a complete blood count, electrolyte panel, liver function tests, and urinalysis. Daily weights and intake and output should also be recorded. Several medications have been used with success and these include ondansetron, methylprednisolone, and droperidol. Vitamin B_6 and ginger have also been used. Once the vomiting ceases, these patients may be given small meals of clear liquids that are advanced as tolerated. An outpatient course of antiemetics is commonly needed. Despite seemingly adequate treatment, up to one third of discharged patients require readmission for similar symptoms.

Appropriately treated, HG is associated with favorable outcomes for both the mother and her fetus. However, rarely, life threatening conditions such as Wernicke's encephalopathy, central pontine myelinolysis, cerebral artery vasospasm, pneumomediastinum, and Boorhaeve's syndrome have been reported.

Pre-Eclampsia/Eclampsia

Definition and Epidemiology

Pre-eclampsia, a hypertensive disease of pregnancy is common and found in 5% of all pregnancies. It manifests as a triad of hypertension, proteinuria, and edema. The risk of developing pre-eclampsia is increased in nulliparas, females with chronic hypertension, pregestational diabetes, multifetal gestation, positive family history, very young or advanced maternal age, and previous episodes. Pre-eclampsia does not usually involve the liver. However, its dreaded progression to HELLP demonstrates liver involvement.

Etiology

The etiology of pre-eclampsia is unknown but may be related to uteroplacental ischemia, which may then trigger maternal endothelial injury and subsequently the coagulation cascade. There may also be a genetic component suggested by the elevated risk of pre-eclampsia when there exists a positive family history. Earlier onset of disease is associated with greater risk to the mother and fetus compared with near term presentations. The etiology may vary with time of presentation.

Diagnosis

Pre-eclampsia associated hypertension is defined as a rise in systolic blood pressure (BP) of 30 mmHg or diastolic BP of 15 mmHg from baseline or any BP above 140/90 mmHg. Significant proteinuria is considered to be above 300 mg over 24 hours. Edema of the hands and face is often observed. Increased uric acid may reflect impaired tubular function decreasing uric acid clearance. Low platelet count with increased platelet activation is common. Pre-eclampsia usually manifests during the second half of the second trimester through the third trimester.

Treatment/Management

Delivery of the fetus is the only definitive treatment for pre-eclampsia and is standard beyond 36 weeks of gestation. Vaginal delivery is preferred when possible. Between 28 and 32 weeks, "expectant management" should be undertaken. As part of this management, hypertension must be controlled with a medication safe for use in pregnancy. Methyldopa is one such antihypertensive agent. In emergency situations, hydralazine may be used. To prevent progression to eclampsia in which seizures are typical, prophylactic MgSO4 should be administered. If MgSO4 is contraindicated, phenytoin may be used. Steroids may accelerate fetal lung maturity in the event that early delivery is required. They should be tapered after delivery to avoid a rebound decrease in platelet count. Additionally, the patient must be monitored intensively for 24 to 72 hours after delivery as serious complications including eclampsia, HELLP, cerebral hemorrhage, DIC, and renal failure may ensue. Pre-eclampsia recurs in 20% to 42% of pregnancies (see Table 10-2).

Hemolysis, Elevated Liver Tests, Low Platelets

Definition and Epidemiology

Three to 10% of cases of pre-eclampsia progress to HELLP, the syndrome of hemolysis, elevated liver tests, and low platelets, first described by Weinstein in 1982. This condition may be a more severe form of pre-eclampsia with a similar etiology. HELLP complicates 0.5% of all live births. It is a serious disease, resulting in maternal mortality of approximately 2% and fetal mortality of around 33%. There may be an increased risk in white and multiparous females.

Etiology

Liver damage in HELLP may be cytokine mediated or a result of abnormally activated neutrophils. The systemic vascular abnormalities may be due to overactivity of the coagulation and complement cascades. Ultimately, endothelial and microvascular injury may result in microangiopathic hemolytic anemia (MAHA), abnormal hepatic biochemical tests, and decreased platelet counts that characterize HELLP. There may also be an endothelial excess of procoagulants and vasoconstrictors (thromboxane, endothelin) over anticoagulants and vasodilators (prostacyclin, nitric oxide). This imbalance may trigger the disseminated intravascular coagulation seen in 20% to 40% of HELLP.

Diagnosis

HELLP is associated with symptoms of right upper quadrant abdominal pain and malaise. Additionally, over half of the patients report nondependent edema, nausea, and vomiting. In contrast to pre-eclampsia, less than 20% of patients are hypertensive at diagnosis. Ten percent of patients have little or no proteinuria. There is often no correlation between presence of proteinuria, degree of hypertension, and other laboratory findings. HELLP may manifest anytime between the midsecond trimester and several days postpartum. Seventy percent of cases occur between 27 and 32 weeks, and 20% of cases present postpartum. The differential diagnosis of HELLP includes ITP (Idiopathic Thrombocytopenic Purpura), SLE (Systemic Lupus Erythematosus), HUS (Hemolytic Uremic Syndrome), TTP (Thrombotic Thrombocytopenic Purpura), and AFLP. The diagnosis of HELLP is best made using clinical judgment in combination with laboratory tests. When HELLP is suspected, laboratory tests should be obtained every 6 to 8 hours. Laboratory values suggesting hemolysis include increased bilirubin and LDH>600 IU/L. Decreased haptoglobin is a very sensitive marker of HELLP and is found in the overwhelming majority of cases. This decreased haptoglobin precedes the reduction of platelet count. There are some cases of HELLP in which haptoglobin is falsely normal as in the case of inflammatory conditions. In this situation, all acute phase proteins are elevated. Therefore, it may be helpful to measure C reactive protein in addition to looking for signs of infection. Haptoglobin values normalize 24 to 30 hours postpartum.

Moderate increases in transaminases of 200 to 700 IU/L (3 times the upper limit of normal) and platelet counts below 100,000 per mL also support the diagnosis of HELLP. The severity of thrombocytopenia correlates with the degree of liver dysfunction. The platelet count should normalize in 6 to 11 days postpartum, but should trend upward within 4 days of delivery. Liver enzyme abnormalities generally resolve 3 to 5 days postpartum. Finding a positive D dimer in the setting of pre-eclampsia signifies an elevated risk of HELLP. A prolonged prothrombin time is not usually part of HELLP, unless disseminated intravascular coagulation is present.

Biopsy is rarely needed to diagnose HELLP, but would be expected to show periportal hemorrhage and fibrin deposition with hepatocellular necrosis.

Treatment/Management

As with pre-eclampsia, delivery of the fetus is the only definitive treatment for HELLP. There are several systems designed to classify the severity of HELLP, most notably the Mississippi triple classification. Platelet count is less than 50, 100, and

150 thousand in classes I, II, and III, respectively. The lowest antepartum platelet count should be used in classification. Additional laboratory values such as LDH above 1400, AST greater than 150, uric acid greater than 7.8 and decreased platelets are correlated with increased maternal morbidity.[3] These systems help weigh the risks of early delivery against morbidity and mortality of expectant management. For example, Class I HELLP should be treated with delivery at 34 weeks gestation. Some authorities advocate delivery as early as 32 weeks or when fetal lung maturity can be demonstrated. Steroids may be given prior to delivery to accelerate fetal lung maturity and postpartum. Intravenous administration of 40 mg methyprednisolone or 10 mg dexamethasone every 12 hours prior to delivery is the usual dose. Fluids should be administered to avoid acute renal failure. However, one must proceed with caution to avoid pulmonary edema in the setting of large volume shifts. Platelet transfusion is appropriate at counts under 30,000 or 50,000 when prior to delivery or surgery. Fresh frozen plasma may be given when fibrinogen is less than 100 mg/mL, suggestive of DIC. Low molecular weight heparin may also be used with caution when the fibrinogen is greater than or equal to 200 and platelets are greater than 100,000. Most cases of HELLP worsen immediately postpartum. However, the abnormalities should resolve within 72 hours. HELLP is known to recur in approximately 5% of pregnancies. However, recurrence rates 5 times higher than that value have been reported. Therefore, subsequent pregnancies are considered high risk and should be managed as such.

Most maternal deaths related to HELLP are the result of intracerebral hemorrhage, cardiopulmonary arrest, DIC, acute respiratory distress syndrome (ARDS), acute renal failure, sepsis, hypoxic encephalopathy, and hepatic hemorrhage. Sibai et al described serious maternal complications excluding DIC in 45.4% of cases in a study of 443 cases of HELLP. Twenty one percent of cases resulted in DIC, a relatively common complication of HELLP. Placental abruption, intrauterine hypoxia, growth retardation, and prematurity are among the major sources of morbidity for the fetus.

Complications of HELLP

Ruptured hepatic hematoma is a complication found in 2% of cases of HELLP. Factors contributing to increased risk of rupture include multiparity and older age. Symptoms of shock with right upper quadrant pain combined with transaminases above 1000 IU/L, fever, and coagulopathy suggest rupture, which usually involves the right lobe. Due to the potential disastrous consequences of rupture, an upper abdominal ultrasound should be performed when a patient reports right upper quadrant pain postpartum, even when there are no symptoms of pre-eclampsia or HELLP prior to delivery. The diagnosis of rupture is suggested when a hyperechoic mass or areas within a mass are seen on ultrasound.

Treatment of suspected hepatic rupture consists of volume resuscitation with intravenous fluids and packed red blood cell transfusion, arterial embolization, and surgical evacuation. Liver transplant may be considered in severe cases. Abscess formation and pleural effusions may further complicate rupture. Hepatic infarction during pregnancy is almost always associated with antiphospholipid antibody syndrome often in the setting of HELLP. Diagnosis of hepatic infarction can be aided by CT or MRI. Signs overlap with that of rupture and may include fever, significant transaminase elevations, and anemia.

Intercurrent Liver Disease in Pregnancy

Liver diseases that occur in the nonpregnant patient may also present in the pregnant patient. Some of these conditions are worsened or precipitated by pregnancy, such as cholelithiasis, Budd Chiari syndrome, hepatitis E (HEV), and *Herpes simplex* hepatitis. Others, for instance, hepatitis A (HAV) and hepatitis B (HBV) run their typical course. However, the diagnosis and management of any of these conditions in the pregnant female warrant special consideration as the health of the fetus is also involved.

Cholelithiasis

Cholelithiasis is present in 6% of pregnancies. Gallbladder emptying slows in the second trimester and may contribute to the formation of gallstones. Pregnant patients present with symptoms similar to their nonpregnant counterparts. However, in pregnant women an increase in alkaline phosphatase is less helpful in diagnosis due to the expected increase of this enzyme due to placental production.

Complications of cholelithiasis are uncommon occurring in 0.16% of pregnant patients. If surgery is necessary, it is more safely performed in the second trimester, when the gravid uterus has not extended as far upward into the abdominal cavity as later in pregnancy and risk of preterm labor is lowest. Endoscopic retrograde cholangiopancreatography and sphincterotomy can be safely performed with careful attention to radiation exposure to the fetus, although pancreatitis is a very rare complication.

Budd-Chiari Syndrome

Budd-Chiari syndrome, or hepatic venous outflow obstruction, is seen more often in hypercoagulable states, pregnancy being among them. In contrast to observations in the Western world, pregnancy is amongst the most common causes of Budd-Chiari in the far East. It carries a poor prognosis. Liver associated enzymes, duration of illness, clinical course, and liver histology are used in classifying symptomatic patients into subgroups with different prognoses. Symptoms include abdominal pain, distention, and jaundice, which is often accompanied with signs such as ascites and tender hepatomegaly.

Pulsed Doppler ultrasound, venography, and liver biopsy are also helpful in diagnosis. MRI has recently been gaining utility in diagnosis of Budd-Chiari syndrome. Liver biopsy shows characteristic histological changes of centrizonal congestion and necrosis with a normal periportal area in the early stage. As the disease progresses, centrizonal fibrosis occurs, ultimately leading into cirrhotic changes.

Treatment includes delivery followed by liver transplant in severe cases. Medical management alone with diuretics, anticoagulants, and thrombolytic agents is generally insufficient. Balloon angioplasty, stenting, and portosystemic shunting have been used successfully in the treatment of Budd-Chiari in nonpregnant individuals. There is one reported case in the literature of a portacaval shunt placement at 18 weeks gestation. After delivery of a healthy newborn at 31 weeks, this patient developed progressive liver failure for which she underwent transplant and died 10 months later.[12] Regardless of immediate treatment modality, all patients will require lifelong anticoagulation.

Acute Viral Hepatitis

Viral hepatitis as a whole is the most common cause of jaundice in pregnancy. However, each type of viral hepatitis in the pregnant patient differs in treatment and risk.

Hepatitis A

The course of HAV is similar to that of nonpregnant females. Perinatal transmission from mother to fetus is exceedingly uncommon. Most physicians feel it is safe to administer the HAV vaccine and immunoglobulins to a pregnant female. The newborn should also receive 0.5 mg immune serum globulin immediately after delivery. Breastfeeding is safe. There may be an increased risk of preterm labor if HAV is contracted during the third trimester though this risk is not confirmed.

Hepatitis B

The course of HBV is largely unaltered by pregnancy. However, perinatal transmission from mother to fetus is an important issue. The presence of HBVe antigen correlates with increased transmission rates. Patients negative for HBVe antigen, but antibody positive have vertical transmission rates of 10%, whereas patients with positive HBVe antigen have rates as high as 90%. Transmission of acute HBV is rare in the first trimester, but increases to approximately 6% and 67% in the second and third trimesters, respectively. Prophylaxis of the newborn with HBV immunoglobulin and a 3-injection schedule of HBV vaccine at birth, and then 1 month and 6 months later reduce infection rates in the offspring to less than 3%.[13]

Hepatitis E and *Herpes Simplex* Hepatitis

HEV and *Herpes simplex* hepatitis may follow a more severe course in pregnant women, especially when contracted in the third trimester. Fulminant hepatic failure occurs in up to 58% of HEV and mortality may be as high as 10% to 20%. Hepatitis E is endemic to the Middle East, Asia, and Africa and is not encountered in the United States. Pregnant women should be advised to travel to these areas with caution.

Without treatment, herpetic hepatitis related mortality is high. A vesicular rash is usually present and suggests the diagnosis. But, absence of this rash does not rule out the disorder. Aminotransferases may be elevated to 6000. However, jaundice is uncommon. Culture of the vesicular fluid, serologic testing, and liver histology help to distinguish herpetic hepatitis from other severe liver disorders associated with pregnancy. If this condition is suspected, the patient should receive acyclovir. Early delivery is not felt to be necessary.

Drug-Induced Liver Damage

Pregnancy does not confer increased susceptibility to toxin-induced liver damage. In fact, pregnant patients generally take few medications due to the possibility of teratogenicity (Table 10-4). However, many prescription and nonprescription medications, especially herbal products, do pose a risk of hepatotoxicity and should be considered in the differential of abnormal liver enzymes in a pregnant female. Treatment is the same for both pregnant and nonpregnant individuals and consists of withdrawing the offending agent and administering supportive care.

Table 10-4

MEDICATIONS FOR TREATMENT OR AMELIORATION OF SYMPTOMS IN LIVER DISEASE

Drug	*Category*	*Use*
Azathioprine	D	Autoimmune hepatitis
Prednisone	B	Autoimmune hepatitis
Lactulose	B	Hepatic encephalopathy
Neomycin	C	Hepatic encephalopathy
Acyclovir	B	Herpes simplex
Interferon alpha 2b	C	Hepatitis C and B
Interferon alpha 2a	C	Hepatitis C
Ribavarin	X	Hepatitis C
Octreotide	B	Varices
Propranolol	C, D (2nd, 3rd trimesters)	Varices
Cholestyramine	C	ICP
Ursodeoxycholic acid	B	ICP
Phenobarbital	D	ICP
SAMe (s-adenosyl methionine)	NA	ICP
Zinc acetate	A	Wilson's
Trientine	C	Wilson's
Penicillamine	D	Wilson's
Tetrathiomolybdate	D	Wilson's
Cyclosporine	C	Post-transplant
Hepatitis B immunoglobulin	C	Hepatitis B
Hepatitis B vaccine	C	Hepatitis B
Lamivudine	C	Hepatitis B
Immune serum globulin	C	Hepatitis A
Hepatitis A vaccine	C	Hepatitis A
Pyridoxine	A	Nausea/Vomiting
Doxylamine	B	Nausea/Vomiting
Cyclizine	B	Nausea/Vomiting
Meclizine	B	Nausea/Vomiting
Dimenhydrinate	B	Nausea/Vomiting
Diphenhydramine	B	Nausea
Metoclopramide	B	Nausea/Vomiting
Scopolamine	C	Nausea/Vomiting
Promethazine	C	Nausea/Vomiting
Prochlorperazine	C	Nausea/Vomiting

continued

Table 10-4 (continued)

MEDICATIONS FOR TREATMENT OR AMELIORATION OF SYMPTOMS IN LIVER DISEASE

Drug	*Category*	*Use*
Chlorpromazine	C	Nausea/Vomiting
Trimethobenzamide	C	Nausea/Vomiting
Droperidol	C	Vomiting
Ondansetron	B	Nausea/Vomiting
Dexamethasone	C	ICP
Hydroxyzine	C	ICP
Methyldopa	B	Pre-eclampsia
Magnesium sulfate	B	Pre-eclampsia
Phenytoin	D	Eclampsia
Charcoal	C	Photocutaneous porphyria
Beta carotene	C	Photocutaneous porphyria
Chloroquine	C	Photocutaneous porphyria

The Food and Drug Administration (FDA) classifies certain drugs for use during pregnancy with safety ratings of A, B, C, D, or X:

A = Well-controlled studies show no fetal risk.

B = Animal studies show no risk but human studies are inadequate, or animal studies show some risk but the risk is not supported by human studies.

C = Animal studies show risk but human studies are lacking, or there are no studies in humans or animals.

D = Definite fetal abnormalities in human studies, but potential benefits may outweigh risks.

X = Risks outweigh potential benefits.

METASTASES TO LIVER

A palpable liver is abnormal during pregnancy since the liver is pushed up farther into the chest by the expanding uterus. If the liver can be palpated, imaging and labs are required to rule out metastatic disease. Abdominal or back pain, abnormal liver enzymes, and even frank hepatic failure may be present. The possibility of rupture should be explored when abdominal pain occurs in a patient with known liver metastases. The most common cancers to metastasize to the liver during pregnancy are colon, breast, pancreas, and gestational trophoblastic disease.

CHRONIC LIVER DISEASE IN PREGNANCY

Females with chronic liver disease have relatively low rates of pregnancy due in part to the older age and anovulatory state often associated. Cirrhosis decreases fertility. However, in noncirrhotic portal hypertension, liver function and fertility are preserved.

Cirrhosis

Cirrhosis decreases fertility in proportion to degree of hepatic dysfunction. When portal hypertension is present, it may worsen due to the expansion of total blood volume. There is also an increased risk of splenic artery aneurysm rupture. Changes in both the portal and systemic circulation are most notable in the second stage of labor, the time of greatest maternal hemorrhagic risk. Endoscopy should be performed in known cirrhotics prior to pregnancy to assess for the presence of varices and then the subsequent risk of bleeding. A large proportion of patients with varices bleed at some point during pregnancy. However, prophylactic banding, medications, or shunt procedures are generally not felt necessary. When there is evidence of active variceal bleeding, treatment with endoscopic band ligation and octreotide is indicated. Ligation should continue at 1 to 2 week intervals until varices are obliterated. Vasopressin is contraindicated during pregnancy due to its contractile effects on the uterus.[14]

An attempt should be made to treat the underlying cause of portal hypertension. Despite various treatment measures, the risk of spontaneous abortion is 20% and perinatal mortality is 11% to 18% in cirrhotics.

Hepatitis C

The course of hepatitis C (HCV) is generally unaltered by pregnancy. Vertical transmission of HCV is reported to be between 6% and 10%. This rate increases when the mother is coinfected with human immunodeficiency virus (HIV) and HCV RNA is greater than 1 million copies per mL.

Treatment of HCV with interferon and ribavarin should be discontinued during pregnancy due to potential for teratogenicity from ribavirin. It is not necessary to perform a cesarean section for the sole purpose of preventing vertical transmission of HCV. Patients may be advised that breastfeeding poses no additional risk to the newborn of perinatal transmission.

Autoimmune Hepatitis

Autoimmune hepatitis is chronic hepatitis with varying severity that usually affects young women. Women with autoimmune hepatitis receiving appropriate treatment may become pregnant. However, there is an increased risk of pre-eclampsia, premature delivery, low birth weight, and fetal loss in females with autoimmune hepatitis. Flare-ups of liver disease have been described in pregnant women who were previously in remission. Alternately, there have been cases of remission occurring while pregnant. In either case, a clear causal link has not been established.

Prednisone is considered safe for use in pregnancy. In contrast, azathioprine is a potential teratogen, but there are many reported cases of its safe use in pregnant women with inflammatory bowel disease. At doses used in the treatment of autoimmune hepatitis, azathioprine is generally considered safe to use during pregnancy. Withdrawal of treatment altogether may lead to disease recurrence and should, therefore, be avoided.

Wilson's Disease

Wilson's disease (WD) is an autosomal recessive disorder of copper metabolism that usually manifests as neurologic disease and chronic hepatitis with or without cirrhosis. With the use of appropriate chelating therapy, it is possible to become pregnant. However, fetal loss and mortality is a known risk of pregnancies complicated by portal hypertension. Therefore, these patients must be monitored closely.

Treatment with penicillamine and trientene should be continued during pregnancy despite the association of cutis laxa, a connective tissue disorder, in the newborn with exposure to penicillamine. However, penicillamine should be discontinued prior to episiotomy or other surgery due to potential risk of hemorrhage and impaired wound healing. Therapy may be restarted as soon as the wound has healed. A cesarean section should be not performed routinely, rather when obstetrically indicated.

Inherited Hyperbilirubinemia

Dubin Johnson sydrome, an autosomal recessive disease of conjugated hyperbilirubinemia may worsen. Patients may become jaundiced. Treatment is generally not required since spontaneous recovery upon delivery is the norm. Pregnancy is not known to affect Gilbert's syndrome, a benign disorder of unconjugated hyperbilirubinemia caused by a defect in the promotor region of the gene for bilirubin UDP-glucoronyltransferase.

Postliver Transplant

Fertility may be regained following liver transplant, but the risk for preterm labor, hypertensive disease, and abnormal liver enzymes may be increased. Immunosuppressants are not known to be teratogenic. However, cyclosporine levels may be altered during pregnancy and should, therefore, be monitored closely. Females who wish to become pregnant after transplant should be advised to wait at least 6 months, and preferably longer, to reduce risk of cytomegalovirus transmission and rejection during pregnancy, which is of concern and thus the need to proceed with extreme caution. Antibiotic prophylaxis should be given at time of delivery. No elevated incidence of birth defects has been demonstrated.[20]

References

1. Bacq Y, Zarka O, Brechot J-F, et al. Liver function tests in normal pregnancy: a prospective study of 103 pregnant women and 103 matched controls. *Hepatology.* 1996;23:1030-1034.
2. Reyes H, Wegmann ME, Segovia N, et al. HLA in Chileans with intrahepatic cholestasis of pregnancy. *Hepatology.* 1982;2:463-466.
3. Treem W, Shoup M, Hale D, et al. Acute fatty liver of pregnancy, hemolysis, elevated liver enzymes, and low platelets syndrome and long chain 3-hydroxyacyl-coenzyme A dehydrogenase deficiency. *Am J Gastroenterol.* 1996;91:2293-2300.
4. Vanjak D, Moreau R, Roche-Sicot J, Soulier A, Sicot C. Intrahepatic cholestasis of pregnancy and acute fatty liver of pregnancy. An unusual but favorable association? *Gastroenterology.* 1991;100:1123-1125.
5. Frigo P, Lang C, Reisenberger K, Hirsch AM. Hyperemesis gravidarum associated with Helicobacter Pylori seropositivity. *Obstet Gynecol.* 1999;91:615-617.

6. Martin JN J, Rinehart BK, May WL, et al. The spectrum of severe preeclampsia: comparative analysis by HELLP syndrome classification. *Am J Obstet Gynecol.* 1999;180:1373-1384.
7. Eliakim R, Abulafia O, Sherer DM. Hyperemesis Gravidarum: a current review. *Am J Perinatol.* 2000;17:207-218.
8. Sandhu BS, Sanyal AJ. Pregnancy and liver disease. *Gastroenterol Clin N Am.* 2003;32:407-436.
9. Sibai BM, Ramadan MK, Chari RS, Friedman SA. Pregnancies complicated by HELLP syndrome (hemolysis, elevated liver enzymes, and low platelets): subsequent pregnancy outcome and long-term prognosis. *Am J Obstet Gynecol.* 1995;172(1 Pt 1):125-129.
10. Sullivan CA, Magann EF, Perry KG Jr, et al. The recurrence risk of the syndrome of hemolysis, elevated liver enzymes, and low platelets (HELLP) in subsequent gestations. *Am J Obstet Gynecol.* 1994;171:940-943.
11. Vigil-De Gracia P, Lavergne JA. Acute fatty liver of pregnancy. *Int J Gynaecol Obstet.* 2001;72:193-195.
12. Grant WJ, McCashland T, Botha JF, et al. Acute Budd-Chiari syndrome during pregnancy: surgical treatment and orthotopic liver transplantation with successful completion of the pregnancy. *Liver Transpl.* 2003;9:976-979.
13. Aravelo J. Hepatitis B in pregnancy. *West J Med.* 1989;150:668-674.
14. Reily CA. Liver disease in the pregnant patient. *Am J Gastroenterol.* 1999;94:1728-1732
15. Rioseco AJ, Ivankovic MB, Manzur A, et al. Intrahepatic cholestasis of pregnancy: a retrospective case-control study of perinatal outcome. *Am J Obstet Gynecol.* 1994;170: 890-895.
16. Sheehan HL. The pathology of acute yellow atrophy and delayed chloroform posoning. *J Obstet Genaecol Br Empire.* 1940;47:49.
17. Sibai BM, Ramadan MK, Usta I, et al. Maternal morbidity and mortality in 442 pregnancies with hemolysis, elevated liver enzymes, and low platelets (HELLP syndrome). *Am J Obstet Gynecol.* 1993;169:1000-1006.
18. Weinstein L. Syndrome of hemolysis, elevated liver enzymes and low platelet count: a severe consequence of hypertension in pregnancy. *Am J Obstet Gynecol.* 1982;142:159-167.
19. Ch'ng CL, Morgan M, Hainsworth I, Kingham JG. Prospective study of liver dysfunction in pregnancy in Southwest Wales. *Gut.* 2002;51:876-880.
20. Armenti VT, Herrine SK, Radomski JS, Moritz MJ. Pregnancy after liver transplantation. *Liver Transpl.* 2000;6:671-685.

Suggested Readings

Bacq Y. Acute fatty liver in pregnancy. *Gastroenterol Clin Biol.* 1997;21:109-115.

Cruickshank D, Wigton T, Hays P. Maternal physiology in pregnancy. In: Gabb S, Nieby J, Simpson J, editors. *Obstetrics: normal and problem pregnancies.* New York: Churchill Livingstone; 1996:91-109.

Fagan EA. Intrahepatic cholestasis of pregnancy. *Clin Liver Dis.* 1999;3:603-632.

Knox TA, Olans LB. Liver disease in pregnancy. *N Eng J Med.* 1996;335:569-576.

Lee WM. Pregnancy in patients with chronic liver disease. *Gastroenterol Clin N Am.* 1992;21:889-903.

Misra S, Sanyal AJ. Pregnancy in a patient with portal hypertension. *Clin Liver Dis.* 1999;3:147-162.

Periera SP, O'Donahue J, Wendon J, Williams R. Maternal and perinatal outcome in severe pregnancy related liver disease. *Hepatology.* 1997;26:1258-1262.

Reinus J, Leikin E. Viral hepatitis in pregnancy. *Clin Liver Dis.* 1999;3:115-130.

chapter 11

Postoperative Jaundice

Jayanta Choudhury, MD and Arun J. Sanyal, MD

Synopsis

Abnormal liver chemistry tests (LCTs) are common after surgery. Patients with a history of liver disease require careful medical assessment and management of their disease before surgery and close follow-up afterwards. Evaluation of postoperative cholestasis requires a careful review of the medical record in combination with blood tests, noninvasive and invasive medical imaging, and liver biopsy when appropriate. Postoperative jaundice can be subdivided into disorders associated with bilirubin overproduction, hepatocellular injury, intrahepatic or extrahepatic cholestasis, and miscellaneous conditions. Commonly, there may be multiple mechanisms responsible for jaundice in a given patient. Diagnosis and management of postoperative jaundice are directed towards the underlying disease process.

Introduction

Twenty-five percent to 75% of patients who undergo surgery develop abnormal liver chemistry tests (LCTs) postoperatively.[1] Whereas postoperative jaundice is unusual in patients without liver disease, 47% of patients with cirrhosis will become icteric.[2] Patients with chronic liver diseases who may be at risk for hepatic decompensation require careful medical assessment and management of their underlying liver disease before surgery, and close follow-up afterwards. Elective surgery poses minimal risk for patients with no clinical evidence of liver disease; mild elevations of aminotransferases or cholestatic liver enzymes are typical. Gastroenterologists and hepatologists are frequently called upon to evaluate a patient who develops abnormal LCTs postoperatively. A careful history and physical examination in conjunction with an assessment of the type of surgery performed, number of blood products transfused, perioperative hemodynamic parameters, and medications (including anesthetics) used is mandatory for all patients. The physician should also inquire about the pattern and timing of LCT abnormalities in patients who undergo surgery, and the use of total parenteral nutrition (TPN) during the perioperative and postoperative periods. Any patient with abnormal LCTs should also be carefully screened for infections. Judicious use of noninvasive and invasive medical imaging and liver biopsy may be required in selected cases.

Postoperative LCT aberrations can occur as a consequence of many different disorders.[1-8] Isolated unconjugated hyperbilirubinemia can arise as a consequence of hemolytic diseases, hemolysis of transfused red blood cells, resorption of hematomas, or Gilbert's syndrome. Ischemic liver injury usually occurs within the first few days after surgery and is characterized by markedly abnormal aminotransferases in combination with a significantly elevated lactic acid dehydrogenase (LDH).[9] The severity of injury is largely dependent upon the degree and duration of ischemia. Patients with significant ischemic injury can also develop conjugated hyperbilirubinemia. As in patients with ischemic liver injury, strikingly elevated aminotransferases are seen in patients who develop viral or drug-induced hepatitis in the postoperative period; however unlike ischemic injury, LCT abnormalities usually arise 2 to 3 weeks or later after surgery. Benign postoperative cholestasis is characterized by hyperbilirubinemia that develops shortly after surgery and rises progressively over 2 to 3 weeks.

Postoperative LCT abnormalities can be categorized into 1 of 4 groups: disorders of increased bilirubin production, hepatocellular diseases, cholestatic disorders, and preexisting liver diseases. As mentioned above, disorders of increased bilirubin production are associated with underlying hemolytic states, resorbing hematomas, drug-induced hemolytic disorders, valvular prostheses, or blood transfusions. Ischemic liver injury, medication effects, sepsis, anesthetics, TPN, and viral hepatitis produce hepatocellular injury postoperatively. Postoperative cholestasis can be subdivided into intrahepatic and extrahepatic disorders. Benign postoperative cholestasis, sepsis, and medications account for most cases of intrahepatic cholestasis, whereas common bile duct stones, acalculous and calculous cholecystitis, pancreatitis, and bile duct strictures are responsible for most cases of extrahepatic cholestasis. Pre-existing chronic liver diseases or inherited disorders of bilirubin metabolism such as Gilbert's and Dubin-Johnson syndromes can also give rise to LCT abnormalities postoperatively. Most cases of postoperative jaundice resolve spontaneously, but a few are life-threatening and require prompt diagnosis and treatment.

Preoperative Assessment

A careful preoperative assessment is imperative for all patients with suspected acute or chronic liver diseases.[10-12] Physicians should inquire about alcohol consumption and high-risk activities that presage alcoholic liver disease and viral hepatitis respectively. Patients should also be questioned about a family history of liver disease. In addition, the physician should carefully assess for peripheral stigmata of acute or chronic liver disease such as jaundice, gynecomastia, spider angiomata, ascites, hepatosplenomegaly, lower extremity edema, and encephalopathy. Routine laboratory investigation often includes a complete blood count, coagulation profile, electrolytes, and LCTs. In selected patients, other tests may include viral and autoimmune serologies, as well as screening for Wilson's disease (WD), α-1 antitrypsin deficiency, hereditary hemochromatosis, and nonalcoholic steatohepatitis with ceruloplasmin, α-1 antitrypsin level and phenotype, iron indices, and a lipid profile respectively. Abdominal ultrasound, computed tomography (CT), and magnetic resonance imaging (MRI) are useful noninvasive tests to screen for gallstones, dilated bile ducts, or

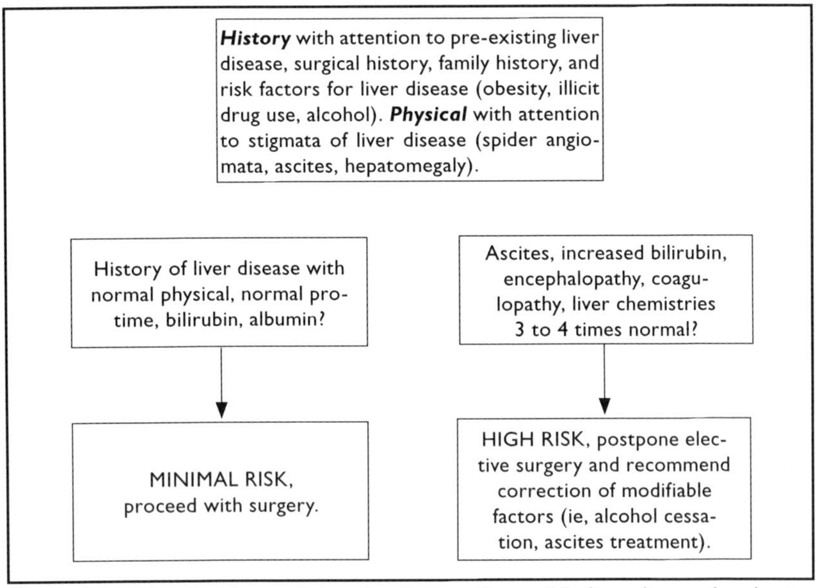

Figure 11-1. Preoperative work-up of patients with possible liver disease for elective surgery.

portal hypertension. Magnetic resonance cholangiopancreatography (MRCP) and endoscopic retrograde cholangiopancreatography (ERCP) are useful for patients with suspected extrahepatic cholestatic disorders. Liver biopsy is occasionally required when the etiology of liver disease is not clear or when the degree of liver impairment requires assessment prior to elective surgery. In addition to a thorough history, physical examination, and diagnostic evaluation, the consultant should also review the surgical procedure to be performed.

Patients with liver disease can be subdivided into minimal and increased operative risk (Figure 11-1). Those at minimal risk are without symptoms and have a normal physical examination. The aminotransferases are usually less than 4 times the upper limit of normal or there may be an isolated elevation of the alkaline phosphatase or gamma glutamyl transpeptidase. Alcoholic fatty liver, mild chronic hepatitis, and drug-induced liver injury fall into this group. Patients with isolated unconjugated hyperbilirubinemia frequently have underlying Gilbert's syndrome, which poses no increased risk for surgery. An evaluation is warranted if the LCTs remain elevated postoperatively. Both acute and chronic liver diseases can be associated with increased operative risk. Patients with acute viral hepatitis are at risk for significant morbidity and perioperative mortality, especially if the aminotransferases are greater than 4 times the upper limit of normal and the bilirubin is elevated. Elective surgery should be postponed for at least 1 month after normalization of LCTs, and emergency surgery should only be performed, albeit at increased risk, if absolutely required. It is preferable that patients with alcoholic hepatitis be abstinent for 1 to 3 months and the bilirubin be normal before elective surgery. Severe chronic hepatitis with piecemeal, bridging, or multilobular necrosis and cirrhotic liver disease increases the operative risk for both elective and emergency surgery. Patients can be stratified into different categories of risk based upon hepatic synthetic reserve, and the Child's classification is often used to determine the severity of liver disease.[12-17] Child's class A cirrhosis is associated with 10% mortality for elective surgery; there are no particular restrictions for this group. Even though mortality may be as high as 30% for patients with Child's class B liver disease, most will tolerate elective surgery with careful preoperative preparation; however, major hepatic resections should be avoided to minimize the chance of worsening hepatic function. Patients with Child's class C cirrhosis pose the greatest challenge for elective surgery. Mortality rates of 75% are commonly quoted for patients with cryptogenic cirrhosis who undergo abdominal surgery (eg, portosystemic shunt, biliary tract procedures, hepatic resection, surgery for complicated gastroduodenal ulcer, colonic resections, surgery for small bowel obstruction, and pancreatic surgery).[14] Laparascopic procedures have been well tolerated in patients with Child's class A and B cirrhosis with minimal mortality.[12] Frequently, patients are jaundiced and have evidence of markedly impaired hepatic reserve before surgery. Under normal circumstances, the hepatic artery supplies one-third of the blood flow to the liver, whereas two-thirds is supplied by the portal vein. Patients with cirrhosis and portal hypertension are more dependent upon hepatic arterial flow. Hypotension, anesthetics administered during surgery, and hypoxemia result in decreased hepatic blood flow and oxygenated blood to the liver. Consequently, patients with marginal hepatic reserve are at risk for further decompensation. Sepsis, gastrointestinal bleeding, and multisystem organ failure frequently develop postoperatively in Child's class C patients. Other comorbidities that increase operative risk include renal failure, chronic obstructive pulmonary disease, preoperative infections or gastrointestinal bleeding, and male gender.[13] Hepatic resections should not be performed in this group of patients. If elective surgery is required for patients with Child's class C liver disease, it is imperative that the patient's condition be optimized beforehand. Treatment of ascites, spontaneous bacterial peritonitis, and encephalopathy should be undertaken with the intent of improving the Child's class before surgery. Careful attention to renal function, nutritional status, fluid balance, and vital signs is also essential.

Etiology of Postoperative Jaundice

Figure 11-2 presents a guide to diagnosis and treatment of the most common causes of postoperative jaundice.

Bilirubin Overproduction

Bilirubin overproduction accounts for a minority of cases of postoperative jaundice; most cases occur within the first 2 weeks of surgery (Table 11-1). A normal healthy liver conjugates 250 mg of bilirubin per day derived from senescent red blood cells; however, the liver has the capacity to conjugate more. For this reason, jaundice will not develop unless bilirubin production exceeds three times normal. Other factors including underlying chronic liver disease, hepatic ischemia, sepsis, anesthetic effects, and impaired renal reserve in combination with increased bilirubin production can result in postoperative jaundice. Conditions identified with increased pigment load include hemolysis of transfused red blood cells (10% of red cells greater than 2 weeks old are destroyed within 24 hours of transfusion), resorption of hematomas, underlying hemolytic diseases (G6PD deficiency, sickle cell diseases, thalassemias, autoimmune

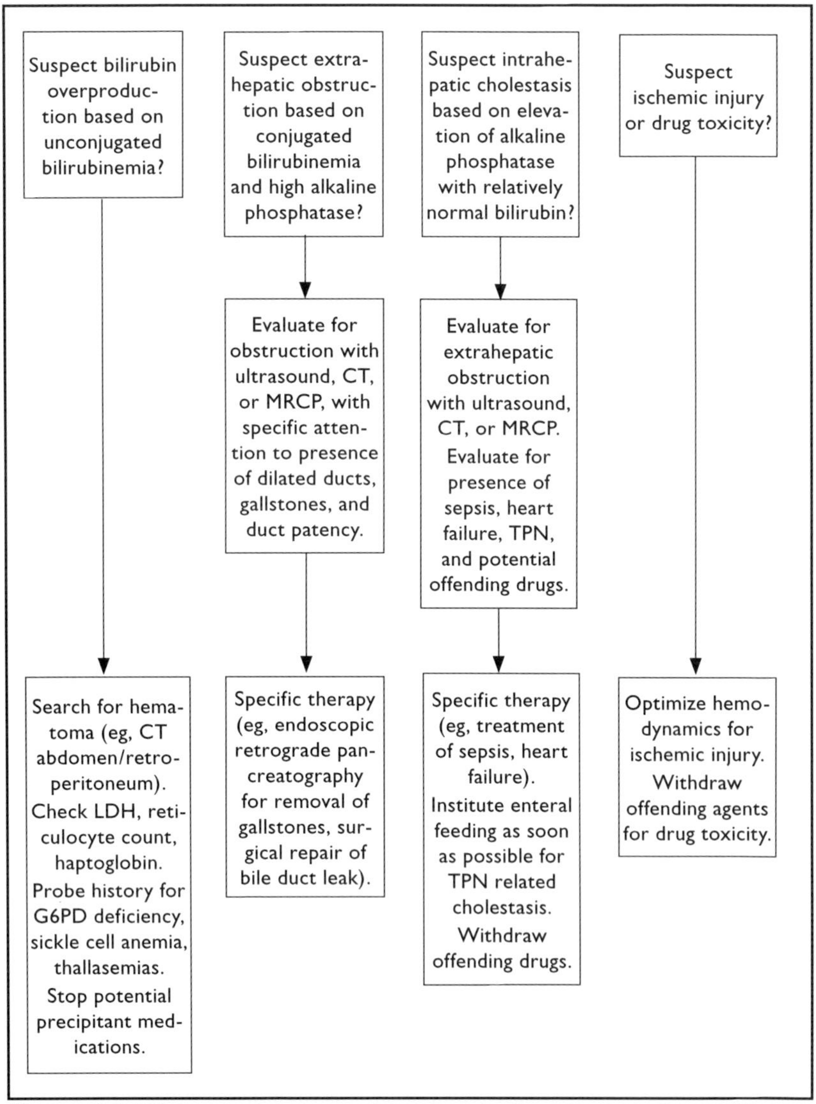

Figure 11-2. Work-up and treatment of postoperative liver chemistry abnormalities.

hemolytic anemia), mechanical heart valves, infections, and medications. A diagnosis of bilirubin overproduction is based upon an elevated reticulocyte count, unconjugated hyperbilirubinemia (bilirubin <5 mg/dL), elevated aspartate aminotransferase (AST) and LDH, reduced haptoglobin, and schistocytes on peripheral blood smear. The alanine aminotransferase (ALT) and alkaline phosphatase are not significantly elevated in disorders of bilirubin overproduction.

Table 11-1

DIFFERENTIAL DIAGNOSIS OF POSTOPERATIVE JAUNDICE BASED ON TIME ELAPSED SINCE SURGERY

Less Than 2 Weeks	*Greater Than 2 Weeks*
Ischemia	Benign postoperative jaundice
Benign postoperative jaundice	TPN-associated fatty liver
Bile leak*	TPN-associated cholestasis
Acalculous cholecystitis	Cytomegalovirus infection*
Hepatic artery thrombosis*	Acute viral hepatitis (including recurrent disease)
	Acute rejection*
	Acalculous cholecystitis

*Post-liver transplant complication

INTRAHEPATIC DISORDERS

HEPATOCELLULAR NECROSIS

Ischemic Liver Injury

Ischemic liver injury is a common cause for postoperative LCT abnormalities and jaundice.[9,18-20] Injury usually occurs within 1 day to 2 weeks of surgery and can occur as a consequence of many different conditions. Cardiogenic and noncardiogenic shock and respiratory failure are common causes. Patients who undergo cardiovascular bypass surgery are also at risk for ischemic liver injury. Inadvertent ligation of the hepatic artery at the time of cholecystectomy is a rare cause of hepatic necrosis. The pathogenesis of ischemic liver injury is multifactorial. Hypotension in association with a reduction in splanchnic, portal venous, and hepatic arterial blood flow can lead to ischemic injury as a consequence of reduced hepatic perfusion; restoration of hepatic blood flow can damage the liver through ischemic-reperfusion injury. Anesthetics are commonly associated with a reduction in hepatic blood flow that can contribute to hepatic injury perioperatively.[21] Chronic passive hepatic congestion in the setting of right heart failure in combination with reduced hepatic perfusion as a consequence of left heart failure may increase the risk of hepatic ischemia over that of left heart failure alone.[9,18] The diagnosis of ischemic liver injury is based upon markedly elevated aminotransferases to greater than 5 to 100 times the upper limit of normal in combination with a markedly elevated LDH. The alkaline phosphatase is usually less than or equal to 2 times the upper limit of normal. Patients with significant ischemic liver injury can develop subfulminant or fulminant liver failure with progressive hyperbilirubinemia, encephalopathy, coagulopathy, hypoglycemia, and renal failure. Even though a diagnosis of ischemic liver injury is usually based upon clinical criteria, liver biopsy is occasionally recommended to exclude other causes for abnormal LCTs. Typical findings on biopsy include centrilobular sinusoidal congestion with necrosis; panlobular necrosis may be seen in biopsies of patients with more extensive liver injury. Aminotransferases promptly return to normal in most cases after correction of the underlying process, but on occasion they may be elevated for 3 to 10 days. Hyperbilirubinemia can develop later and may persist for several weeks given that these patients are critically ill and multiple factors may be involved in the pathogenesis of jaundice. Optimizing cardiac output and treatment of underlying diseases are standards of care. Mortality can be as high as 75% and is generally attributable to other nonhepatic comorbid conditions. Other disorders that must be considered in the differential diagnosis of markedly abnormal aminotransferases include drug-induced liver injury and viral hepatitis; however, most aminotransferase elevations occur later than that of ischemic liver injury.

Viral Hepatitis

Viral hepatitis is a rare cause of postoperative jaundice. Acquisition of viral hepatitis before surgery is more common than that acquired through blood product transfusions. The onset of hepatic injury is ordinarily seen 2 weeks after surgery and is manifested by a progressive rise in aminotransferases exceeding 10 times the upper limit of normal. The alkaline phosphatase and LDH are only mildly increased. With severe injury, patients can become icteric and coagulopathic. HAV and HAB serologies and HCV RNA analysis by polymerase chain reaction (PCR) are suggested for patients suspected of having acute viral hepatitis.

Drug-Induced Hepatitis

Drug-induced liver injury most commonly occurs as a consequence of idiosyncratic mechanisms; most reactions develop 2 weeks after surgery. Volatile anesthetics can injure the liver through different mechanisms.[21,22] Almost all agents have been associated with transient liver dysfunction in 25% to 75% of patients. LCTs are most commonly less than 2 times the upper limit of normal; however, mortality rates of 10% to 30% have been reported for patients who develop significant hepatic dysfunction as a consequence of anesthetic administration. Ischemic injury as a result of reduced splanchnic and hepatic blood flow and oxygenation, and ischemic-reperfusion injury can lead to hepatic dysfunction in the postoperative period. Anesthetic metabolites can also directly injure the liver or bind to hepatocyte macromolecules and act as haptens to cause hepatic injury. Immunologic or hypersensitivity reactions are usually seen with repeated administration of anesthetics over short intervals and are commonly associated with eosinophilia.

Halothane has been classically associated with severe hepatic injury.[23,24] Risk factors for halothane hepatitis include age over 30 years, female gender, obesity, genetic factors, multiple exposures, and short intervals between exposures (usually less than 3 months). Patients with halothane-induced liver injury can present with fever and jaundice within 2 weeks of a single exposure. Other clinical manifestations include skin rash, arthralgias, and mild tender hepatomegaly. With subsequent exposures, fever and significant jaundice can develop within 1 to 11 days, and 5 to 7 days respectively. Aminotransferases are markedly elevated in patients who have received multiple exposures to halothane. Progressive liver injury resulting in acute liver and renal failure is a potential consequence. Panlobular and multifocal spotty necrosis, submassive confluent zonal necrosis, and massive necrosis can be seen on liver biopsies of patients with halothane hepatitis. Patients with massive hepatic necrosis typically have involvement of the entire lobule with lymphocytes, neutrophils, plasma cells, and eosinophils.

Halothane hepatitis can be subdivided into mild/moderate or severe liver injury. Mild/moderate injury usually develops 1 to 3 days after exposure and is thought to occur as a consequence of direct hepatotoxicity. Patients with mild disease exhibit moderate increases in aminotransferases with cholestasis, and liver biopsy demonstrates centrilobular necrosis with a mild mononuclear infiltrate. After multiple exposures, massive hepatic necrosis with eosinophilia occurs in 1 in 7000 cases.[23] Immunologic mechanisms are thought to be important in the pathogenesis of severe liver injury.[22,23,25] Trifluroacetyl (TFA) chloride is a metabolite of halothane that binds covalently to the endoplasmic reticulum of the hepatocyte.[22] Following creation of the TFA protein complex, immune responses are elicited that may promote liver injury. Patients with severe liver injury are critically ill with aminotransferases over 10 times the upper limit of normal, conjugated and unconjugated hyperbilirubinemia, and coagulopathy. The alkaline phosphatase is usually less than 2 times the upper normal limit.

As with halothane, methoxyflurane can cause liver injury. Obese females are at higher risk. Fever and jaundice generally develop within 14 days of a single exposure; however, the latent period is shorter for patients with prior exposure to either halothane or methoxyflurane. Markedly elevated aminotransferases, jaundice, and eosinophilia are common, and findings on liver biopsy are similar to that of halothane. Mortality for patients with severe hepatitis approaches 60%. Treatment includes withdrawal of the anesthetic and supportive care.

Isoflurane, enflurane, sevoflurane, and desflurane have rarely been associated with hepatic injury.[26-29] The ability of anesthetics to cause injury is directly proportional to their ability to undergo biotransformation. Rates of biotransformation for halothane, enflurane, sevoflurane, and isoflurane/desflurane are 20%, 2%, 1%, and 0.2%, respectively. For this reason, anesthetics such as isoflurane and sevoflurane infrequently cause drug-induced liver injury. All halogenated anesthetics exhibit cross reactivity and increase the risk of liver injury for patients with prior anesthetic exposure. Liver dysfunction ordinarily develops within 2 to 3 weeks of surgery with clinical features similar to that of halothane and methoxyflurane. Of the other anesthetics mentioned above, evidence for injury is greatest for enflurane. Fever develops within 3 days of enflurane administration and is commonly associated with anorexia, nausea, and vomiting. Jaundice and eosinophilia ensue within 3 to 19 days, and acute liver failure with encephalopathy, coagulopathy, and renal failure can develop with severe hepatic injury. Mortality rates of 21% have been reported.[28] LCTs return to normal within 3 to 4 weeks in patients who survive.[28] Two-thirds of patients with enflurane-induced hepatotoxicity have been previously exposed to either halothane or enflurane.[28] Typical findings on liver biopsy include centrilobular necrosis with ballooning degeneration of centrilobular and mid-zonal regions, and fatty change. Biopsies of patients with severe injury reveal massive panlobular necrosis. Liver injury from isoflurane, sevoflurane, and desflurane is infrequent; previous sensitization to either halothane or enflurane increases the risk.[26-27]

Many other medications administered during the perioperative and postoperative periods have rarely been associated with abnormal LCTs and jaundice. Sulfonamides, penicillin, tetracycline, rifampin, isoniazid, nitrofurantoin, fluconazole, methyldopa, phenytoin, and acetaminophen can cause liver injury. Most cases of injury occur between 2 weeks and 12 months. Presenting features include fever, pruritus, arthralgias, skin rash, and eosinophilia. Mild to moderately increased aminotransferases, bilirubin, and prothrombin time are frequently seen. As with the halogenated anesthetics, severe injury is associated with acute liver failure and the development of encephalopathy and coagulopathy. The differential diagnosis for drug-induced liver injury includes ischemic and viral hepatitis; however, ischemic liver injury usually occurs earlier and viral hepatitis may occur at the same time, although it is rarely seen in the postoperative period.

Postliver Transplantation

Hepatocellular necrosis of the allograft can be seen in patients who undergo liver transplantation. The differential diagnosis of abnormal LCTs in transplant patients depends on the time period after transplantation: first 3 days, 3 to 14 days, and beyond 14 days. Primary graft nonfunction and hepatic artery thrombosis are the most common causes for markedly abnormal aminotransferases during the first 3 days of transplantation; either scenario can result in graft failure and necessitate retransplantation. Portal vein and inferior vena caval thrombosis occurs in 1% to 3% of patients and can present with hepatic infarction and acute liver failure or complications attributable to portal hypertension. Unlike acute cellular or chronic rejection, hyperacute rejection is rarely seen in liver transplantation, but can be associated with markedly abnormal LCTs in the immediate postoperative period. Acute cellular rejection, recurrent viral hepatitis, hepatic artery thrombosis, bile leak, and drug toxicity are the most common causes for LCT abnormalities 3 to 14 days after transplantation. Between 14 days and 3 months, opportunistic infection with cytomegalovirus (CMV) needs to be considered in transplant patients with elevated aminotransferases or jaundice. However, acute cellular rejection, HCV, and drug effects also cause allograft dysfunction during this period. Noninvasive medical imaging (sonography, CT or MR scanning), cholangiography, and/or liver biopsy may be necessary to sort out the different causes for LCT abnormalities in transplant patients.

Intrahepatic Cholestasis

Cholestasis is defined as impairment in bile flow that can result from either intrahepatic or extrahepatic disorders. Patients frequently present with acholic stools, bilirubinuria, and pruritus. The alkaline phosphatase and bilirubin are usually greater than 3 times the upper limit of normal; the aminotransferases are only mildly elevated. Patients can also have a prolonged prothrombin time either secondary to fat malabsorption and vitamin K deficiency, or as a consequence of end stage biliary cirrhosis. The prothrombin time will correct with parenteral vitamin K in patients with vitamin K malabsorption. Canalicular bile plugs, centrilobular cholestasis with bile staining, and steatosis are characteristically seen on liver biopsy.

Benign Postoperative Cholestasis

Benign cholestasis, with or without jaundice, is commonly seen in patients following surgery.[30-32] Even though LCTs are frequently abnormal, jaundice is seen in less than 1% of cases. Benign postoperative cholestasis is a multifactorial process. Critically ill trauma or burn patients, with or without pre-existing liver or cardiovascular diseases, can present with jaundice postoperatively. Prolonged intra-abdominal or cardiothoracic surgery with passive hepatic congestion may also contribute to cholestasis. Increased pigment load (multiple blood transfusions, resorption of hematomas) decreased hepatic perfusion (all halogenated anesthetics, hypotension, passive hepatic congestion), hypoxemia, and infection with gram positive and negative organisms can result in cholestasis.

Benign postoperative cholestasis is customarily associated with a progressive rise in conjugated bilirubin within the first 2 to 10 days of surgery. The total bilirubin is usually between 10 and 40 mg/dL, the aminotransferases are less than 5 times the upper limit of normal, and the alkaline phosphatase is between 2 and 4 times the upper limit of normal in most patients. In patients without cirrhosis, the prolonged prothrombin usually corrects with parenteral administration of vitamin K. Abdominal ultrasound should be performed to exclude extrahepatic biliary obstruction. Liver biopsy is generally not required for diagnosis of this condition as it is often based on clinical features. However, if a biopsy is performed, nonspecific features include canalicular bile stasis and casts, dilated biliary canaliculi, mild centrilobular necrosis, minimal inflammation, varying degrees of hepatic congestion, and mild focal fatty change. Treatment is largely supportive. Restoration of blood volume, treatment of underlying infection, and the discontinuation of offending medications are important adjunctive measures. Mortality is generally attributable to other comorbidities and multisystem organ failure, and not cholestasis. Jaundice may not resolve for several weeks to months as often these patients are quite ill and have other contributing factors such as renal failure and transfusion requirements that exacerbate the process.

Infection

Infection must be considered in the differential diagnosis of intrahepatic cholestasis after surgery.[33-38] Aerobic gram positive and negative or anaerobic infections associated with appendicitis, diverticulitis, pyelonephritis, pneumonia, endocarditis, and pelvic or soft tissue infections can precede or coincide with postoperative cholestasis. Cholestasis can arise as a result of direct bacterial invasion of the liver, hemolysis, or endotoxin production with impairment in bilirubin and bile salt transport. Patients with cholestasis or jaundice attributable to infections typically present with fever and leucocytosis, positive blood cultures, and jaundice within several days of bacteremia. The total bilirubin is usually between 5 and 50 mg/dL and the alkaline phosphatase is generally between 2 and 3 times the upper limit of normal. The aminotransferases of patients with cholestasis of sepsis are usually only mildly abnormal. As with benign postoperative cholestasis, the underlying cholestasis associated with infections is frequently overshadowed by the underlying disease. A diagnosis of septic cholestasis is most commonly based upon clinical criteria; however, liver biopsy may be required if the cause for underlying LCT abnormalities is not clear. Centrilobular or midzonal cholestasis with bile plugs, nonspecific portal or parenchymal lymphocytic infiltrates, Kupffer cell hyperplasia, and steatosis are characteristically present. Mortality in this group approaches 90% and is usually attributable to the underlying disease and not intrahepatic cholestasis. The primary therapeutic aim is to treat the underlying infection.

Medications

A variety of medications in the postoperative period can result in cholestasis. Erythromycin, antiemetics, chlorpromazine, methyltestosterone, and TPN can lead to impairment in bile flow. Increased total bilirubin and alkaline phosphatase are typical. Treatment includes withdrawal of the offending medication and supportive care.

Postliver Transplantation

Drug toxicity, viral hepatitis, sepsis, opportunistic infections, and preexisting cholestatic liver diseases (eg, primary biliary cirrhosis or primary sclerosing cholangitis) are associated with intrahepatic cholestasis after transplantation. HBV and HCV can cause fibrosing cholestatic hepatitis that can lead to graft failure.[39,40] Cholestatic liver injury from HBV is thought to occur as a consequence of a high level of viral replication and direct cytopathic injury. Likewise, HCV can produce a similar lesion due to a high level of circulating virus. Typical findings on liver biopsies of patients with fibrosing cholestatic HCV include canalicular cholestasis, portal lymphocytic infiltration, lymphoid aggregates, mild steatosis, ballooning degeneration of centrilobular hepatocytes, bile ductular proliferation, and bridging fibrosis. Liver failure may ensue as an aftermath of progressive liver injury. Biliary strictures, benign postoperative cholestasis, CMV hepatitis, sepsis, and medication effects must be considered in the differential diagnosis of cholestasis after transplantation. The role of antiviral therapy for cholestatic hepatitis C in the transplant patient remains to be defined.

Extrahepatic Cholestasis

Extrahepatic disorders rarely cause postoperative jaundice, but they should be considered in any patient presenting with cholestasis. Causes of extrahepatic cholestasis include upper abdominal surgery, acalculous cholecystitis, complications from liver transplantation, postoperative pancreatitis, and unrecognized pre-existing liver disease (eg, PSC).

Upper Abdominal Surgery

Patients who undergo upper abdominal surgery are at risk for extrahepatic biliary obstruction and postoperative jaundice.[41-48] Bile duct injury and retained common bile duct stones following cholecystectomy or other upper abdominal operations can result in postoperative cholestasis; biliary injury is more commonly associated with jaundice than retained stones. Bile duct transection or leak can give rise to postoperative cholestasis. Common sites of injury include the common hepatic duct, confluence of the hepatic ducts, right hepatic or common bile ducts, and the secondary biliary radicals.

Patients with retained common bile duct stones, biliary strictures, or leaks can present with epigastric or right upper quadrant pain, fever, and jaundice within 2 to 14 days of surgery. Bacterial cholangitis can present with superimposed sepsis. Bile ascites or secondary biliary cirrhosis can arise as a consequence of a bile leak or stricture respectively. Mild to moderate increases in total bilirubin, aminotransferases, and alkaline phosphatase are common and usually occur within the first 2 weeks of surgery.

Abdominal ultrasound and CT scanning are excellent tests for evaluating biliary obstruction, bile leaks, or bilomas. MRCP is appropriate for cholestatic patients with multiple comorbidities to exclude extrahepatic obstruction when the index of suspicion for biliary obstruction is low. ERCP should be considered when there is a high index of suspicion of biliary pathology. Patients with retained common duct stones are at risk for cholangitis. Consequently, sphincterotomy with removal of retained stones is indicated either prior to or following cholecystectomy in most patients; however, ERCP with sphincterotomy and stone removal without cholecystectomy is appropriate for elderly patients who are at high risk for surgery. ERCP with insertion and exchange of single or multiple stents every 3 months is the initial treatment of choice for biliary strictures with success rates approaching 90%. The mean duration of treatment for the endoscopic approach is 12 months. For patients with strictures that are not amenable to endoscopic therapy, percutaneous biliary intervention with placement of biliary drains is another viable alternative. Roux-en-Y hepaticojejunostomy should be reserved for patients who fail either endoscopic or radiologic attempts, and for patients with transected bile ducts. Liver transplantation is occasionally required for patients who develop secondary biliary cirrhosis as a consequence of prolonged extrahepatic biliary obstruction. The management of bile leaks and bilomas usually requires endoscopic and radiologic intervention. Percutaneous drainage of bilomas in combination with endoscopic biliary drainage and broad-spectrum antibiotics are usually sufficient for bile leaks.

Acalculous Cholecystitis

Acalculous cholecystitis is a rare cause of cholestasis and jaundice.[49,50] Risk factors include male gender, major surgery (eg, abdominal, cardiovascular, gynecologic, orthopedic, and head and neck), trauma, burns, TPN >3 months, mechanical ventilation with positive end expiratory pressure (PEEP), narcotics, and renal failure. Bile stasis, increased gallbladder wall pressure, hypotension, gallbladder ischemia, and bacterial invasion contribute to gallbladder injury in this group. Patients with acalculous cholecystitis are critically ill in the intensive care unit recovering from major surgery. Fever, right upper quadrant pain, leucocytosis, and nonspecific LCT abnormalities develop 3 to 30 days postoperatively. The aminotransferases and alkaline phosphatase are mildly increased with or without an elevation of the total bilirubin. Abdominal ultrasound demonstrates gallbladder wall thickening and distension, pericholecystic fluid, and intramural gas with fragmentation or gangrene of the gallbladder. Like sonography, CT scanning can also show a thickened gallbladder wall with pericholecystic fluid. Radionuclide cholescintigraphy has too many false positives and negatives to be of clinical use. Treatment of patients with acalculous cholecystitis includes broad-spectrum antibiotics and open or laparoscopic cholecystectomy, whereas percutaneous or open cholecystostomy may be preferable for acutely ill patients who may not tolerate cholecystectomy. Mortality may be as high as 70% and is usually attributable to sepsis in the setting of either a gangrenous or emphysematous gallbladder with or without perforation and empyema. Other comorbid events include ischemic cardiovascular events and respiratory or renal failure that can also contribute to mortality in patients with acalculous cholecystitis.

Postliver Transplantation

Extrahepatic biliary obstruction must be considered in any patient presenting with cholestasis and jaundice after transplantation.[51] Ten to 20% of patients develop a biliary complication within 6 months of surgery. Biliary leaks or stones, anastomotic and nonanastomotic strictures, and sphincter of Oddi dysfunction can produce cholestasis. Anastomotic strictures are seen in the early and late postoperative periods and are usually the result of faulty surgical technique. Nonanastomotic strictures develop later and may be seen in the setting of hepatic artery thrombosis, prolonged cold ischemia time, ABO blood group incompatibility, opportunistic infections, or recurrent PSC. Sphincter of Oddi dysfunction is associated with dilated donor and recipient bile ducts. Abdominal sonography and/or CT scanning should be ordered in transplant patients presenting with cholestasis to exclude extrahepatic biliary obstruction. Therapeutic options include balloon dilation with stenting for patients with biliary strictures; anastomotic strictures are more amenable to endoscopic treatment than nonanastomotic strictures. Sphincterotomy with stone extraction and sphincterotomy alone are appropriate for patients with common duct stones and sphincter of Oddi dysfunction respectively.

Miscellaneous Causes

Genetic Disorders of Bilirubin Metabolism

Gilbert's syndrome is a genetic disorder of bilirubin metabolism. Reduced expression of UDP glucuronosyltransferase can result in unconjugated hyperbilirubinemia within 2 weeks of surgery; total bilirubin is frequently less than 4 mg/dL. Other LCTs are usually normal. Stress and fasting during the perioperative and postoperative periods are contributing factors.

As with Gilbert's syndrome, the Dubin-Johnson syndrome is a familial affliction of bilirubin metabolism. Patients with Dubin-Johnson syndrome have a isolated conjugated hyperbilirubinemia that is exacerbated with the stress of surgery.

Total Parenteral Nutrition

TPN is an uncommon cause for postoperative liver dysfunction.[52-54] Prematurity, sepsis, ileal disease or resection, inflammatory bowel disease, and bacterial overgrowth are risk factors for hepatotoxicity. Excessive nonprotein kilocalories (eg, glucose and lipids) and amino acids can also predispose to injury. Patients with nutritional deficiencies and/or hormonal imbalances may also be at risk.

Short-term administration (<90 days) is associated with fatty liver, cholestasis, and nonspecific triaditis. Fatty liver usually develops within the first 2 weeks of TPN administration and is the most benign lesion. Patients frequently have hepatomegaly and vague right upper quadrant pain. Fatty liver is more commonly seen with dextrose as the sole caloric source; coadministration of lipids as an additional source of non-protein kilocalories is recommended to reduce the chance of hepatic steatosis. Moderately increased aminotransferases and a mildly increased alkaline phosphatase are typically seen in patients with fatty liver. With mild disease, periportal fat is appreciated on liver biopsy, whereas centrilobular or panlobular involvement can be seen with more extensive injury. Cholestatic liver disease is rare with short-term administration of TPN, but is more commonly seen in premature or low weight for age children. Prematurity of the biliary secretory apparatus contributes to pericentral and periportal cholestasis, ductular proliferation, and mild portal triaditis. TPN cholestasis in adults generally develops after 3 weeks of administration and is commonly associated with progressive elevation in the alkaline phosphatase and total bilirubin. Lipid emulsions can also predispose the liver to cholestatic injury. Nonspecific triaditis can be seen within the first 90 days of TPN and is characterized by an increase in the aminotransferases.

Long-term administration (>6 months) is linked with steatohepatitis and cholestasis, ductular proliferation, and micronodular cirrhosis.[52] A progressive rise in the aminotransferases, alkaline phosphatase, and total bilirubin is typical of patients receiving long-term TPN.

Other complications of TPN include cholelithiasis and acalculous cholecystitis. Pigment gallstones are more common than cholesterol stones and patients with symptomatic disease usually require cholecystectomy. Acalculous cholecystitis usually occurs after 3 months of TPN. As described above, either cholecystectomy or cholecystostomy is recommended for this group. Early enteral feeding with or without parenteral cholecystokinin is recommended to promote gallbladder motility and to minimize the chance of symptomatic disease.

Most LCT abnormalities are mild and reversible and do not warrant a change in the TPN formula. Excessive carbohydrate nonprotein kilocalories should be avoided, lipid should be added as an additional source of calories, and the TPN should be cycled if possible over 10 to 12 hours. All of the disorders discussed above must be considered in the differential diagnosis of LCT abnormalities in patients who are receiving TPN. Abdominal sonography, CT or MR scanning, cholangiography, and liver biopsy should be considered where appropriate. Combined liver and small bowel transplantation is acceptable therapy for patients with extensive small intestinal disease and progressive irreversible liver injury as a consequence of TPN.

Summary

Abnormal LCTs after surgery are common, and consultants are frequently called upon to evaluate critically ill patients with abnormal tests. All patients undergoing consideration for elective surgery and a history of either acute or chronic liver disease require careful evaluation beforehand. A thorough history and physical examination, complete blood count, routine electrolytes, LCTs, and a coagulation profile should be ordered. For patients with marginal hepatic reserve, it is important that patient well-being be maximized before any elective operation. The type of surgery to be performed should also be reviewed.

All patients with postoperative jaundice should be evaluated for a prior history of liver disease. The consultant should also review the surgical procedure performed, anesthetics administered, other medications used, and whether blood products were given during the perioperative and postoperative periods. The pattern and timing of LCT abnormalities may also give a clue to the underlying disorder. As in the preoperative assessment, a routine complete blood count, electrolyte panel, LCTs, and coagulation profile should be ordered.

Unconjugated hyperbilirubinemia can develop as a consequence of blood transfusions, underlying hemolytic disorders, resorbing hematomas, drug effects, or Gilbert's syndrome. A haptoglobin, reticulocyte count, LDH, and Coomb's test should be considered in patients with unconjugated hyperbilirubinemia. Treatment is directed towards the underlying condition.

Conjugated hyperbilirubinemia can occur as a result of either intrahepatic or extrahepatic disorders. Markedly abnormal aminotransferases and LDH in conjunction with a normal abdominal ultrasound suggest ischemic liver injury, drug-induced hepatitis, or viral infections of the liver. Treatment entails restoration of hepatic perfusion, removal of offending medications, and supportive care or antivirals respectively.

Extrahepatic biliary obstruction must be considered in all patients with conjugated hyperbilirubinemia. Abdominal sonography is the best screening test to assess for obstruction. Patients with common bile duct stones usually require ERCP with sphincterotomy and stone removal. Biliary strictures or leaks may require ERCP with balloon dilation of strictures or stent placement for strictures and leaks; percutaneous drainage of bilomas in combination with broad-spectrum antibiotics is recommended for patients with bile leaks and large intraabdominal fluid collections. Surgery may be required for patients with strictures or leaks not amenable to either endoscopic or percutaneous intervention, or for patients who have transected bile ducts after laparoscopic cholecystectomy. Medication effects, benign postoperative jaundice, sepsis, TPN, and acalculous cholecystitis are responsible for intrahepatic cholestasis and conjugated hyperbilirubinemia. Treatment includes removal of offending drugs, supportive care, broad-spectrum antibiotics with drainage of infected fluid collections, adjustment of TPN, and either cholecystectomy or cholecystostomy respectively.

References

1. LaMont JT, Isselbacher KJ. Current concepts of postoperative hepatic dysfunction. *Conn Med.* 1975;39(8):461-464.
2. LaMont JT. Postoperative juandice. *Surg Clin North Am.* 1974;54(3):637-45.
3. Molina EG, Reddy KR. Postoperative jaundice. *Clin Liver Dis.* 1999;3(3):477-488.
4. LaMont JT, Isselbacher KJ. Postoperative jaundice. *N Engl J Med.* 1973;288(6):305-307.
5. Becker SD, Lamont JT. Postoperative jaundice. *Semin Liver Dis.* 1988;8(2):183-190.
6. Evans C, Evans M, Pollock AV. The incidence and causes of postoperative jaundice. A prospective study. *Br J Anaesth.* 1974;46(7):520-525.
7. Green RM, Crawford JM. Hepatocellular cholestasis: pathobiology and histological outcome. *Semin Liver Dis.* 1995;15(4):372-389.
8. Van Thiel DH, Lester R. Postoperative jaundice. Mechanism, diagnosis and treatment. *Surg Clin North Am.* 1975;55(2):409-418.
9. Giallaourakis CC, Rosenberg PM, Friedman LS. The liver in heart failure. *Clin Liver Dis.* 2002;6(4):947-967.
10. Bizouarn P, Ausseur A, Desseigne P, et al. Early and late outcome after elective cardiac surgery in patients with cirrhosis. *Ann Thorac Surg.* 1999;67(5):1334-1338.
11. Whitcomb FF, Trey C, Braasch JW. Preoperative preparation of the jaundiced patient. A review of current practice. *Surg Clin North Am.* 1970;50(3):663-682.
12. Rizvon MK, Chou CL. Surgery in the patient with liver disease. *Med Clin North Am.* 2003;87(1):211-227.
13. Ziser A, Plevak DJ, Wiesner RH, Rakela J, Offord KP, Brown DL. Morbidity and mortality in cirrhotic patients undergoing anesthesia and surgery. *Anesthesiology.* 1999;90(1):42-53.
14. Garrison RN, Cryer HM, Howard DA, Polk HC, Jr. Clarification of risk factors for abdominal operations in patients with hepatic cirrhosis. *Ann Surg.* 1984;199(6):648-655.
15. Kanel GC, Kaplan MM, Zawacki JK, Callow AD. Survival in patients with postnecrotic cirrhosis and Laennec's cirrhosis undergoing therapeutic portacaval shunt. *Gastroenterology.* 1977;73(4 Pt 1):679-683.
16. Bloch RS, Allaben RD, Walt AJ. Cholecystectomy in patients with cirrhosis. A surgical challenge. *Arch Surg.* 1985;120(6):669-672.

17. Friedman LS, Maddrey WC. Surgery in the patient with liver disease. *Med Clin North Am.* 1987;71(3):453-476.
18. Seeto RK, Fenn B, Rockey DC. Ischemic hepatitis: clinical presentation and pathogenesis. *Am J Med.* 2000;109(2):109-113.
19. Johnson RD, O'Connor ML, Kerr RM. Extreme serum elevations of aspartate aminotransferase. *Am J Gastroenterol.*1995;90(8):1244-1245.
20. Gibson PR, Dudley FJ. Ischemic hepatitis: clinical features, diagnosis and prognosis. *Aust NZ J Med.* 1984;14(6):822-825.
21. Ngai SH. Effects of anesthetics on various organs. *N Engl J Med.* 1980;302(10):564-566.
22. Brown BR, Jr., Gandolfi AJ. Adverse effects of volatile anaesthetics. *Br J Anaesth.* 1987;59(1):14-23.
23. Farrell G, Prendergast D, Murray M. Halothane hepatitis. Detection of a constitutional susceptibility factor. *N Engl J Med.* 1985;313(21):1310-1314.
24. Benjamin SB, Goodman ZD, Ishak KG, Zimmerman HJ, Irey NS. The morphologic spectrum of halothane-induced hepatic injury: analysis of 77 cases. *Hepatology.* 1985;5(6):1163-1171.
25. Dawson B, Adson MA, Dockerty MB, et al. Hepatic function tests: postoperative changes with halothane or diethyl ether anesthesia. *Mayo Clin Proc.* 1966;41(9):599-607.
26. Nishiyama T, Yokoyama T, Hanaoka K. Liver and renal function after repeated sevoflurane or isoflurane anaesthesia. *Can J Anaesth.* 1998;45(8):789-793.
27. Brunt EM, White H, Marsh JW, Holtmann B, Peters MG. Fulminant hepatic failure after repeated exposure to isoflurane anesthesia: a case report. *Hepatology.* 1991;13(6):1017-1021.
28. Lewis JH, Zimmerman HJ, Ishak KG, Mullick FG. Enflurane hepatotoxicity. A clinicopathologic study of 24 cases. *Ann Intern Med.* 1983;98(6):984-992.
29. Lambert DH. Isoflurane and hepatic dysfunction. *Anesth Analg.* 1985;64(4):458-460.
30. Kantrowitz PA, Jones WA, Greenberger NJ, Isselbacher KJ. Severe postoperative hyperbilirubinemia simulating obstructive jaundice. *N Engl J Med.* 1967;276(11):590-598.
31. Chu CM, Chang CH, Liaw YF, Hsieh MJ. Jaundice after open heart surgery: a prospective study. *Thorax.* 1984;39(1):52-56.
32. Collins JD, Bassendine MF, Ferner R, , et al. Incidence and prognostic importance of jaundice after cardiopulmonary bypass surgery. *Lancet.* 1983;1(8334):1119-1123.
33. Moseley RH. Sepsis-associated jaundice. *Hepatology.* 1996;24(4):969-970.
34. Levinson MJ. Jaundice in the intensive care unit. *Hosp Pract (Off Ed).* 1993;28(3A):51-4, 57-60.
35. Gottlieb JE, Menashe PI, Cruz E. Gastrointestinal complications in critically ill patients: the intensivists' overview. *Am J Gastroenterol.* 1986;81(4):227-238.
36. Neale G, Caughey DE, Mollin DL, Booth CC. Effects of intrahepatic and extrahepatic infection on liver function. *Br Med J.* 1966;5484:382-387.
37. Miller DJ, Keeton DG, Webber BL, Pathol FF, Saunders SJ. Jaundice in severe bacterial infection. *Gastroenterology.* 1976;71(1):94-97.
38. Carrico CJ, Meakins JL, Marshall JC, Fry D, Maier RV. Multiple-organ-failure syndrome. *Arch Surg.* 1986;121(2):196-208.

39. Cotler SJ, Taylor SL, Gretch DR, et al. Hyperbilirubinemia and cholestatic liver injury in hepatitis C-infected liver transplant recipients. *Am J Gastroenterol.* 2000;95(3): 753-759.
40. Lau JY, Bain VG, Davies SE, et al. High-level expression of hepatitis B viral antigens in fibrosing cholestatic hepatitis. *Gastroenterology.* 1992;102(3):956-962.
41. Lee VS, Chari RS, Cucchiaro G, Meyers WC. Complications of laparoscopic cholecystectomy. *Am J Surg.* 1993;165(4):527-532.
42. Davidoff AM, Pappas TN, Murray EA, et al. Mechanisms of major biliary injury during laparoscopic cholecystectomy. *Ann Surg.* 1992;215(3):196-202.
43. Contractor QQ, Dubian MK, Boujemla M, Contractor TQ. Endoscopic therapy after laparoscopic cholecystectomy. *J Clin Gastroenterol.* 2001;33(3):218-221.
44. Costamagna G, Pandolfi M, Mutignani M, Spada C, Perri V. Long-term results of endoscopic management of postoperative bile duct strictures with increasing numbers of stents. *Gastrointest Endosc.* 2001;54(2):162-168.
45. Lillemoe KD, Melton GB, Cameron JL, et al. Postoperative bile duct strictures: management and outcome in the 1990s. *Ann Surg.* 2000;232(3):430-441.
46. Loinaz C, Gonzalez EM, Jimenez C, et al. Long-term biliary complications after liver surgery leading to liver transplantation. *World J Surg.* 2001;25(10):1260-1263.
47. Himal HS. Common bile duct stones: the role of preoperative, intraoperative, and postoperative ERCP. *Semin Laparosc Surg.* 2000;7(4):237-245.
48. Righi D, Cesarani F, Muraro E, et al. Role of interventional radiology in the treatment of biliary strictures following orthotopic liver transplantation. *Cardiovasc Intervent Radiol.* 2002;25(1):30-35.
49. Frazee RC, Nagorney DM, Mucha P, Jr. Acute acalculous cholecystitis. *Mayo Clin Proc.* 1989;64(2):163-167.
50. Orlando R, 3rd, Gleason E, Drezner AD. Acute acalculous cholecystitis in the critically ill patient. *Am J Surg.* 1983;145(4):472-476.
51. Rerknimitr R, Sherman S, Fogel EL, et al. Biliary tract complications after orthotopic liver transplantation with choledochocholedochostomy anastomosis: endoscopic findings and results of therapy. *Gastrointest Endosc.* 2002;55(2):224-231.
52. Baker AL, Rosenberg IH. Hepatic complications of total parenteral nutrition. *Am J Med.* 1987;82(3):489-497.
53. Fisher RL. Hepatobiliary abnormalities associated with total parenteral nutrition. *Gastroenterol Clin North Am.* 1989;18(3):645-666.
54. Chung C, Buchman AL. Postoperative jaundice and total parenteral nutrition-associated hepatic dysfunction. *Clin Liver Dis.* 2002;6(4):1067-1084.

chapter 12

Nonviral Infections of the Liver

Mical S. Campbell, MD and Thomas Faust, MD

Introduction

Patients with infections of the liver can present a difficult and fascinating diagnostic puzzle. Diagnosis usually requires a careful history and physical examination. Sometimes travel history, occupation, and recreational exposures provide clues. For example, an amebic abscess may be suspected in a patient with fever and right upper quadrant abdominal pain who has recently traveled to Mexico. A variceal bleed in an Egyptian patient with no stigmata of chronic liver disease may prompt consideration of schistosomiasis. Careful clinical evaluations are required because there is no routine panel of tests that can reliably lead to a diagnosis. For example, fecal ova and parasite testing will not diagnose acute fascioliasis because immature flukes causing the disease do not produce eggs. Serology for brucella in a patient with hepatosplenic suppurative brucellosis is not part of any routine panel. The knowledge required to reliably arrive at the correct diagnosis is extensive. The essential aspects needed to recognize and manage nonviral infections of the liver are presented in this chapter.

Pyogenic Liver Abscess

Patients with pyogenic liver abscesses often have an insidious illness with nonspecific symptoms. Symptoms may precede diagnosis by 2 to 4 weeks or longer. Recognizing the clinical scenario in which a pyogenic liver abscess could develop is critical to considering the diagnosis. The median age reported in most recent case series is between 55 and 65 years. There are no significant ethnic, geographic, or gender differences in patients with pyogenic liver abscess, although some authors have reported a slight male predominance. Clues to the presence of a pyogenic liver abscess may be found in a patient's history. For example, a patient who has recently been treated for cholangitis due to a common bile duct stone may develop cough, fever, and vague abdominal pain. While it is possible that the patient has developed a respiratory infection, the patient may instead have a pyogenic liver abscess as a consequence of biliary tract infection. Cough may result from diaphragmatic irritation by an underlying liver abscess.

Pyogenic liver abscesses usually arise from infections elsewhere in the body. Most but not all recent case series have identified the biliary tract as the most common source of pyogenic liver abscesses. A large series from Johns Hopkins (incidence of 20 per 100,000 hospital admissions) showed that whereas earlier cases were most commonly caused by benign biliary disease, recent cases were more often due to malignant biliary obstruction.[1]

Any infected organ drained by the portal venous system may spread infection to the liver. Common sources of infection include diverticulitis, appendicitis, and pancreatitis. In early case series, appendicitis was the most common cause. Inflammatory bowel disease has also been associated with pyogenic liver abscesses. In contrast to the Hopkins series, a 2002 UK case series showed that a majority of hepatic abscesses were caused by spread via the portal venous system from an abdominal visceral source of infection. The UK study had a remarkably low rate of cryptogenic abscesses; 92% of all investigated patients yielded a source. Interestingly, of the few patients diagnosed as cryptogenic, 25% developed colon cancer within 2 years of follow-up.[2]

Infectious thrombosis, or pylephlebitis, of the portal vein is associated with liver abscesses in over 50% of cases. Pylephlebitis can complicate any intraabdominal infection, including female genital tract infections, bowel perforation, appendicitis, and diverticulitis. It is diagnosed by finding portal vein thrombosis in association with bacteremia. Intravascular air may also be demonstrated. Often the affected patient has sepsis. Mortality can be as high as 50%, although more recent data suggest a mortality rate between 10% and 32%. Diagnostic and treatment options include the identification of a hypercoagulable state, heparin, and broad-spectrum intravenous antibiotics to cover gram positive and negative organisms, as well as anaerobes. Not all authorities recommend the use of heparin because the risk of bowel infarction in the setting of pylephlebitis is rare. In addition to the above, treatment of the underlying focus of infection must be instituted.

Hepatocellular carcinoma can develop into a liver abscesses. Furthermore treatment of hepatocellular carcinoma with hepatic artery catheterization procedures has been associated with the development of pyogenic liver abscesses. One case series of 211 patients showed that 3 patients developed an abscess following hepatic intraarterial embolization and/or chemotherapy.[3] Hepatic abscesses have also been reported following blunt or penetrating trauma.

Pyogenic liver abscesses are more common and more often fatal among cirrhotic patients. A population-based Danish study showed that the age standardized incidence rate of pyogenic liver abscesses was 15.4 times higher in cirrhotic patients. Furthermore patients with cirrhosis were 4 to 5 times more likely to die within 30 days of diagnosis.[4]

Pyogenic liver abscesses are cryptogenic in up to 40% of cases. Cryptogenic abscesses are sometimes associated with systemic illnesses such as diabetes, cancer, and cirrhosis. Some authors have speculated about the role of oral flora and transient bacteremia in causing these abscesses.

Clinicians cannot rely on the presence of risk factors to consider the diagnosis because the underlying cause is often not known prior to diagnosing a pyogenic liver abscess. Cholangiocarcinoma, common bile duct stones, or diverticulitis are frequently discovered after the diagnosis of a pyogenic liver abscess. Causes of pyogenic liver abscesses are listed in Table 12-1.

Table 12-1

CAUSES OF PYOGENIC LIVER ABSCESSES

Examples	*Mechanism*
Choledocholithiasis, malignancy, parasites	Biliary tree
Diverticulitis, appendicitis, inflammatory bowel disease, pancreatitis, pylephlebitis	Portal venous spread
Blunt, penetrating trauma	Trauma
Chemoembolization of hepatocellular carcinoma, line sepsis	Hepatic arterial spread
Diabetes mellitus, cancer, cirrhosis	Cryptogenic

The history and physical examination plus laboratory investigation may provide clues to the diagnosis of pyogenic liver abscess; however, they are often nonspecific. Fever is the most reliable symptom and is present in about 90% of patients with liver abscess. Abdominal pain is also common. Other symptoms may include malaise, anorexia, nausea, vomiting, diarrhea, chest pain, and cough; however, they are nonspecific and not reliably present. Physical examination may reveal right upper quadrant tenderness in more than half of cases. Sometimes hepatomegaly, rales, and decreased breath sounds at the lung bases are present. The presence of jaundice should raise questions about biliary obstruction and alternative diagnoses such as choledocholithiasis, biliary strictures, and the jaundice of sepsis. Laboratory investigation commonly reveals an infiltrative pattern of liver associated enzymes with an isolated elevation of alkaline phosphatase.[5] Up to 33% of patients with pyogenic liver abscesses may have entirely normal liver associated enzymes. An elevated white blood cell count and positive blood cultures are present in 90% and 50%, respectively, of patients with hepatic abscesses (Table 12-2).

Radiologic imaging is key to diagnosing liver abscesses. Ultrasound has over 90% sensitivity and computed tomography (CT) has nearly 100% sensitivity for detecting liver abscesses. Intravenous contrast allows visualization of rim enhancement around the abscess on CT scanning. Over 50% of abscesses are solitary, and most affect the right lobe of the liver. Ten percent of patients present with only left lobe involvement.

Given the high prevalence of biliary causes for hepatic abscess, endoscopic retrograde cholangiopancreatography (ERCP) could perhaps be diagnostically useful. One study found that ERCP revealed a biliary source (stones, strictures, or neoplasms) in 24% of patients; however, only 13% of patients had therapeutic inverventions at the time of ERCP.[6] Magnetic resonance cholangiopancreatography (MRCP) may be useful to screen for which patients should undergo ERCP.

In the past, surgical treatment was the standard of care. At present, percutaneous aspiration and/or drainage is performed, and broad-spectrum antibiotics are administered to cover gram positive and negative organisms. Surgery is reserved for refractory cases or when an operation is required to manage an underlying abdominal infection. In practice, percutaneous aspiration may not be able to remove all purulent material

Table 12-2

FINDINGS MOST COMMONLY ASSOCIATED WITH PYRGENIC LIVER ABSCESS

Findings	*Frequency (%)*
Fever	90
Abdominal pain	50
Elevate white blood cell count	90
Elevated alkaline phosphatase	80
Positive blood culture	50

from small abscesses, abscesses with a thick rind, or those with viscous material. In these cases, antibiotics will allow resolution of any residual abscess material. A common question is whether to place a drainage catheter at the time of percutaneous aspiration. Although there are no randomized controlled trials addressing this issue, most studies have shown similar, very high rates of success (over 90%) from either approach. Drainage catheters can become clogged and may need to be readjusted. On the other hand, multiple aspirations may be required if a drainage catheter is not placed. One study showed a 97% success rate with aspiration alone. One-half of patients required only one aspiration, one quarter required two aspirations, and one quarter required three or more.[7]

Cultures recovered from aspiration most commonly show polymicrobial infection. Bacteria include *Klebsiella pneumoniae, Escherichia coli (E. Coli), streptococci, Staphylococcus aureus,* and *Bacteroides* species. One study showed that candida can be seen in one-quarter of patients. This is important, as antifungal agents are not typically part of empiric antibiotic regimens. At times, purulent material from percutaneous drainage catheters is sent for culture. Unfortunately, these culture results are often misleading. One study compared culture results of fluid sent from an existing drain with that from a fresh percutaneous aspiration. In 44% of cases, antibiotic choice based on cultures from an existing drainage catheter would have been excessive or inadequate.[8]

Broad-spectrum antibiotics should be initiated empirically. As culture results become available, antibiotic selection can be refined. Initial antibiotic choices include a third generation cephalosporin with metronidazole or clindamycin, broad-spectrum penicillin with an aminoglycoside, imipenem alone, or a quinolone with metronidazole. In cases in which it is initially unclear whether an abscess is amebic or pyogenic, metronidazole may be included. Antibiotics are usually given intravenously for 2 to 3 weeks and then orally to finish a 6-week course. At that point, the liver can be reimaged to assure that abscesses have resolved and no further intervention is required.

Several case series of successful treatment of liver abscesses by antibiotics alone without drainage have been reported. A meta-analysis of 176 liver abscesses shows that 81% of patients were successfully treated with antibiotics alone. The most important predictor of treatment failure was abscess diameter greater than 5 cm.[9] However, most studies allowed initial diagnostic aspirations and it is not clear if these "diagnostic" aspirations may have been sufficient to resolve the abscess. At present, antibiotics alone cannot generally be recommended.

Mortality in most case series has ranged from 10% to 20%. A number of predictors of mortality have been identified and vary from study to study. The most consistent predictor of a poor prognosis is the presence of underlying malignancy.

In summary, pyogenic liver abscesses usually result from biliary or intra-abdominal infections. Fever, abdominal pain, and abdominal tenderness are common. Laboratory studies often show an elevated white blood cell count, an elevated alkaline phosphatase, and positive blood cultures. The diagnosis is usually established after imaging of the liver followed by percutaneous aspiration of the abscess. Empiric antibiotics should be started immediately, and surgery is usually reserved for refractory cases. Prognosis has improved recently, with mortality rates generally between 10% and 20%.

Amebic Liver Abscess

Entamoeba histolytica (*E. histolytica*) is the cause of amebic liver abscess. It is a protozoa spread through ingestion of contaminated food. Amebiasis is prevalent where sanitation and hygiene are poor. Endemic areas include Mexico, parts of Central and South America, eastern and southern Africa, and India. *E. histolytica* usually causes no symptoms, but may cause dysentery. Liver abscesses result when organisms traverse the bowel wall and ascend the portal vein towards the liver. Under a light microscope, *E. histolytica* appears identical to its cousin *Entamoeba dispar* (E. dispar). *E. dispar* is about 10 times as prevalent as *E. histolytica*. *E. dispar* does not cause disease in humans, does not give false positive *E. histolytica* serology, and does not require treatment.

Patients with an amebic liver abscess usually present between 20 and 40 years of age. There is a striking male predominance (male to female ratio of over 7 to 1). Eliciting a travel history is crucial. Patients with amebic liver abscess have usually traveled to or migrated from an endemic area. Whereas more than one month of exposure is usually required for travelers to acquire amebic dysentery, only a few days are needed for travelers to be at risk for amebic liver abscesses. After returning from an endemic area, almost all patients with amebic abscess will present within 8 to 20 weeks. One case series of 57 patients from San Francisco found that up to one-fourth of patients with amebic liver abscess had no history of travel to an endemic area. Two-thirds of those patients were found to have severe immunosuppression, the most common causes being HIV and tuberculosis.[10]

Symptoms from amebic liver abscesses are similar to but usually more acute than those from pyogenic liver abscesses. Symptoms are usually present for less than 10 days before patients seek medical attention. In contrast patients with pyogenic liver abscess often have an insidious course. Fever and abdominal pain occur in 80% to 90% of patients with amebic liver abscesses. Nausea, diarrhea, weight loss, and cough are sometimes but not reliably present. Amebic dysentery is only infrequently associated with amebic liver abscess. In fact, diarrhea is present or has preceded amebic abscess in less than one-third of cases, and dysentery is associated with less than 10% of patients presenting with amebic liver abscesses. Ova and parasite examination reveals the presence of *E. histolytica* in less than 20% of patients with amebic liver abscess.

On physical examination patients with amebic liver abscess frequently (80% to 90%) have right upper quadrant tenderness. As is the case with pyogenic liver abscess, the alkaline phosphatase and white blood cell count are elevated in about 80% to 90%

Table 12-3

TREATMENT OF AMEBIC LIVER ABSCESS

Drug	*Dosage*	*Side Effects*
Metronidazole	750 mg PO tid x 10 days	Disulfiram-like reaction to alcohol, peripheral neuropathy, nausea, metallic taste
Chloroquine	600 mg PO qd x 2 days, then 300 mg PO qd x 14 to 21 days	Abdominal discomfort, seizures, retinopathy, hearing loss
Iodoquinol (luminal agent)	650 mg PO tid x 20 days	Optic neuritis
Paromomycin (luminal agent)	500 mg PO tid x 7 days	Diarrhea, nausea

of cases. Mild anemia is also frequent, and eosinophilia is usually not present. Even though jaundice is infrequent, it can occasionally develop as a consequence of biliary tract compression by a large amebic abscess.

Both ultrasound and CT scanning are very sensitive for detecting amebic abscesses. Acute amebic liver abscesses are multiple in 50% of cases, whereas chronic amebic liver abscesses are often solitary right lobe lesions. Studies comparing radiological features of pyogenic liver abscesses with amebic liver abscesses have failed to define radiological criteria that can reliably distinguish the two diseases. Often a combination of serologic and clinical characteristics are required to make the distinction.

Serology for *E. histolytica* must be carefully interpreted. In the first 7 to 10 days of infection, serologies may be negative. In the appropriate clinical setting, serologies need to be repeated before ruling out an amebic liver abscess. In endemic areas, up to 25% of people may have a positive serologic test indicating past infection. A positive serology is more useful in travelers, who are unlikely to have had prior exposure to *E. histolytica*. Given the high sensitivity (over 95%), a negative serology can rule out infection if sufficient time has elapsed from time of infection.

Amebic liver abscesses are treated with antibiotics (Table 12-3). Metronidazole is effective in over 90% of amebic infections. No cases of drug resistance have been reported. Metronidazole, 750 mg PO tid, is given for 10 days. Possible side effects include a disulfiram-like reaction to alcohol, metallic taste, nausea, and neuropathy. Chloroquine is a second line option. Response to treatment need only be assessed clinically. Resolution of amebic abscesses on radiological studies may in some cases take many months, and treatment decisions should not be changed if the patient is doing well clinically. Administration of luminal agents (iodoquinol and paromomycin) should follow to eradicate *E. histolytica* residing in the colon.

In contrast to pyogenic liver abscesses, amebic liver abscesses generally do not require drainage. Aspiration is mainly reserved when the diagnosis is not certain. Clinical features and Entamoeba serology usually allow diagnosis without aspiration. Refer to Table 12-4 for a comparison of features of amebic and pyogenic liver abscesses.

Table 12-4

Comparison of Amebic and Pyogenic Liver Abscesses

Feature	*Amebic Abscess*	*Pyogenic Abscess*
Average age (years)	20 to 40	55 to 65
Gender	Up to 90% male	Males equal females
Geographic	Immigrant or traveler	No geographic factor
Underlying cause	Immunosuppression rarely	Biliary tree pathology, intra-abdominal infection, trauma, hepatic artery catheterization, cryptogenic
Onset of symptoms	Acute	Insidious
Symptoms	Fever	Fever
Lab investigations	Leukocytosis Elevated alkaline phosphatase Positive *E. histolytica* serology	Leukocytosis, Elevated alkaline phosphatase Positive blood cultures (50% of patients)
Imaging studies	US and CT accurate; cannot reliably distinguish amebic from pyogenic abscess	US and CT accurate
Treatment	Antibiotics (include luminal agent) Aspiration not required	Antibiotics Aspiration ± drainage Follow-up imaging to show abscess resolution

If needed, percutaneous aspiration of amebic liver abscesses can be safely performed. Typically the fluid recovered from patients with amebic liver abscess will not show the presence of *E. histolytica*. The fluid is frequently described as appearing like anchovy or chocolate paste. Percutaneous aspiration is generally recommended when: diagnostic uncertainty exists, clinical worsening occurs despite antibiotics, and in cases where rupture appears imminent. Predictors of rupture include left lobe abscesses, abscesses larger than 5 cm, and failure to respond to treatment after 5 to 7 days.

Mortality from amebic abscesses is about 3%. The major complication is rupture. Rupture can occur into the peritoneum, pleural space, or into the pericardial space. Amebic abscesses may also develop in the brain and the skin. One prospective study of 135 patients with amebic liver abscess reported a mortality of 17.7% . Independent predictors of death were serum bilirubin greater than 3.5 mg/dL, encephalopathy, size and number of abscesses, and serum albumin less than 2.0 g/dL. There was an extremely long delay of 2 years between onset of symptoms and diagnosis. It is questionable whether the above study is generalizable to the Western world.

In short, amebic liver abscesses are caused by *E. histolytica*. Infection occurs mainly in young male travelers or recent immigrants. Patients commonly have acute onset of symptoms, usually fever and abdominal pain. Serology for *E. histolytica* is typically positive. Generally aspiration of abscess contents is not required. First line treatment is a course of metronidazole followed by a luminal agent.

Hepatic Schistosomiasis

Over 200 million people are infected with schistosomiasis, which results in approximately 200,000 deaths annually. The vast majority of affected people resides in tropical and subtropical regions and are asymptomatic. In the United States, 400,000 people who have emigrated from or traveled to endemic areas are infected. Patients with schistosomiasis cannot infect others. Although travelers can develop schistosomiasis after even a brief exposure, they are unlikely to develop chronic complications. Complications are more common among people living in endemic areas because they tend to have higher worm and egg burdens. In endemic areas, late childhood and early adolescence account for the highest prevalence rates.

Schistosomes are flat, unsegmented blood flukes classified as trematodes. Cercariae are the larval form. They live in fresh water and can penetrate intact human skin to cause infection. Inside humans, they become schistosomulae and migrate through the bloodstream into the heart and lungs. *S. haematobium* resides in the vesical venous plexus and causes bladder disease. *S. mansoni, S. japonicum, S. mekongi,* and *S. intercalatum* live in the mesenteric venules and cause liver or intestinal disease. Disease is caused by the inflammatory reaction to Schistosoma eggs. Eventually eggs find their way into the stool and fresh water. Eggs mature in fresh water snails to complete the life cycle.

Clinical syndromes parallel the migration of parasites and eggs through the body. Within one day of exposure to infested fresh water, cercarial dermatitis may develop at the site where cercariae have penetrated the skin. Four to 8 weeks after exposure, egg deposition in blood vessels may cause Katayama fever. The syndrome is a serum sickness-like illness caused by circulating immune complexes. Symptoms include fever, chills, myalgias, arthralgias, malaise, and headache. Eosinophilia and hepatosplenomegaly are common. With time, eggs may erode from the mesenteric venules into the intestine, causing bleeding, ulceration, and scarring. Symptoms may mimic inflammatory bowel disease. Eggs may also be carried by the portal circulation to the liver. Less commonly, eggs may be carried by the circulatory system to the spinal cord and cause transverse myelitis. Eggs which reach the brain may lead to epilepsy. When eggs travel to the lungs, pulmonary hypertension and cor pulmonale can result. Worms may be a source of recurrent *salmonella bacteremia* and hepatic abscesses.

Eggs induce granulomas and fibrosis within branches of the portal vein. After 5 to 15 years, presinusoidal hypertension develops, which places patients at risk for the development of esophageal and gastric varices. Splenomegaly and cytopenias may also develop. Given the lack of intrasinuosoidal portal hypertension, ascites does not usually occur. Stigmata of chronic liver disease, including spider angiomata, testicular atrophy, gynecomastia, and plamar erythema are typically absent. Furthermore, liver function and liver associated enzymes are usually normal. Because schistosomiasis patients generally have preserved hepatic function, they tend to tolerate variceal bleeding relatively well.

A small percentage of patients with schistosomiasis develop either compensated or decompensated cirrhosis. Most cirrhotic patients with schistosomiasis are coinfected with hepatitis B (HBV) or hepatitis C (HCV). It is likely that viral hepatitis, not schistosomiasis, is responsible for cirrhosis in patients with schistosomiasis. Some but not all studies show that viral hepatitis may have a syngergistic effect with schistosomal infection in causing cirrhosis. One Egyptian study followed 126 patients infected with hepatitis C and/or schistosomiasis for a mean of 62 months. No patient infected with schistosomiasis alone developed Child's class C cirrhosis, and mortality was 3%. Fifteen percent of patients infected with hepatitis C alone had Child's class C cirrhosis and a mortality rate of 12%. Forty-eight percent of coinfected patients had Child's class C cirrhosis with a 48% mortality.[12]

Diagnosis of schistosomiasis can be made in a number of different ways. Stool samples have a sensitivity between 50% and 90%. Rectal biopsies are more sensitive. Serology for schistosomiasis has sensitivity and specificity over 90%, but cannot distinguish active from past infection. Serology is most useful in ruling out schistosomiasis in a traveler to an endemic region. Ultrasound has also been used to assess for fibrous thickening around the portal vein and its branches.

Praziquantel effectively eradicates infection in 85% to 90% of patients. Furthermore it can reverse the changes of presinusoidal portal hypertension. Infections with *S. japonicum*, *S. mekongi*, and *S. intercalatum* can be treated with praziquantel 60 mg/kg PO given in 2 to 3 divided doses on the same day. Patients with *S. mansoni* infections require only 40 to 50 mg/kg. Side effects of the medication include abdominal discomfort, nausea, and headache. Resistance has been described in Senegal and Egypt. After treatment, eggs may continue to be excreted for a few months, though they will not necessarily be viable. Generally proof of cure requires follow-up stool studies 3 to 6 months after treatment.

Apart from eradication of schistosomes, treatment must also focus on managing the complications of portal hypertension. Acute variceal bleeding is managed with esophageal band ligation, sclerosis, and vasoconstrictors (octreotide, terlipressin, or vasopressin). Rebleeding may be prevented with β-blocker therapy and esophageal banding. Transjugular intrahepatic portosystemic shunting (TIPS) may be considered, but given the adequate hepatic reserve, this treatment may not be preferred. Surgical shunts may be the best option for patients with variceal bleeding refractory to endoscopic and medical therapy. A randomized controlled trial of 94 patients in Brazil examined proximal splenorenal shunts, distal splenorenal shunts, and esophageal devascularization with splenectomy. There was no difference in rebleeding after a mean of 85 months follow-up, but patients with a proximal shunt were much more likely to develop hepatic encephalopathy than those who received a distal shunt (39.3% vs 14.8%). No patient who underwent devascularization with splenectomy developed encephalopathy.[13]

In summary, hepatic schistosomiasis is a common, usually asymptomatic infection of tropical and subtropical regions. Presinusoidal portal hypertension may develop which can lead to variceal bleeding. Generally ascites and cirrhosis do not develop unless patients are coinfected with HBV or HCV. Praziquantel is an effective treatment for most patients.

Echinococcosis

The larval stage of the tapeworm *Echinococcus* can cause two types of human disease. Cystic echinococcosis is caused by *E. granulosus.* It is typically a solitary slowly-growing hepatic cyst with potential for rupture and secondary complications. *E. granulosus* occurs mainly in sheep-raising areas where canines eat the viscera of infected sheep. *E. multilocularis* causes alveolar echinococcosis, an aggressive disease which often behaves like a malignancy. *E. multilocularis* occurs in only the northern hemisphere, often in arctic areas.

Although most *E. granulosus* infections are acquired in childhood, the disease usually does not present until the fourth decade or later, as cystic lesions are usually slow-growing. In fact, most infections are asymptomatic. Approximately 80% of cases present as a solitary hepatic cyst, most commonly involving the right lobe. Less frequently, multiple cysts can be seen within the liver or in extrahepatic sites. As cysts grow larger than 5 to 10 cm, patients may begin to experience right upper quadrant abdominal discomfort and nausea. Depending on location, cystic rupture may cause anaphylactic reactions, pulmonary symptoms, peritonitis, biliary obstruction, and pancreatitis. The serum alkaline phosphatase is frequently elevated, and eosinophilia is a common, but not reliable feature. Stool ova and parasite examinations are always negative.

Diagnosis can usually be made from the patient history and medical imaging. Serology can be helpful, but has variable sensitivity. One case series showed that a CT scan alone made the correct diagnosis of *E. granulosus* infection in 96% of cases.[14] Ultrasound or CT scan may reveal a smooth, round cyst; internal septation and hydatid sand are often visualized as well. Cysts that appear heavily calcified are usually nonviable, and treatment may not be required. Generally aspiration should be avoided because spillage of cyst contents can precipitate an anaphylactic reaction. However, aspiration has been safely performed in cases where there is difficulty distinguishing cystic echinoccosis from an abscess or cancer.

First line therapy for cystic echinococcosis remains surgery, usually without the infusion of a protoscolicidal agent. Experience is accumulating with an ultrasound-guided percutaneous technique called PAIR (Puncture, Aspiration, Injection, Reaspiration). Whether surgery or PAIR is performed, albendazole (10 to 15 mg/kg per day in 2 divided doses) is given several days before and 2 months following treatment. Side effects of albendazole are generally mild and include alopecia, abdominal pain, nausea, and modestly increased serum hepatic transaminases. Medical therapy alone has been studied and is not generally recommended. An Italian study of 448 patients showed that medical therapy alone induced initial degenerative changes in 74% of cysts, but 25% of those later increased in size. In only 10% did cysts completely resolve.[15]

Alveolar echinococcosis, caused by *E. multilocularis,* is much less common than cystic echinococcosis. Irregular lesions spread aggressively within and outside of the liver. The clinical manifestations are similar to that of an aggressive malignancy. Mortality in untreated patients with this form of echinococcosis is 90% within 10 years. First line therapy is surgery followed by 2 years of albendazole or mebendazole.

Clonorchiasis and Opisthorchiasis

Clonorchis sinensis and opisthorchis species are parasitic flukes (trematodes). Infection is most common in the Far East, Southeast Asia, and parts of the former

Soviet Union. Infection is acquired from the ingestion of undercooked fish in endemic areas. Cases have been reported in nonendemic areas due to the importation of fish products. Generally infections are asymptomatic. Worm burden tends to increase with age, and most who develop symptoms present after the age of 30.

One to 4 weeks after ingesting eggs, a serum sickness-like illness can result with fever, eosinophilia, malaise, abominal pain, arthralgias, and myalgias. Chronic infection may result in episodic right upper quadrant pain, nausea, anorexia, and diarrhea. Adult flukes live in the bile ducts and may be a nidus for stone formation. Furthermore, worms may initiate biliary ductal inflammation and fibrosis, resulting in strictures and cholangiocarcinoma. Patients may develop relapsing bacterial cholangitis due to the presence of pigment stones in irregularly dilated and strictured ducts. Hepatic abscesses may secondarily develop.

Diagnosis of clonorchiasis and opisthorchiasis can be made by stool ova and parasite examination. The serum alkaline phosphatase may be elevated, and eosinophilia is variably present. Serology may be helpful. Ultrasound, CT scan, and ERCP may also be suggestive. Treatment with praziquantel (75 mg/kg in three divided doses for 1 day) is highly effective.

Fascioliasis

Fasciola hepatica is a liver fluke (trematode) that occurs in temperate sheep-rearing areas throughout the world. Humans acquire infection when they ingest fresh water plants (eg, watercress) that have become contaminated with sheep or cattle feces. Immature flukes migrating through hepatic parenchyma are responsible for acute illness. Typically fascioliasis presents for up to 3 months with fever, nausea, abdominal pain, hepatomegaly, and eosinophilia. Occasionally hemobilia, subcapsular hematomas, or extrahepatic masses may occur. Whereas stool examination for ova and parasites is typically negative, serologic tests are usually diagnostic. CT scanning may show characteristic tortuous tracks indicative of worm migration. Mature fasciola parasites reside in the biliary system. Unlike acute infection, chronic infection is associated with characteristic ova detectable by stool examination. Even though chronic infection is generally asymptomatic, biliary obstruction can occur. Unlike other trematode infections, fascioliasis is not effectively treated by praziquantel. Acute and chronic fascioliasis are most commonly treated with bithionol (available from the CDC) for up to 30 days.

Other Parasitic Infections of the Liver

A number of parasites, including protozoa, flukes, tapeworms, and roundworms may affect the liver. Refer to Table 12-5.

Malaria is caused by a protozoa transmitted by mosquitoes in tropical regions. Approximately 2.7 million deaths occur annually because of malaria. Before erythrocytic infection occurs, replication of the parasite takes place in hepatocytes. In Plasmodium vivax and ovale infections, inactive forms of the parasite may remain inactive in the liver for years. Hepatitis, hepatomegaly, and splenomegaly are common features of malaria. Some medications used for the treatment of malaria, including quinine, mefloquine, sulfadioxine-pyrimetheme, and amodiaquone, can cause hepatotoxicity. Rare cases of fulminant liver failure from *Plasmodium falciparum* infections have been reported.

Table 12-5

Hepatic Parasites

Organism; Classification	Distribution; Transmission	Signs and Symptoms	Diagnosis	Treatment
Entameoba histolytica (amebic abscess); Protozoa	Tropics; Fecal-oral	Fever and abdominal pain	Medical imaging, serology	Metronidazole plus luminal agent
Schistosoma mansoni, japonicum, mekongi, intercalatum; Blood fluke (trematode)	Tropics, subtropics; Fresh water with infected snails	Cercarial dermatitis, Katayama fever, Presinusoidal portal hypertension with varices and splenomegaly, no ascites	Stool O&P Rectal biopsy	Praziquantel Treatment of varices
Echinococcus granulosus, multilocularis; Larval tapeworm (cestode)	Sheep-raising areas (*E. granulosus*) North hemisphere, arctic (*E. multilocularis*); Contaminated soil	*E. granulosus*: Slowly growing hepatic or extrahepatic cyst. Rupture and anaphylaxis *E. multilocularis*: aggressive spread	CT Serology (Stool O&P not useful)	Surgery (or PAIR) with albendazole before and after
Clonorchis sinensis, Opisthorchis species; Liver fluke (trematode)	Far East, Southeast Asia, former USSR; Undercooked fish products	RUQ pain, nausea, anorexia, biliary stones, strictures, dilatation of bile ducts, cholangiocarcinoma	Stool O&P CT/US ERCP	Praziquantel

continued

Table 12-5 (continued)

HEPATIC PARASITES

Organism; Classification	*Distribution; Transmission*	*Signs and Symptoms*	*Diagnosis*	*Treatment*
Fasciola hepatica; Liver fluke (trematode)	Temperate sheep-raising areas; Contaminated fresh water plants (watercress)	Fever, nausea, hepatomegaly, eosinophilia	CT (tortuous tracks) Serology (Stool O&P negative during acute phase)	Bithionol
Plasmodium species (malaria); Protozoa	Tropics; Infected mosquito	Hemolysis, fever, CNS involvement, hepatitis, hepatosplenomegaly	Blood smear	Variable (Chloroquine, atovaquone-proguanil, mefloquine, others)
Trypanosoma brucei (African trypanosomiasis, sleeping sickness); Protozoa	Africa; Tsetse fly	Fever, malaise, headache, lymphadenopathy, CNS involvement, stupor, splenomegaly	Parasite in blood, lymph node, or CSF	Variable (pentamidine, eflornithine, suramin, or melarsoprol)
Trypanosoma cruzi (Chagas' disease, American trypanosomiasis); Protozoa	South and Central America; Reduviid bug (kissing bug)	Megacolon, megaesophagus, cardiomyopathy Early: hepatitis, hepatomegaly Late: hepatic congestion from cardiomyopathy	Serology, medical imaging, clinical features	Nifurtimox, Benznidazole

continued

Table 12-5 (continued)

HEPATIC PARASITES

Organism; Classification	*Distribution; Transmission*	*Signs and Symptoms*	*Diagnosis*	*Treatment*
Leishmania species (Kala-Azar); Protozoa	Tropical regions Seen with HIV coinfection (southern. Europe); Sandfly	Skin infection, lymphadenopathy, massive hepatosplenomegaly, fevers, cachexia, pancytopenia, hypergammaglobulinemia	Bone marrow biopsy	Variable (pentavalent antimony, pentamidine, amphotericin B, others)
Toxocara canis, catis (visceral larva migrans); Roundworm (nematode)	Common in USA; Soil contaminated with dog or cat feces	Young children with fever, hepatomegaly, respiratory symptoms, ocular involvement, eosinophilia	Serology (Stool O&P not useful)	Generally not required
Capillaria hepatica; Roundworm (nematode)	Worldwide, rare; Infested soil	Symptoms identical to visceral larva migrans	Serology negative for toxocara	Unknown (albendazole?)

Splenomegaly is a common finding in *African trypanosomiasis,* also known as sleeping sickness. The tsetse fly is the vector responsible for transmission. Fever, malaise, headache, lymphadenopathy, psychiatric changes, and stupor can arise in patients infected with African trypanosomiasis.

Chagas' diasease or *American trypanosomiasis,* is caused by a protozoa transmitted by the reduviid bug (kissing bug). Hepatosplenomegaly and mildly abnormal liver associated enzymes are common in the acute phase. With the development of cardiomyopathy, passive liver congestion is commonly seen with chronic disease. Other gastrointestinal manifestations include megacolon and megaesophagus.

Leishmaniasis is caused by protozoan parasites transmitted by the sandfly in tropical regions. Infection can be localized to the skin or spread throughout the reticuloendothelial system. *Kala-azar* refers to severe visceral leishmaniasis. It is associated with massive splenomegaly, moderate hepatomegaly, fever, cachexia, pancytopenia, and hypergammaglobulinemia. Liver histopathology can show granulomas or severe fibrosis. Modest increases in hepatic transaminases and alkaline phosphatase are common. Diagnosis is usually made by bone marrow biopsy, though splenic aspiration is a highly sensitive test (>95%). Pentavalent antimony compounds, pentamadine, or amphotericin B can be used for treatment. Leishmaniasis can be seen in patients with HIV infection and CD4+ counts less than 200/mm^3, especially in southern Europe. Typically, HIV patients require long-term treatment, as relapse is common after treatment discontinuation.

Toxocara canis and catis are nematodes (roundworms) that cause *visceral larva migrans*, usually in young children who ingest contaminated soil. The infection is common in the United States. Larvae migrating through the liver and systemic circulation cause fever, hepatomegaly, respiratory symptoms, ocular involvement, and eosinophilia. Treatment is generally not required for this self-limited disease. Hepatic capillariasis causes an identical syndrome and can be suspected when toxocara serology is negative.

Liver Dysfunction in Systemic Bacterial Infection

Cholestasis can occur in response to sepsis or bacteremia. Case series have shown that hyperbilirubinemia may develop in 6% to 54% of patients with positive blood cultures.[16] Transaminases are variably elevated, but usually less than 3 times the upper limit of normal; higher elevations suggest alternative diagnoses such as shock liver and toxic drug effects. Cholestasis may precede or occur in the absence of documented bacteremia. Furthermore, abnormalities in liver associated enzymes may not occur until sepsis begins to resolve. Gram negative bacterial infections cause cholestasis through the release of bacterial endotoxins and lipopolysaccharides. Cytokines are subsequently released, resulting in hepatocyte dysfunction. Mortality is determined by the underlying infection. Persistent or worsening hyperbilirubinemia may indicate ongoing infection. Treatment is primarily directed towards the underlying illness. Other therapies, such as ursodeoxycholic acid and anti-TNF alpha antibody, have not proven to be effective.

Hepatologists are often asked to see critically ill patients in the intensive care unit with sepsis and hepatic dysfunction. Factors that may contribute to hepatic dysfunction in septic patients include the severity and duration of the infection, the concomitant administration of total parenteral administration, and location of the infection. Further investigation may reveal underlying chronic liver disease, which increases the risk of developing jaundice in response to sepsis.

The differential diagnosis of cholestasis and/or jaundice in a septic patient includes gallstone disease, acalculous cholecystitis, hemolysis, and toxic effects from medications and total parenteral nutrition. Abdominal CT scan is often useful to evaluate for hepatobiliary diseases and intraabdominal infections. Liver biopsy is generally not useful in cholestasis related to sepsis; histology shows cholestasis without other findings. Biopsy may be indicated when the differential diagnosis is not straight-forward.

Systemic Bacterial Infections Involving the Liver

A number of different bacterial infections cause systemic infections which may variably affect the liver. Diagnosis often depends upon a knowledge of predisposing factors and clinical manifestations.

Typhoid fever is caused by the gram negative rod Salmonella choleraesuis (serotype typhi and paratyphi). Typically the infection occurs in travelers to or immigrants from Southeast Asia, India, Africa, and South America. Patients are often younger than 30. They present with fever, flu-like symptoms, and often constipation. Abdominal pain and Rose spots (erythematous macules usually on the trunk) often develop in the second week. By the third week, untreated patients may develop complications of intestinal perforation or bleeding. Diagnosis is usually made by blood culture, which is positive in 40% to 80% of cases. Stool culture is much less sensitive, and bone marrow biopsy can usually provide the diagnosis in patients with negative blood cultures.

Abnormalities in hepatic transaminases and alkaline phosphatase are very common, though usually mild. In a minority of cases, salmonella hepatitis may develop, which resembles acute viral hepatitis. Features which distinguish typhoid fever from viral hepatitis include a higher fever, relative bradycardia, a left shift of the white blood cell count, a higher alkaline phosphatase level, lower peak transaminase levels, and an ALT to LDH ratio of less than 5.[17] Some cases have even presented as fulminant hepatic failure. With the emergence of multidrug resistant species, modern antibiotic choices for treatment of typhoid fever include a fluoroquinolone or a third generation cephalosporin.

Leptospirosis is a spirochetal zoonosis caused by Leptospirosa interrogans. It occurs more commonly in the tropics, though it can occur worldwide. In the United States the highest case rate occurs in Hawaii. A person with skin abrasions or cuts may acquire leptospirosis after either an occupational or recreational exposure to contaminated water. Usually the illness presents with fever, myalgias, and headache. Conjunctival suffusion is common and a clue to diagnosis. Occasionally patients have aseptic meningitis. Serum creatine phophokinase levels are often elevated. Hepatosplenomegaly and modest elevations in serum transaminases are common, occurring in up to 40% of patients. Weil's syndrome is a severe, icteric form of leptospirosis, which occurs in about 5% to 10% of cases. The illness can present as multiorgan failure with jaundice and hepatocellular dysfunction, acute renal failure, and gastrointestinal tract hemorrhage. Myocarditis and the acute respiratory distress syndrome may also occur. Diagnosis of leptospirosis is usually made by serology. Treatment options include doxycycline or penicillin for 1 to 2 weeks.

Brucellosis is a zoonotic gram negative coccobacillary infection caused by Brucella melitensis and other Brucella species. It is acquired from contact with infected sheep, goats, and cattle or ingestion of raw cheese and unpasteurized milk. Typically brucellosis presents with fever, malaise, fatigue, and weight loss, and it is often a fever of unknown origin. Sacroiliitis and orchitis may also occur. Modest elevations in liver associated enzymes (particularly alkaline phosphatase) occur in up to 50% of cases. Hepatosplenomegaly is frequently found, and granulomatous hepatitis may be seen on liver biopsy. A chronic hepatosplenic suppurative form of brucellosis has been reported; abscesses with calcium densities can be seen in the liver and spleen. This form of brucellosis is rare and is likely a reactivation of prior infection, similar to what occurs in patients with tuberculosis.[18] Diagnosis of brucellosis is made by blood culture and/or serology. Treatment includes doxycycline 100 mg PO twice daily for 6 weeks plus either streptomycin 1 gm IM daily for 2 to 3 weeks or rifampin 600 to 900 mg PO once daily for 6 weeks. The rare patient with brucella hepatic abscess will require percutaenous or surgical drainage in addition to antibiotics.

Q fever is transmitted by the plemorphic rod Coxiella burnetti. Transmission usually results from occupational exposure to infected livestock. Although Q fever is usually asymptomatic, it can present as a flu-like illness, pneumonia, and/or hepatitis. Chronic cases may result in endocarditis. The hepatitic manifestation of Q fever usually involves modest elevations of serum transaminases and alkaline phosphatase; hyperbilirubinemia and jaundice are rare. Antinuclear and antismooth muscle antibodies are often associated with the infection. Biopsies may show granulmoatous hepatitis with doughnut ring granulomas; the granuloma has a central clear space and a fibrin ring. Diagnosis of Q fever is generally made by serology, and treatment is with doxycycline 100 mg PO bid for 14 days.

Conclusion

A wide range of organisms can infect the liver. Pyogenic liver abscesses are diagnosed by imaging the liver and percutaneous aspiration with gram stain and culture. Amebic liver abscesses can be distinguished from pyogenic abscesses by a more acute presentation, younger patient age, travel history, and positive serology for *E. histolytica*. Schistosomiasis causes presinusoidal portal hypertension with the potential for variceal bleeding; ascites and decompensated cirrhosis usually develop only in the presence of coinfection with viral hepatitis. Echinococcosis can usually be diagnosed by serology and CT scan. Experience with a percutaneous aspiration treatment technique is accumulating. Clonorchis and opisthorchis can cause obstructive jaundice and cholangiocarcinoma. Serious bacterial infections may cause hepatocyte dysfunction and jaundice. Excellent clinical judgement, appropriate biochemical and serologic tests, as well as medical imaging are required for diagnosing the great diversity of hepatic infections. Judicious use of antibiotics in conjunction with either percutaneous or surgical drainage are recommended depending upon the nature of the underlying infection.

References

1. Huang C-J, Pitt HA, Lipsett PA, et al. Pyogenic hepatic abscess: changing trends over 42 years. *Ann Surg.* 1996;223:600-607.
2. Mohsen AH, Green ST, Read RC, et al. Liver abscess in adults: ten years experience in a UK centre. *Q J Med.* 2002;95:797-802.
3. Wong E, Khardori N, Carrgsco CH, et al. Infectious complications of hepatic artery catheterization procedures in patients with cancer. *Rev Infect Dis.* 1991;13:583-589.

4. Molle I, Thulstrup AM, Vilstrup H, et al. Increased risk and case fatality rate of pyogenic liver abscess in patients with liver cirrhosis: a nationwide study in Denmark. *Gut.* 2001;48:260-263.
5. Man KC, Tat SF, Edward CSL, et al. Pyogenic liver abscess: an audit of experience over the past decade. *Arch Surg.* 1996;131:148-152.
6. Lam Y-h, Wong SK-h, Lee DW-h, et al. ERCP and pyogenic liver abscess. *Gastrointest Endosc.* 1999;50:340-344.
7. Ch Yu S, Hg Lo R, Kan PS, et al. Pyogenic liver abscess: treatment with needle aspiration. *Clin Radiol.* 1997;52:912-916.
8. Everts RJ, Heneghan JP, Adholla PO, et al. Validity of cultures of fluid collected through drainage catheters versus those obtained by direct aspiration. *J Clin Microbiol.* 2001;39:66-68.
9. Bamberger DM. Outcome of medical treatment of bacterial abscesses without therapeutic drainage: review of cases reported in the literature. *Clin Infect Dis.* 1996; 23:592-603.
10. Seeto RK, Rockey DC. Amebic liver abscess: epidemiology, clinical features, and outcome. *West J Med.* 1999;170:104-109.
11. Sharma MP, Dasarathy S, Verma N, et al. Prognostic markers in amebic liver abscess: a prospective study. *Am J Gastroenterol.* 1996;91:2584-2588.
12. Kamal S, Madwar M, Bianchi L, et al. Clinical, virological, and histopathological features: long-term follow-up in patients with chronic hepatitis C co-infected with S. mansoni. *Liver.* 2000;20:281-289.
13. Raia S, Da Silva LC, Gayotto LCC, et al. Portal hypertension in schistosomiasis: a long-term follow-up of a randomized trial comparing three types of surgery. *Hepatology.* 1994;20:398-403.
14. Munzer D. New perspectives in the diagnosis of Echinococcus disease. *J Clin Gastroenterol.* 1991;13:415-423.
15. Franchi C, di Vico B, Tegg A. Long-term evaluation of patients with Hydatidosis treated with benzimidazole carbamates. *Clin Infect Dis.* 1999;29:304-309.
16. Moseley RH. Sepsis and cholestasis. *Clin Liver Dis.* 1999;3:465-475.
17. El-Newihi HM, Alamy ME, Reynolds TB. Salmonella hepatitis: analysis of 27 cases and comparison with acute viral hepatitis. *Hepatology.* 1996;24:516-519.
18. Ariza J, Pigrau C, Canas C, et al. Current understanding and management of chronic hepatosplenic suppurative brucellosis. *Clin Infect Dis.* 2001;32:1024-1026.

Bibliography

Amman RW, Eckert J. Cestodes: echinococcus. *Gastro Clin N Am.* 1996;25:655-689.

Bica I, Hamer DH, Stadecker MJ. Hepatic schistosomiasis. *Infect Dis Clin North Am.* 2000;14:583-604.

Hughes MA, Petri WA. Amebic liver abscess. *Infect Dis Clin North Am.* 2000;14:565-582.

Johannsen EC, Sifri CD, Madoff LC. Pyogenic liver abscesses. *Infect Dis Clin North Am.* 2000;14:547-563.

chapter 13

Hepatopulmonary Syndrome

Josh Levitsky, MD and Timothy McCashland, MD

Introduction

Hepatopulmonary syndrome (HPS) is a clinical triad of liver disease, hypoxemia, and intrapulmonary vasodilation. Although HPS typically occurs in patients with cirrhosis, it may also be seen in patients with portal hypertension due to presinusoidal or postsinusoidal etiologies. The two types of HPS are distinguished by the presence or absence of significant arteriovenous malformations. The characteristic clinical presentation (dyspnea, orthodeoxia, cyanosis, and clubbing) is usually present. The diagnosis is determined by the following criteria: hepatic dysfunction or portal hypertension, hypoxemia (or an elevated alveolar-arterial [A-a] gradient), and suspected intrapulmonary shunting on echocardiography or radionuclide imaging. Only a few nonsurgical treatments have been successful in small studies. Liver transplantation (LT) is the mainstay of therapy for HPS and usually results in complete resolution of intrapulmonary shunting. This chapter will provide an overview of the epidemiology, pathophysiology, diagnosis, and treatment of HPS.

Epidemiology and Natural History

The prevalence of HPS in patients with liver disease is reported to be 4% to 27.6%.[1-10] The highest percentage (27.6%) has been reported in patients with Budd-Chiari syndrome, while lower percentages are typically seen in patients with presinusoidal portal hypertension.[7,9,10] These variations are likely due to the use of different methods for diagnosing HPS. While up to 50% of patients with chronic liver disease have abnormal contrast echocardiography suggesting intrapulmonary shunting, only 5% to 13% are actually hypoxemic.[1] Also, hypoxemia in patients with liver disease is often due to causes other than intrapulmonary vasodilation or HPS.[11] Therefore, the actual prevalence of HPS in patients with liver disease is unknown due to the lack of standardized diagnostic criteria.

Portal hypertension of any etiology can lead to the development of HPS (Table 13-1). The vast majority have cirrhosis with sinusoidal portal hypertension.[12] Almost two-

Table 13-1

REPORTED CAUSES OF HEPATOPULMONARY SYNDROME

Presinusoidal Portal Hypertension
Extrahepatic portal vein obstruction
Noncirrhotic portal fibrosis
Congenital portosystemic shunts
Sinusoidal Portal Hypertension
Cirrhosis
Noncirrhotic hepatic injury:
• Chronic graft-vs-host disease
• Acute hepatitis A and B
• Autoimmune hepatitis
Postsinusoidal Portal Hypertension
Budd-Chiari syndrome
Inferior vena-cava obstruction

thirds of patients with cirrhosis and HPS have well compensated liver disease (Child's A) at the time of diagnosis.[3] Patients with HPS and Child's C cirrhosis do very poorly and have expected survivals in the range of weeks to months.[8]

The natural history and outcome of HPS depends on the severity of liver disease and whether or not LT is an option. One study reported an overall mortality of 41% at a mean of 2.5 years after initial diagnosis.[13] Without transplantation, the median survival in patients with HPS has been reported to be significantly lower (10.6 months) than in patients without HPS (40.8 months), especially in patients with Child's C cirrhosis and HPS.[8] The outcome of LT for HPS will be reviewed in later sections.

PATHOPHYSIOLOGY

The underlying mechanism of hypoxemia in HPS involves intrapulmonary shunting through dilated pulmonary vessels and arteriovenous communications. Casts of the pulmonary vasculature in patients who die with cirrhosis show multiple vascular plexuses beneath the pleura, especially in the lower lung zones. Dilated vascular channels found in the pulmonary parenchyma, rather than the pleura, are thought to contribute most to the development of hypoxemia.[14] Direct portopulmonary venous anastomoses, present in up to 20% of patients with cirrhosis, are not believed to play a major role in the pathogenesis of HPS.

The two types of HPS are differentiated by their structural features. Type I HPS, the more common form, is characterized by diffuse, "sponge-like" precapillary and capillary dilation. The degree of intrapulmonary shunting is typically not severe; hypoxemia can usually be reversed by inhaled oxygen. Type II HPS, however, is characterized by direct arteriovenous malformations (AVMs) that bypass alveoli and

Table 13-2

DIAGNOSTIC CRITERIA FOR HEPATOPULMONARY SYNDROME

Must include all of the following:

1. Chronic liver disease or portal hypertension of any etiology
2. Hypoxemia:
   a. PaO_2 <70
      and/or
   b. A-a gradient >20
3. Evidence of intrapulmonary vascular shunting:
   a. Delayed (>3 cardiac cycles) visualization of agitated saline on echocardiography
      and/or
   b. >5% extrapulmonary uptake of technetium-labeled macroaggregated albumin

cause severe hypoxemia poorly responsive to supplemental oxygen. In both types, the normal vascular response to hypoxia, vasoconstriction, is blunted, resulting in persistent vasodilation and shunting.

The most accepted theory for the pathogenesis of HPS is that portosystemic shunting leads to vascular mediators bypassing metabolism in the liver and entering the pulmonary circulation, causing vasodilation. Evidence for this is suggested in pediatric patients who have anomalous hepatic vein return into the left atrium and pulmonary AVMs; surgically correcting the venous drainage into the right heart leads to resolution of AVMs.[15] This "vascular mediator" theory is hindered by the fact that resolution of HPS is not immediate after LT. Vascular remodeling and reversal of HPS after LT may take months to occur.

The main pulmonary vasodilator implicated in HPS is nitric oxide (NO), which is produced by nitric oxide synthase (NOS). Studies involving rat models of HPS have shown that bile duct ligation causes increased NOS levels, enhanced NO activity in pulmonary arteries, and intrapulmonary vasodilation similar to HPS.[16-18] In humans, exhaled NO levels are higher in patients with HPS than in those without HPS and significantly decrease after LT.[19,20] Treatment with inhibitors of NOS has led to improvements in hypoxemia in a small number of patients.[21,22] Other potential vascular mediators, such as endothelin-1, progesterone, and estradiol, may play a role in the pathogenesis of HPS, but have not undergone extensive laboratory or clinical investigation.[23,24]

DIAGNOSIS

The diagnosis of HPS is suspected in any patient with portal hypertension who complains of dyspnea (especially in the standing position), has digital clubbing and cyanosis on physical examination, and is hypoxemic on blood gas analysis. The diagnostic criteria are listed in Table 13-2. An algorithm for establishing the diagnosis of HPS is shown in Figure 13-1.

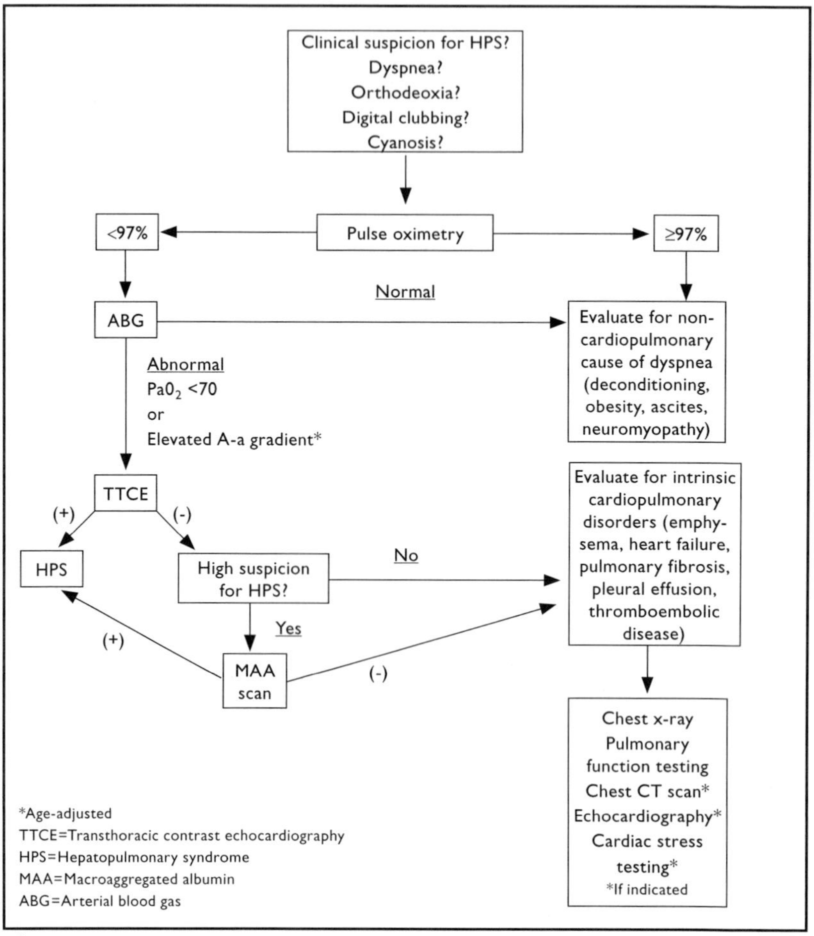

Figure 13-1. Algorithm for the diagnosis of hepatopulmonary syndrome.

Signs and Symptoms

Most patients with HPS have pulmonary symptoms due to hypoxemia. Orthodeoxia (worsening dyspnea and hypoxemia while upright) is the pathognomonic symptom experienced by up to 80% of patients with HPS.[25] The cause of orthodeoxia is likely due to increased shunting in the lower lung zones commonly affected by vasodilation in HPS. Although rare, patients may have a history of paradoxical embolic phenomenon due to venous clots bypassing the pulmonary circulation and directly entering the systemic circulation. Physical examination may be normal, but signs of chronic hypoxemia (cyanosis, digital clubbing) and vasodilation (spider angiomata, bounding pulses) are often present.[5,7] Polycythemia may be present due to severe hypoxemia.[26]

Baseline Testing

Pulse oximetry should be performed in any patient suspected of having HPS. Room air oxygen saturation of <97% is highly sensitive (96%) and can be used as initial screening before proceeding with further testing. Because the specificity of pulse oximetry for diagnosing HPS is low (76%), an arterial blood gas measurement should be performed in patients with pulse oximetry <97% to determine the PaO_2 and A-a gradient. Either a PaO_2 <70 or an A-a gradient greater than 20 must be present to entertain the diagnosis of HPS. Performing imaging studies for intrapulmonary shunting in the absence of hypoxemia is not warranted. A PaO_2 <70 has a positive predictive value for diagnosing HPS of 93%.[27]

Some patients with HPS may also have abnormal pulmonary function tests and chest radiography due to other diseases (emphysema, asthma, hepatic hydrothorax). Chest radiography in patients with HPS may show lower lung zone reticulonodular opacities consistent with dilated lung vessels.[28] However, abnormal findings on chest radiographs in these patients should be further evaluated with helical CT imaging in order to exclude other pulmonary diseases.

Diagnostic Imaging

The most commonly utilized diagnostic test for HPS is contrast echocardiography. In this procedure, agitated saline is given intravenously during echocardiography. The diagnosis of intrapulmonary shunting is confirmed by the visualization of bubbles in the left heart after more than three cardiac cycles. Immediate (<3 cardiac cycles) visualization is more consistent with intracardiac shunting. Transesophageal contrast echocardiography (TECE) has a higher detection rate of intrapulmonary shunting than transthoracic contrast echocardiography (TTCE).[29] However, given the higher expense, required procedure time, and complication rate associated with TECE, TTCE is more widely used as the primary diagnostic test. TECE may be considered in situations where the index of suspicion for HPS is high but other imaging tests (TTCE, lung perfusion scan) are nondiagnostic.

Intrapulmonary shunting can also be detected by radionuclide lung perfusion scanning using technetium-labeled macroaggregated albumin (MAA). Abnormal extrapulmonary uptake (>5%) of MAA is indicative of intrapulmonary shunting. MAA scanning is less sensitive than TTCE and seldom used during initial evaluation for HPS.[30-31] The MAA scan is useful in three possible scenarios: 1) high suspicion for HPS despite negative contrast echocardiography, 2) diagnosis of intrapulmonary shunting in the presence of intrinsic cardiopulmonary disease, and 3) quantifying shunt fraction to determine severity, progression or resolution of HPS.[32]

Alternative Diagnostic Measures

While thin section chest CT imaging is accurate in measuring the degree of pulmonary vascular dilation in patients with HPS,[33] more data are needed prior to universally recommending its use. Angiography is the best way to structurally evaluate the pulmonary vasculature and differentiate type I and type II HPS. However, it is the most invasive and expensive of all imaging modalities, utilizes intravenous contrast, and can be normal in patients with HPS.

Response to 100% oxygen may predict the severity of intrapulmonary shunting. However, it does not separate HPS from other cardiopulmonary etiologies. Given the lack of specificity, response to 100% oxygen is not used in the standard diagnostic criteria for HPS.

Treatment

Nonsurgical

In general, medical therapies for HPS have been unsatisfactory. All of the studies performed are either case reports or small pilot trials and have included a small number of patients in total. Various treatments, such as phenylephrine/isoproterenol, almitrine, indomethacin, aspirin, PGF, somatostatin analogues, cyclophosphamide/prednisone, antibiotics, and plasma exchange, have resulted in only minimal improvement in HPS.

Somewhat more promising are agents such as garlic powder, methylene blue, and NOS inhibitors. In a pilot trial of 15 patients with HPS, 40% had significant improvements in $Pa0_2$ after 6 months of garlic powder.[34] Methylene blue, an inhibitor of NO-stimulated guanylate cyclase, has been shown to temporarily increase oxygenation and pulmonary vascular resistance in patients with HPS.[35] Long-term data on methylene blue is not available. Lastly, treatment with NOS inhibitors (NG-nitro-L-arginine methyl ester, NG–monomethyl-L-arginine) in two patients resulted in decreased exhaled NO and variable improvements in oxygenation.[21,22] Overall, medical therapies have not become standard of care and should only be used in experimental trials.

Interventional radiology procedures (eg, transjugular intrahepatic portosystemic shunting (TIPS) and coil embolotherapy) have also produced mixed results in small numbers of patients with HPS. Since portal hypertension is necessary for the development of HPS, it has been hypothesized that reduction of portal pressures after TIPS may improve the manifestations of HPS. Of the 5 patients reported in the literature, 4 had improved symptoms and oxygenation after TIPS.[36-40] Coil embolotherapy can be attempted in patients with large pulmonary AVMs who do not respond to 100% oxygen.[41] One case report showed improvement in a patient with type I HPS.[42] Although TIPS and embolotherapy could be used to "bridge" patients prior to LT, larger randomized studies are needed to strengthen these recommendations.

Liver Transplantation

The only known effective cure for HPS is LT. Since the first report of resolution of shunting and hypoxemia after LT,[43] subsequent studies involving over 100 patients have supported this outcome. In the mid 1980s, it was considered an absolute contraindication to perform LT in patients with severe hypoxemia ($Pa0_2$ <50). Because the severity of HPS is now considered an indicator of the need for transplantation, views have been modified to include most of these patients for transplant listing. However, LT is not always successful. Some patients have prolonged or chronic hypoxemia despite transplantation.

This raises an important question: which subset of patients with HPS should not be listed for transplantation? Although significant long-term data and randomized controlled trials are lacking, inferences can be made from the retrospective data comparing pre-operative severity of HPS and post-transplant outcomes. In 1997, a review of 81 liver transplant recipients with HPS reported that 30% of patients with pretransplant room air $Pa0_2$<50 died after LT, while only 4% of patients with $Pa0_2$>50 died.[44] Other studies have shown that preoperative $Pa0_2$ in patients with HPS did not affect postoperative mortality.[45-46] This highlights the concern for using $Pa0_2$ as a single measure to determine who should or should not be listed for transplantation, although patients with $Pa0_2$<50 are likely at higher risk.

Response to 100% oxygen and degree of shunt fraction can also be used to risk stratify patients prior to transplantation. Inability to correct hypoxemia with 100% oxygen is associated with severe shunting which may not reverse after LT. This diagnostic predictor has not been evaluated extensively in clinical trials. Perhaps the best test to identify the highest risk patients is MAA scanning. One study involving three groups (shunt fraction <20%, 20% to 40%, >40%) of patients undergoing living-related transplantation for HPS showed a 1-year survival of 80%, 66.7%, and 48%, respectively.[47] The high mortality rate after LT in patients with shunt fractions greater than 40% is worrisome.

In summary, while further studies are needed to clarify the role of these tests, the presence of severe hypoxemia ($Pa0_2$<50), high shunt fraction (>40%) via MAA scanning, and/or nonresponse to 100% oxygen may identify patients at highest risk for undergoing LT. Fortunately, only one case of recurrent HPS after transplantation has been reported in the literature.[48] Careful decision-making regarding listing these patients for LT is essential in improving post-transplantation outcomes.

Future Directions

The future in HPS investigation includes further clarifying the role of vascular mediators in the pathogenesis of HPS, developing nonsurgical treatments, and improving definitions of criteria for transplant listing. Investigation into NO and other potential mediators could lead to improved understanding of the pathophysiology of HPS and further options for medical therapy. The most promising nonsurgical treatments (garlic, methylene blue, NOS inhibitors, TIPS) require more extensive evaluation through randomized, controlled trials before widespread use is recommended. Lastly, improved efforts at risk stratifying patients prior to LT would likely lead to listing patients who have the best chance of survival following transplantation.

References

1. Krowka MJ. Hepatopulmonary syndrome: recent literature (1997 to 1999) and implications for liver transplantation. *Liver Transpl.* 2000;6(4 Suppl 1):S31-S35.
2. Stoller JK, Lange PA, Westveer MK, et al. Prevalence and reversibility of the hepatopulmonary syndrome after liver transplantation. The Cleveland Clinic experience. *West J Med.* 1995;163(2):133-138.
3. Abrams GA, Nanda NC, Dubovsky EV, Krowka MJ, Fallon MB. Use of macroaggregated albumin lung perfusion scan to diagnose hepatopulmonary syndrome: a new approach. *Gastroenterology.* 1998;114(2):305-310.
4. Abrams GA, Sanders MK, Fallon MB. Utility of pulse oximetry in the detection of arterial hypoxemia in liver transplant candidates. *Liver Transpl.* 2002;8(4):391-396.
5. Martinez GP, Barbera JA, Visa J, et al. Hepatopulmonary syndrome in candidates for liver transplantation. *J Hepatol.* 2001;34(5):651-657.

6. Aller R, Moya JL, Moreira V, et al. Diagnosis of hepatopulmonary syndrome with contrast transesophageal echocardiography: advantages over contrast transthoracic echocardiography. *Dig Dis Sci.* 1999;44(6):1243-1248.
7. Anand AC, Mukherjee D, Rao KS, Seth AK. Hepatopulmonary syndrome: prevalence and clinical profile. *Indian J Gastroenterol.* 2001;20(1):24-27.
8. Schenk P, Schoniger-Hekele M, Fuhrmann V, et al. Prognostic significance of the hepatopulmonary syndrome in patients with cirrhosis. *Gastroenterology.* 2003;125(4): 1042-1052.
9. De BK, Sen S, Biswas PK, et al. Hepatopulmonary syndrome in inferior vena cava obstruction responding to cavoplasty. *Gastroenterology.* 2000;118(1):192-196.
10. Gupta D, Vijaya DR, Gupta R, et al. Prevalence of hepatopulmonary syndrome in cirrhosis and extrahepatic portal venous obstruction. *Am J Gastroenterol.* 2001; 96(12):3395-3399.
11. Mohamed R, Freeman JW, Guest PJ, Davies MK, Neuberger JM. Pulmonary gas exchange abnormalities in liver transplant candidates. *Liver Transpl.* 2002;8(9):802-808.
12. Krowka MJ. Clinical management of hepatopulmonary syndrome. *Semin Liver Dis.* 1993;13(4):414-422.
13. Krowka MJ, Dickson ER, Cortese DA. Hepatopulmonary syndrome. Clinical observations and lack of therapeutic response to somatostatin analogue. *Chest.* 1993; 104(2):515-521.
14. Schraufnagel DE, Kay JM. Structural and pathologic changes in the lung vasculature in chronic liver disease. *Clin Chest Med.* 1996;17(1):1-15.
15. Lee J, Menkis AH, Rosenberg HC. Reversal of pulmonary arteriovenous malformation after diversion of anomalous hepatic drainage. *Ann Thorac Surg.* 1998;65(3):848-849.
16. Chang SW, Ohara N. Pulmonary circulatory dysfunction in rats with biliary cirrhosis. An animal model of the hepatopulmonary syndrome. *Am Rev Respir Dis.* 1992; 145(4 Pt 1):798-805.
17. Fallon MB, Abrams GA, McGrath JW, Hou Z, Luo B. Common bile duct ligation in the rat: a model of intrapulmonary vasodilatation and hepatopulmonary syndrome. *Am J Physiol.* 1997;272(4 Pt 1):G779-G784.
18. Fallon MB, Abrams GA, Luo B, et al. The role of endothelial nitric oxide synthase in the pathogenesis of a rat model of hepatopulmonary syndrome. *Gastroenterology.* 1997;113(2):606-614.
19. Rolla G, Brussino L, Colagrande P, et al. Exhaled nitric oxide and oxygenation abnormalities in hepatic cirrhosis. *Hepatology.* 1997;26(4):842-847.
20. Rolla G, Brussino L, Colagrande P, et al. Exhaled nitric oxide and impaired oxygenation in cirrhotic patients before and after liver transplantation. *Ann Intern Med.* 1998;129(5):375-378.
21. Brussino L, Bucca C, Morello M, et al. Effect on dyspnoea and hypoxaemia of inhaled N(G)-nitro-L-arginine methyl ester in hepatopulmonary syndrome. *Lancet.* 2003;362(9377):43-44.
22. Maniscalco M, Sofia M, Higenbottam T. Effects of an NO-synthase inhibitor L-NMMA in the hepatopulmonary syndrome. *Respiration.* 2001;68(2):226.
23. Vettukattil JJ, Stumper O. Endothelin-1 in the rat bile duct ligation model of hepatopulmonary syndrome: correlation with pulmonary dysfunction. *J Hepatol.* 1999; 31(1):192-193.

24. Aller R, de Luis DA, Moreira V, et al. The effect of liver transplantation on circulating levels of estradiol and progesterone in male patients: parallelism with hepatopulmonary syndrome and systemic hyperdynamic circulation improvement. *J Endocrinol Invest.* 2001;24(7):503-509.
25. Herve P, Lebrec D, Brenot F, et al. Pulmonary vascular disorders in portal hypertension. *Eur Respir J.* 1998;11(5):1153-1166.
26. Garcia-Casasola G, Nacher J, Fernandez C, et al. Severe polycythemia as the first clinical presentation of hepatopulmonary syndrome. *J Clin Gastroenterol.* 2003;37(1): 89-91.
27. Schenk P, Fuhrmann V, Madl C, et al. Hepatopulmonary syndrome: prevalence and predictive value of various cut offs for arterial oxygenation and their clinical consequences. *Gut.* 2002;51(6):853-859.
28. McAdams HP, Erasmus J, Crockett R, et al. The hepatopulmonary syndrome: radiologic findings in 10 patients. *Am J Roentgenol.* 1996;166(6):1379-1385.
29. Vedrinne JM, Duperret S, Bizollon T, et al. Comparison of transesophageal and transthoracic contrast echocardiography for detection of an intrapulmonary shunt in liver disease. *Chest.* 1997;111(5):1236-1240.
30. Abrams GA, Jaffe CC, Hoffer PB, Binder HJ, Fallon MB. Diagnostic utility of contrast echocardiography and lung perfusion scan in patients with hepatopulmonary syndrome. *Gastroenterology.* 1995;109(4):1283-1288.
31. Mimidis KP, Vassilakos PI, Mastorakou AN, et al. Evaluation of contrast echocardiography and lung perfusion scan in detecting intrapulmonary vascular dilatation in normoxemic patients with early liver cirrhosis. *Hepatogastroenterology.* 1998; 45(24):2303-2307.
32. Fallon MB, Abrams GA. Pulmonary dysfunction in chronic liver disease. *Hepatology.* 2000;32(4 Pt 1):859-865.
33. Lee KN, Lee HJ, Shin WW, Webb WR. Hypoxemia and liver cirrhosis (hepatopulmonary syndrome) in eight patients: comparison of the central and peripheral pulmonary vasculature. *Radiology.* 1999;211(2):549-553.
34. Abrams GA, Fallon MB. Treatment of hepatopulmonary syndrome with Allium sativum L. (garlic): a pilot trial. *J Clin Gastroenterol.* 1998;27(3):232-235.
35. Schenk P, Madl C, Rezaie-Majd S, Lehr S, Muller C. Methylene blue improves the hepatopulmonary syndrome. *Ann Intern Med.* 2000;133(9):701-706.
36. Allgaier HP, Haag K, Ochs A, et al. Hepato-pulmonary syndrome: successful treatment by transjugular intrahepatic portosystemic stent-shunt (TIPS). *J Hepatol.* 1995; 23(1):102.
37. Riegler JL, Lang KA, Johnson SP, Westerman JH. Transjugular intrahepatic portosystemic shunt improves oxygenation in hepatopulmonary syndrome. *Gastroenterology.* 1995;109(3):978-983.
38. Selim KM, Akriviadis EA, Zuckerman E, Chen D, Reynolds TB. Transjugular intrahepatic portosystemic shunt: a successful treatment for hepatopulmonary syndrome. *Am J Gastroenterol.* 1998;93(3):455-458.
39. Lasch HM, Fried MW, Zacks SL, et al. Use of transjugular intrahepatic portosystemic shunt as a bridge to liver transplantation in a patient with severe hepatopulmonary syndrome. *Liver Transpl.* 2001;7(2):147-149.
40. Corley DA, Scharschmidt B, Bass N, et al. Lack of efficacy of TIPS for hepatopulmonary syndrome. *Gastroenterology.* 1997;113(2):728-730.

41. Poterucha JJ, Krowka MJ, Dickson ER, et al. Failure of hepatopulmonary syndrome to resolve after liver transplantation and successful treatment with embolotherapy. *Hepatology.* 1995;21(1):96-100.
42. Ryu JK, Oh JH. Hepatopulmonary syndrome: angiography and therapeutic embolization. *Clin Imaging.* 2003;27(2):97-100.
43. Starzl TE, Groth CG, Brettschneider L, et al. Extended survival in 3 cases of orthotopic homotransplantation of the human liver. *Surgery.* 1968;63(4):549-563.
44. Krowka MJ, Porayko MK, Plevak DJ, et al. Hepatopulmonary syndrome with progressive hypoxemia as an indication for liver transplantation: case reports and literature review. *Mayo Clin Proc.* 1997;72(1):44-53.
45. Collisson EA, Nourmand H, Fraiman MH, et al. Retrospective analysis of the results of liver transplantation for adults with severe hepatopulmonary syndrome. *Liver Transpl.* 2002;8(10):925-931.
46. Taille C, Cadranel J, Bellocq A, et al. Liver transplantation for hepatopulmonary syndrome: a ten-year experience in Paris, France. *Transplantation.* 2003;75(9):1482-1489.
47. Egawa H, Kasahara M, Inomata Y, et al. Long-term outcome of living related liver transplantation for patients with intrapulmonary shunting and strategy for complications. *Transplantation.* 1999;67(5):712-717.
48. Avendano CE, Flume PA, Baliga P, Lewin DN, Strange C, Reuben A. Hepatopulmonary syndrome occurring after orthotopic liver transplantation. *Liver Transpl.* 2001;7(12):1081-1084.

chapter **14**

Portopulmonary Hypertension

Josh Levitsky, MD and Timothy McCashland, MD

INTRODUCTION

Portopulmonary hypertension (PPHTN) is a pulmonary vascular disorder in patients with portal hypertension. The clinical presentation and consequences are highly variable, ranging from mild (mean pulmonary artery pressure or MPAP 25 to 35) to moderate (MPAP 36 to 49) or severe pulmonary hypertension (MPAP ≥50) associated with a high mortality with or without liver transplantation. Treatment with intravenous agents that cause pulmonary vasodilation or vascular remodeling has made it possible for some patients with significant PPHTN to successfully undergo orthotopic liver transplantation (OLT). This chapter will review the clinical features, diagnosis, treatment, and prognosis of PPHTN.

EPIDEMIOLOGY

In 1983, a study on approximately 18,000 autopsies initially reported the prevalence of PPHTN to be 0.73%, almost 6-fold greater than that of primary pulmonary hypertension (PPH).[1] The first study to utilize right heart catheterization (RHC) criteria for diagnosis reported a higher prevalence (2%) of pulmonary hypertension in 507 patients with portal hypertension.[2] Another study found similar rates (3.1%) in comparable populations.[3] Even higher percentages (12.5% to 26%) may be seen in patients being evaluated for liver transplantation.[4,5] However, when PPHTN is strictly defined by RHC criteria, the actual prevalence in liver transplant candidates is between 3.5% and 9%.[4,6-8] This higher rate of PPHTN is likely due to the fact that patients being evaluated for OLT generally have more severe liver disease than all other patients with portal hypertension.

In contrast to primary pulmonary hypertension, which predominately affects young females, PPHTN occurs more equally in both sexes and is usually identified in the fifth decade of life or later.[9,10] Any cause of portal hypertension can lead to PPHTN. In fact, nonhepatic causes of PPHTN have been reported, including noncirrhotic portal fibrosis,[11] biliary atresia,[12,13] extrahepatic portal vein obstruction,[14,15] and surgical portosystemic shunts.[16] The extent of liver disease, as measured by Child Pugh score, does not appear to correlate accurately with the severity of PPHTN.[2]

Pathophysiology

The arteriopathic changes seen in PPHTN are remarkably similar to those seen in PPH. Three types of pulmonary artery lesions may be seen: 1) medial hypertrophy, 2) plexogenic pulmonary arteriopathy (a network of slit-like channels in the lumen of a dilated pulmonary artery), and 3) intraluminal thrombosis. Because of the hyperdynamic circulation associated with portal hypertension, these lesions may be the product of shear stress leading to smooth muscle hypertrophy, endothelial cell activation and reactivity to circulating thrombotic factors, and vasoconstriction.[17,18] The predominant lesion, microvascular thrombosis, may also be due to the low-grade consumptive coagulopathy, thrombogenic cytokines, and low antithrombin-III levels seen in patients with chronic liver disease.[18] The end result is obliteration of the arterial lumen, resulting in increased resistance and pulmonary hypertension. Surprisingly, the degree of pathologic changes does not appear to correlate with the severity of pulmonary hypertension.

PPHTN may be caused by systemic vasoconstrictors bypassing metabolism in the liver and entering the pulmonary circulation or an imbalance between pulmonary vasoconstrictors (endothelin-1, thromboxane) and vasodilators (prostacyclin, nitric oxide).[19] Increased thromboxane metabolite levels and decreased nitric oxide levels are found in patients with PPH.[20,21] Subjects with PPHTN have significantly higher levels of endothelin-1 in the pulmonary artery than cirrhotic patients without PPHTN.[22] The simultaneous presence of PPHTN and hepatopulmonary syndrome, a disorder characterized by pulmonary vasodilation, in some patients argues against this imbalance as being the primary pathophysiologic mechanism.[23,24] The results of ongoing research will hopefully clarify the role of these mediators in the pathogenesis of PPHTN.

Diagnosis

Although the majority of patients with PPHTN are asymptomatic, any patient with portal hypertension who develops dyspnea should be evaluated for pulmonary hypertension. The diagnostic criteria and evaluation of PPHTN are shown in Table 14-1 and Figure 14-1, respectively. As shown, excluding other etiologies of pulmonary hypertension is necessary in making a unifying diagnosis of PPHTN. Chest and CT radiography may show nonspecific features of pulmonary hypertension, such as peripheral vascular pruning, engorged pulmonary arteries, and right ventricular enlargement.[25] Helical chest CT imaging or ventilation-perfusion scanning is more commonly used to exclude thromboembolic disease as a cause of pulmonary hypertension.[18] Lastly, pulmonary function testing is useful in the evaluation for other chronic restrictive or obstructive lung diseases that may lead to pulmonary hypertension.

Clinical Presentation

Dyspnea is a common complaint in patients with chronic liver disease. These patients should be assessed for other intrathoracic (hepatopulmonary syndrome, inter-

Table 14-1

Diagnostic Criteria for Portopulmonary Hypertension

1. Portal Hypertension
2. Exclusion of Other Etiology of Pulmonary Hypertension
3. Right Heart Catheterization (must meet all three criteria):
    a. Mean Pulmonary Artery Pressure (MPAP) ≥25 mmHg
    b. Pulmonary Vascular Resistance (PVR) ≥120 dynes-s-cm5
    c. Pulmonary Capillary Wedge Pressure (PCWP) <15 mmHg

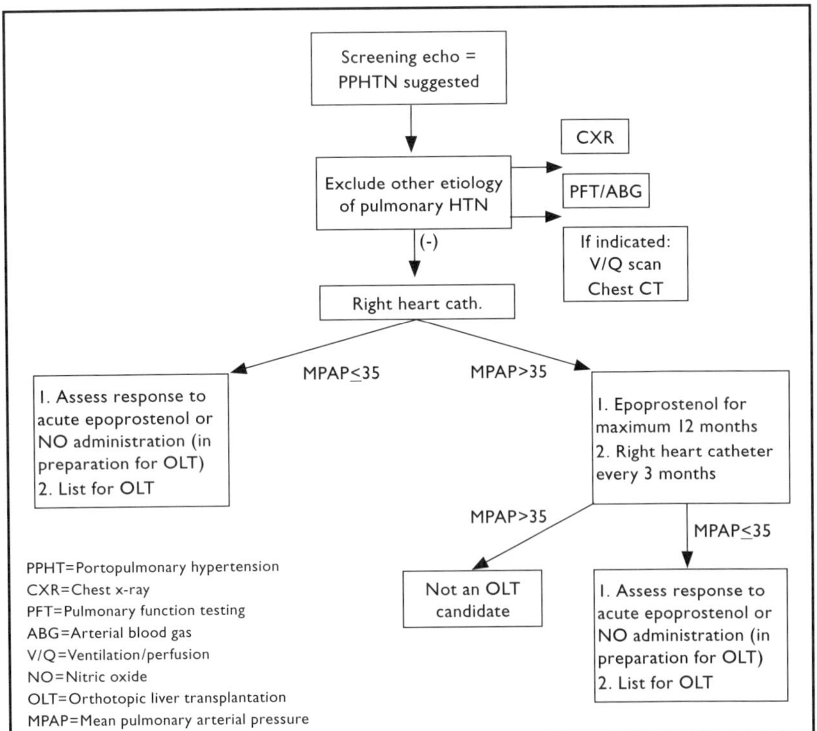

Figure 14-1. Diagnostic and treatment algorithm of portopulmonary hypertension.

stitial lung disease, congestive heart failure, hepatic hydrothorax) and extrathoracic (tense ascites, myopathy, deconditioning) etiologies, even though they may coexist with PPHTN. Other less common symptoms of PPHTN are orthopnea, chest pain, hemoptysis, and syncope. The development of lower extremity edema and ascites is not specific for PPHTN, as many patients with end stage liver disease develop these complications. On physical examination, a loud P2 and palpable right ventricular heave both have a high specificity and low sensitivity for the diagnosis of PPHTN.[26]

PRIMARY DIAGNOSTIC TESTING

Transthoracic echocardiography (TTE) remains the best initial screening test for PPHTN. Significant predictors of pulmonary HTN on TTE are right ventricular dilatation, right ventricular hypertrophy, and an estimated systolic pulmonary artery pressure (SPAP) greater than 40 mmHg.[26] TTE can also assess the degree of right heart dysfunction and tricuspid regurgitation. In a recent study of 165 transplant candidates, the sensitivity and negative predictive value of TTE for the diagnosis of PPHTN were both 100% when using a MPAP of 30 mmHg or greater.[7] Other smaller studies have shown similarly high sensitivities of 91% to 100%.[26-28] Therefore, if pulmonary hypertension is not suggested by TTE, the diagnosis should not be pursued further unless indicated by other clinical evidence.

Despite being an excellent screening test, the positive predictive value of TTE for diagnosing PPHTN is only 30% to 59%.[7,27-28] On RHC, many will not have pulmonary hypertension or have less significant pulmonary pressures than estimated by TTE.[27] The technique of estimating pulmonary pressures by TTE is operator-dependent and depends on finding the tricuspid regurgitant jet and excluding any obstruction to right ventricular outflow. Therefore, patients should not be diagnosed as having PPHTN by TTE alone.

Right heart catheterization is the gold standard for diagnosing PPHTN. Although invasive, RHC determines the severity of pulmonary hypertension, provides wedge pressure measurement to exclude volume-overload states, and assesses the degree of responsiveness of the pulmonary vasculature to vasodilators, such as nitric oxide and epoprostenol, a prostacylin analogue. In patients on chronic epoprostenol therapy, repeat RHC testing is useful in determining if the degree of pulmonary pressure reduction is acceptable for transplant listing. Recent data have also suggested that repeat RHC testing may be indicated for patients with initially mild pulmonary hypertension, as pulmonary hypertension may progress in the waiting period before transplantation.[7]

SUPPLEMENTARY DIAGNOSTIC TESTING

Arterial blood gas (ABG) testing is useful in determining if significant hypocarbia or hypoxemia is present. A PCO_2 <30 mmHg has a relatively high sensitivity and specificity (80% to 90%) for the diagnosis of PPHTN.[29-30] Because of ventilation-perfusion mismatching, patients with PPHTN can have mild hypoxemia when compared to cirrhotic controls, although significant hypoxemia (PaO_2<70 mmHg) is seen in less than 15%.[29-31] In those with significant hypoxemia, a complete evaluation for other causes, including hepatopulmonary syndrome, is warranted. The degree of hypoxemia does not appear to directly correlate with more significant pulmonary hypertension.

Almost all patients with PPHTN have abnormal electrocardiography. The most common changes seen are right axis deviation, right ventricular hypertrophy, and right bundle branch block.[29] Right atrial enlargement and first degree AV block are less common. None of these electrocardiography abnormalities are specific for PPHTN and can be present in various other cardiac and pulmonary disorders.

Dobutamine stress echocardiography (DSE) may be useful in specific situations.[32] An acute volume challenge administered during DSE in patients with PPHTN may determine whether or not the heart can tolerate volume loads during stress, such as those during OLT.[33] However, the value and importance of performing a DSE with volume challenge in the pre-operative evaluation has not been investigated in clinical trials.

PHARMACOTHERAPY

Treatment is warranted in patients with moderate to severe PPHTN (MPAP>35) in an attempt to reduce pulmonary pressures to more acceptable levels (MPAP≤35). In general, the treatments considered for patients with PPHTN are identical to those that have been successful in antecedent studies in patients with primary pulmonary hypertension (PPH).

EPOPROSTENOL

Epoprostenol, a prostacyclin analogue, causes acute vasodilation and has chronic antiproliferative/antiplatelet effects. At the moment, it is the only successful chronic treatment modality for patients with PPHTN, as it has the potential to reverse long-standing pulmonary vascular remodeling. The main drawback is the need for a constant infusion pump (half-life of epoprostenol is 3 to 5 minutes). Patients may develop acute cor pulmonale due to pump malfunction. Other potential adverse effects include hypotension and worsening portal hypertension due to systemic vasodilation, pancytopenia due to progressive splenomegaly, and local or systemic infections from the indwelling catheter.[34-36]

The first report of epoprostenol in the treatment of PPHTN involved four patients who were treated for a range of 6 to 14 months.[37] Long-term administration of epoprostenol resulted in a 29% to 46% decrease in MPAP, 22% to 71% decrease in PVR, and 25% to 75% increase in cardiac output. Of note, all patients had severe PPHTN (MPAP≥50) and, while significant reductions in MPAP occurred, none were less than 40. In one patient, however, epoprostenol was used as a bridge to OLT and was discontinued 3 months after OLT due to resolution of PPHTN.[38] In a series of 10 patients with moderate to severe PPHTN, significant reductions in PVR (47%) and MPAP (16%) and improvements in cardiac output (21%) were seen after long-term epoprostenol.[34] However, six patients died while on therapy, three had progressive portal HTN, and only those with an initial MPAP<50 had reduction in MPAP to 35 or less. Although the numbers are small, epoprostenol has been used successfully in other patients before OLT and in patients with either recurrent or de novo PPHTN after OLT.[31,39-42] Inhaled epoprostenol has been used in one intubated patient with good short-term results.[43] Other prostacyclin analogues currently being investigated in patients with PPH, such as subcutaneous trepoprostinil, oral beraprost, and inhaled iloprost, have not been studied in patients with PPHTN.

Epoprostenol clearly improves PPHTN, but the length of treatment and frequency of monitoring are uncertain. Generally, most of the reported cases were treated with epoprostenol for less than 1 year, usually due to death or transplantation in the interim. The high expense and variable success of epoprostenol treatment probably does not justify treating longer than 1 year. For monitoring, a schedule of every 3 to 6 months of repeat right heart catheterization will allow sufficient time for a treatment response and be conducive to listing patients for transplantation in an expeditious manner.

Nitric Oxide

Nitric oxide (NO) is a potent pulmonary vasodilator that has the advantage of not causing systemic vasodilation and hypotension. Unlike epoprostenol, NO only has acute effects and does not have the potential to reverse the chronic vascular changes of PPHTN. In addition, some studies have shown that inhaled NO has very little effect on MPAP or PVR in patients with moderate to severe PPHTN.[44-45] However, there is some evidence that the reduction of PVR and MPAP with acute inhaled NO is helpful in determining who will respond to chronic epoprostenol therapy and in controlling pulmonary pressures during surgery, such as OLT.[46-48]

Other Pharmacotherapy

A variety of other drugs have been investigated in the treatment of PPHTN. Anticoagulants, such as warfarin, recommended in some patients with PPH may pose a significant risk of bleeding in patients with PPHTN and should only be used when absolutely indicated.[49] During OLT, intravenous nitroglycerin can reduce the MPAP and PVR by an average of 15% and 20%, respectively, although vasopressor medications may be needed to treat hypotension.[8] Interestingly, a 6-month trial of oral isosorbide-5-mononitrate improved pulmonary pressures significantly in one patient with PPHTN.[50] Calcium-channel blockers improve survival in patients with PPH, but little data exist in the treatment of PPHTN. Endothelin-1 antagonists, such as bosentan and sitxsenten, have efficacy in pulmonary hypertension but dose-dependent hepatotoxicity limits their use in PPHTN.[51-52] Phosphodiesterase inhibitors, such as dipyrimadole and sildenafil, are also variably effective in PPH but have not been studied extensively in PPHTN.[53] Lastly, L-arginine increases endogenous NO production, but further studies are needed to determine its effect on PPHTN.[54-55]

Liver Transplantation

Liver transplantation remains the definitive treatment for patients with decompensated cirrhosis and mild PPHTN (MPAP≤35). Rarely, patients require combined heart-lung-liver transplantation for PPHTN, although it appears that the risk of right ventricular failure after OLT is significantly reduced if heart transplantation occurs before OLT.[56-57] The only reported case of a living-related transplant recipient with PPHTN died of right heart failure after transplantation.[58] Improvements in monitoring and control of pulmonary hypertension intra-operatively may reduce morbidity and mortality from OLT in patients with PPHTN.

Selection Criteria

Patients with MPAP≤35 or systolic PAP≤60 have minimal risk to undergo OLT and should be listed without significant concern.[8,59-61] Patients with MPAP of 36 to 49 + PVR >250 or MPAP≥50 have a 50% and 100% postoperative mortality, respectively, and should not be listed unless the MPAP can be typically reduced to 35 or less.[59] Unfortunately, patients with MPAP over 50 do not respond to treatment enough for transplant listing.[37,59] Therefore, select patients who can achieve an MPAP≤35 with epoprostenol treatment should be considered for transplant listing. Those with MPAP>35 should be considered for alternative treatments.

Only a few small studies have reported the outcome of patients with PPHTN who did not undergo OLT. While mild PPHTN typically does not appear to affect long-term outcome, moderate to severe PPHTN, either treated with epoprostenol or untreated, is associated with a high mortality rate (63% to 80%) without OLT.[6,34] The main causes of death in these patients are right heart failure, hepatic deterioration, sepsis, and respiratory failure.

Perioperative Management

Pulmonary pressures are routinely measured intraoperatively. In those with known PPHTN or found to have PPHTN intraoperatively, acute epoprostenol administration is often the first choice to reduce MPAP and PVR. For nonresponse to prostacyclin therapy, inhaled NO or intravenous nitroglycerine, nitroprusside, dobutamine, or diltiazem can be attempted to reduce pressures.[8,46-47] Correcting hypothermia, hypoxia, acidemia, hypercarbia, electrolyte derangements, hypervolemia, and hypovolemia will help lower pulmonary pressures.[62] Vascular clamps should be removed slowly to avoid acute right heart failure in the immediate post-reperfusion time period. Swan-Ganz catheters should continue to monitor pulmonary pressures after OLT, as MPAP may rise in the days following OLT.[63]

Post-Transplant Period

In patients with preoperative MPAP≤35, the immediate and long-term post-transplant period is unlikely to be different than in patients with no PPHTN. Transthoracic echocardiography can be used to screen these patients postoperatively for progression of pulmonary hypertension. However, in patients who needed epoprostenol to achieve an MPAP≤35 prior to OLT, resolution of PPHTN may take weeks to months. They require continued administration of epoprostenol after OLT until pressures are consistently in the normal to mild range. If pulmonary hypertension resolves after OLT, it is unlikely to reoccur in patients with stable graft function. Recurrent or de novo PPHTN has been reported in a small number of patients in the setting of graft dysfunction or failure.[40-42]

Future Directions

The main areas of future research include clarifying pathophysiology of PPHTN and the role of medical and surgical treatments. Further understanding of the potential vascular mediators will provide targets for new drug development. Because the treatment modalities are often borrowed from PPH and applied to PPHTN, newer agents, such as oral vasodilator or antiproliferative drugs, will continue to be developed and investigated in patients with PPHTN. In patients with moderate to severe PPHTN, larger outcome studies need to be performed to refine transplantation criteria and understand pre- and postoperative management. Multidisciplinary teams of hepatologists, surgeons, cardiologists, and pulmonologists need to be developed to assist in decision-making and planning medical or surgical treatments.

References

1. McDonnell PJ, Toye PA, Hutchins GM. Primary pulmonary hypertension and cirrhosis: are they related? *Am Rev Respir Dis.* 1983;127(4):437-441.
2. Hadengue A, Benhayoun MK, Lebrec D, Benhamou JP. Pulmonary hypertension complicating portal hypertension: prevalence and relation to splanchnic hemodynamics. *Gastroenterology.* 1991;100(2):520-528.
3. Yang YY, Lin HC, Lee WC, et al. Portopulmonary hypertension: distinctive hemodynamic and clinical manifestations. *J Gastroenterol.* 2001;36(3):181-186.
4. Castro M, Krowka MJ, Schroeder DR, et al. Frequency and clinical implications of increased pulmonary artery pressures in liver transplant patients. *Mayo Clin Proc.* 1996;71(6):543-551.
5. Starkel P, Vera A, Gunson B, Mutimer D. Outcome of liver transplantation for patients with pulmonary hypertension. *Liver Transpl.* 2002;8(4):382-388.
6. Ramsay MA, Simpson BR, Nguyen AT, et al. Severe pulmonary hypertension in liver transplant candidates. *Liver Transpl Surg.* 1997;3(5):494-500.
7. Colle IO, Moreau R, Godinho E, et al. Diagnosis of portopulmonary hypertension in candidates for liver transplantation: a prospective study. *Hepatology.* 2003;37(2):401-409.
8. Taura P, Garcia-Valdecasas JC, Beltran J, et al. Moderate primary pulmonary hypertension in patients undergoing liver transplantation. *Anesth Analg.* 1996;83(4):675-680.
9. Herve P, Lebrec D, Brenot F, et al. Pulmonary vascular disorders in portal hypertension. *Eur Respir J.* 1998;11(5):1153-1166.
10. Robalino BD, Moodie DS. Association between primary pulmonary hypertension and portal hypertension: analysis of its pathophysiology and clinical, laboratory and hemodynamic manifestations. *J Am Coll Cardiol.* 1991;17(2):492-498.
11. De BK, Pal A, Santra A, et al. Primary pulmonary hypertension in non-cirrhotic portal fibrosis. *Indian J Gastroenterol.* 1997;16(3):85-87.
12. Moscoso G, Mieli-Vergani G, Mowat AP, Portmann B. Sudden death caused by unsuspected pulmonary arterial hypertension, 10 years after surgery for extrahepatic biliary atresia. *J Pediatr Gastroenterol Nutr.* 1991;12(3):388-393.
13. Soh H, Hasegawa T, Sasaki T, et al. Pulmonary hypertension associated with postoperative biliary atresia: report of two cases. *J Pediatr Surg.* 1999;34(12):1779-1781.
14. Tokiwa K, Iwai N, Nakamura K, Shiraishi I, Hayashi S, Onouchi Z. Pulmonary hypertension as a fatal complication of extrahepatic portal hypertension. *Eur J Pediatr Surg.* 1993;3(6):373-375.
15. Klochkov SA, Alekseevskikh I, Seniakovich VM. Histologic changes in the lungs and heart in children with extrahepatic blockade of the portal circulation. *Arkh Patol.* 1996;58(3):54-58.
16. Bernthal AC, Eybel CE, Payne JA. Primary pulmonary hypertension after portocaval shunt. *J Clin Gastroenterol.* 1983;5(4):353-356.
17. Krowka MJ, Edwards WD. A spectrum of pulmonary vascular pathology in portopulmonary hypertension. *Liver Transpl.* 2000;6(2):241-242.
18. Mandell MS. Critical care issues: portopulmonary hypertension. *Liver Transpl.* 2000;6(4 Suppl 1):S36-S43.
19. Fishman AP. Etiology and pathogenesis of primary pulmonary hypertension: a perspective. *Chest.* 1998;114(3 Suppl):242S-247S.

20. Christman BW, McPherson CD, Newman JH, et al. An imbalance between the excretion of thromboxane and prostacyclin metabolites in pulmonary hypertension. *N Engl J Med.* 1992;327(2):70-75.
21. Cella G, Bellotto F, Tona F, et al. Plasma markers of endothelial dysfunction in pulmonary hypertension. *Chest.* 2001;120(4):1226-1230.
22. Benjaminov FS, Prentice M, Sniderman KW, et al. Portopulmonary hypertension in decompensated cirrhosis with refractory ascites. *Gut.* 2003;52(9):1355-1362.
23. Raffy O, Sleiman C, Vachiery F, et al. Refractory hypoxemia during liver cirrhosis. Hepatopulmonary syndrome or "primary" pulmonary hypertension? *Am J Respir Crit Care Med.* 1996;153(3):1169-1171.
24. Mal H, Burgiere O, Durand F, Fartoukh M, Cohen-Solal A, Fournier M. Pulmonary hypertension following hepatopulmonary syndrome in a patient with cirrhosis. *J Hepatol.* 1999;31(2):360-364.
25. Oh YW, Kang EY, Lee NJ, Suh WH, Godwin JD. Thoracic manifestations associated with advanced liver disease. *J Comput Assist Tomogr.* 2000;24(5):699-705.
26. Pilatis ND, Jacobs LE, Rerkpattanapipat P, et al. Clinical predictors of pulmonary hypertension in patients undergoing liver transplant evaluation. *Liver Transpl.* 2000;6(1):85-91.
27. Cotton CL, Gandhi S, Vaitkus PT, et al. Role of echocardiography in detecting portopulmonary hypertension in liver transplant candidates. *Liver Transpl.* 2002;8(11):1051-1054.
28. Torregrosa M, Genesca J, Gonzalez A, et al. Role of Doppler echocardiography in the assessment of portopulmonary hypertension in liver transplantation candidates. *Transplantation.* 2001;71(4):572-574.
29. Kuo PC, Plotkin JS, Johnson LB, et al. Distinctive clinical features of portopulmonary hypertension. *Chest.* 1997;112(4):980-986.
30. Swanson KL, Krowka MJ. Arterial oxygenation associated with portopulmonary hypertension. *Chest.* 2002;121(6):1869-1875.
31. Schott R, Chaouat A, Launoy A, Pottecher T, Weitzenblum E. Improvement of pulmonary hypertension after liver transplantation. *Chest.* 1999;115(6):1748-1749.
32. Kuo PC, Plotkin JS, Gaine S, et al. Portopulmonary hypertension and the liver transplant candidate. *Transplantation.* 1999;67(8):1087-1093.
33. Kuo PC, Schroeder RA, Vagelos RH, et al. Volume-mediated pulmonary responses in liver transplant candidates. *Clin Transplant.* 1996;10(6 Pt 1):521-527.
34. Krowka MJ, Frantz RP, McGoon MD, et al. Improvement in pulmonary hemodynamics during intravenous epoprostenol (prostacyclin): A study of 15 patients with moderate to severe portopulmonary hypertension. *Hepatology.* 1999; 30(3):641-648.
35. Findlay JY, Plevak DJ, Krowka MJ, Sack EM, Porayko MK. Progressive splenomegaly after epoprostenol therapy in portopulmonary hypertension. *Liver Transpl Surg.* 1999;5(5):362-365.
36. McLaughlin VV, Genthner DE, Panella MM, Hess DM, Rich S. Compassionate use of continuous prostacyclin in the management of secondary pulmonary hypertension: a case series. *Ann Intern Med.* 1999;130(9):740-743.
37. Kuo PC, Johnson LB, Plotkin JS, et al. Continuous intravenous infusion of epoprostenol for the treatment of portopulmonary hypertension. *Transplantation.* 1997; 63(4):604-606.
38. Plotkin JS, Kuo PC, Rubin LJ, et al. Successful use of chronic epoprostenol as a bridge to liver transplantation in severe portopulmonary hypertension. *Transplantation.* 1998;65(4):457-459.

39. Tan HP, Markowitz JS, Montgomery RA, et al. Liver transplantation in patients with severe portopulmonary hypertension treated with preoperative chronic intravenous epoprostenol. *Liver Transpl.* 2001;7(8):745-749.
40. Kett DH, Acosta RC, Campos MA, et al. Recurrent portopulmonary hypertension after liver transplantation: management with epoprostenol and resolution after retransplantation. *Liver Transpl.* 2001;7(7):645-648.
41. Rafanan AL, Maurer J, Mehta AC, Schilz R. Progressive portopulmonary hypertension after liver transplantation treated with epoprostenol. *Chest.* 2000;118(5):1497-1500.
42. Koneru B, Fisher A, Wilson DJ, Klein KM, delaTorre AN, Seguel J. De novo diagnosis of portopulmonary hypertension following liver transplantation. *Am J Transplant.* 2002;2(9):883-886.
43. Schroeder RA, Rafii AA, Plotkin JS, et al. Use of aerosolized inhaled epoprostenol in the treatment of portopulmonary hypertension. *Transplantation.* 2000;70(3):548-550.
44. Ramsay MA, Schmidt A, Hein HA, et al. Nitric oxide does not reverse pulmonary hypertension associated with end-stage liver disease: a preliminary report. *Hepatology.* 1997;25(3):524-527.
45. De Wolf AM, Scott V, Bjerke R, et al. Hemodynamic effects of inhaled nitric oxide in four patients with severe liver disease and pulmonary hypertension. *Liver Transpl Surg.* 1997;3(6):594-597.
46. Ramsay MA, Spikes C, East CA, et al. The perioperative management of portopulmonary hypertension with nitric oxide and epoprostenol. *Anesthesiology.* 1999; 90(1):299-301.
47. Findlay JY, Harrison BA, Plevak DJ, Krowka MJ. Inhaled nitric oxide reduces pulmonary artery pressures in portopulmonary hypertension. *Liver Transpl Surg.* 1999;5(5):381-387.
48. Mandell MS, Duke J. Nitric oxide reduces pulmonary hypertension during hepatic transplantation. *Anesthesiology.* 1994;81(6):1538-1542.
49. Rich S. Primary pulmonary hypertension. *Curr Treat Options Cardiovasc Med.* 2000; 2(2):135-140.
50. Ribas J, Angrill J, Barbera JA, et al. Isosorbide-5-mononitrate in the treatment of pulmonary hypertension associated with portal hypertension. *Eur Respir J.* 1999; 13(1):210-212.
51. Rubin LJ, Badesch DB, Barst RJ, et al. Bosentan therapy for pulmonary arterial hypertension. *N Engl J Med.* 2002;346(12):896-903.
52. Barst RJ, Rich S, Widlitz A, Horn EM, McLaughlin V, McFarlin J. Clinical efficacy of sitaxsentan, an endothelin-A receptor antagonist, in patients with pulmonary arterial hypertension: open-label pilot study. *Chest.* 2002; 121(6):1860-1868.
53. Michelakis E, Tymchak W, Lien D, Webster L, Hashimoto K, Archer S. Oral sildenafil is an effective and specific pulmonary vasodilator in patients with pulmonary arterial hypertension: comparison with inhaled nitric oxide. *Circulation.* 2002;105(20):2398-2403.
54. Shiraishi M, Hiroyasu S, Nagahama M, et al. Role of exogenous L-arginine in hepatic ischemia-reperfusion injury. *J Surg Res.* 1997; 69(2):429-434.
55. Nilsson B, Yoshida T, Delbro D, Andius S, Friman S. Pretreatment with L-arginine reduces ischemia/reperfusion injury of the liver. *Transplant Proc.* 1997;29(7):3111-3112.

56. Dennis CM, McNeil KD, Dunning J, et al. Heart-lung-liver transplantation. *J Heart Lung Transplant.* 1996;15(5):536-538.
57. Pirenne J, Verleden G, Nevens F, et al. Combined liver and (heart-)lung transplantation in liver transplant candidates with refractory portopulmonary hypertension. *Transplantation.* 2002;73(1):140-142.
58. Kikuchi H, Ohkohchi N, Orii T, Satomi S. Living-related liver transplantation in patients with pulmonary vascular disease. *Transplant Proc.* 2000;32(7):2177-2178.
59. Krowka MJ, Plevak DJ, Findlay JY, Rosen CB, Wiesner RH, Krom RA. Pulmonary hemodynamics and perioperative cardiopulmonary-related mortality in patients with portopulmonary hypertension undergoing liver transplantation. *Liver Transpl.* 2000; 6(4):443-450.
60. Plevak D, Krowka M, Rettke S, Dunn W, Southorn P. Successful liver transplantation in patients with mild to moderate pulmonary hypertension. *Transplant Proc.* 1993;25(2):1840.
61. Ramsay MA. Perioperative mortality in patients with portopulmonary hypertension undergoing liver transplantation. *Liver Transpl.* 2000;6(4):451-452.
62. Budhiraja R, Hassoun PM. Portopulmonary hypertension: a tale of two circulations. *Chest.* 2003;123(2):562-576.
63. Cheng EY, Woehlck HJ. Pulmonary artery hypertension complicating anesthesia for liver transplantation. *Anesthesiology.* 1992;77(2):389-392.

chapter **15**

Liver Transplantation

Steven-Huy B. Han, MD; Tram T. Tran, MD; and Paul Martin, MD

Introduction

Orthotopic liver transplantation (OLT) is the definitive treatment for patients with end-stage liver failure. An increasing need for donor organs coupled with a static cadaveric donor supply had resulted in an increasing number of waiting list deaths as patients succumb to advancing complications of their liver disease in the face of longer waiting times for OLT prior to the introduction of MELD as the basis for organ allocation (Figure 15-1).

A significant predictor of post-OLT survival is the severity of hepatocellular dysfunction and associated debility at the time of surgery. Patients who have experienced fewer complications of liver disease generally fare better post-OLT than patients who have suffered multiple complications of cirrhosis. However, for the patient who eventually receives an OLT, overall long-term survival is excellent: approximately 85% to 90% at 1 year and 75% at 5 years post-OLT for most indications.

The medical management of OLT has continually evolved since the early 1980s, with the goals shifting from prevention of allograft rejection to prevention and treatment of recurrent disease. Recurrence of hepatitis C virus (HCV) is currently a major challenge as HCV is the most common indication for OLT, and graft reinfection is universal with a lack of effective prophylaxis. Surgical techniques for OLT have also evolved. Innovations such as splitting of cadaveric grafts, the use of so-called marginal grafts from older and nonheart-beating donors, and living-related organ transplantation have all evolved in response to the static supply of deceased donor organs.

Indications

The diagnosis of cirrhosis in the absence of decompensation, per se, is not an indication for OLT in all patients. Indeed, Fattovich and colleagues observed that fewer than 30% of patients with well-compensated cirrhosis due to HCV eventually developed decompensated liver disease (eg, ascites and/or variceal bleeding) at 10 years (Figure 15-2).

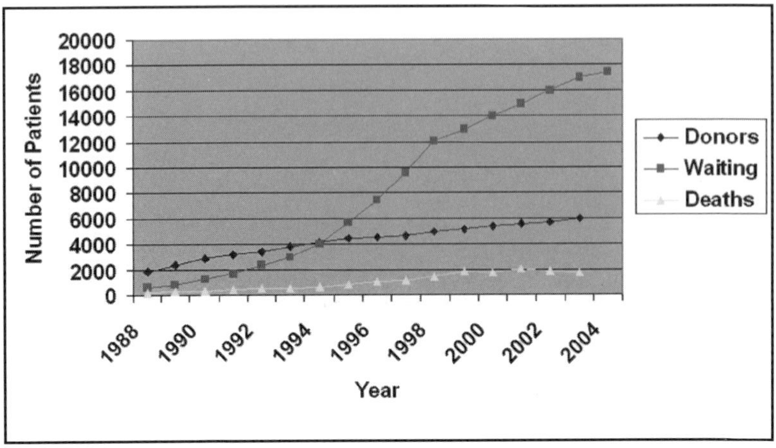

Figure 15-1. UNOS database. Liver transplant recipient waiting list, donors, and waiting list deaths.

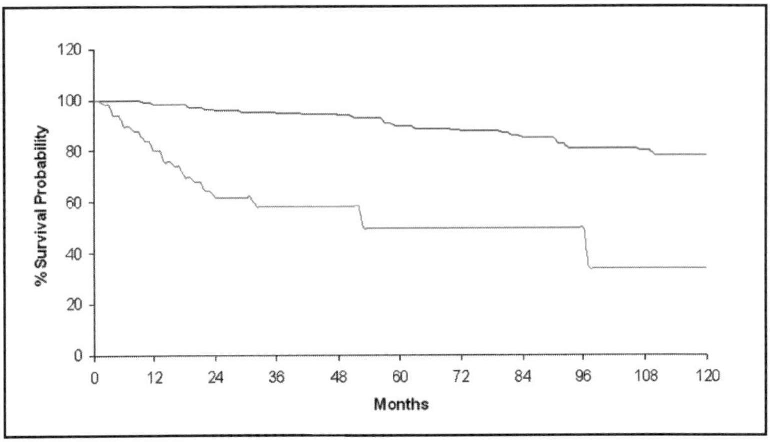

Figure 15-2. Probability of survival with compensated and decompensated hepatitis C cirrhosis. Curve A represents the probability of survival after diagnosis in patients with compensated hepatitis C cirrhosis. The 5-year probability rate was 91%. Curve B represents the probability of survival after the appearance of the first major complication in patients with decompensated hepatitis C cirrhosis. The 5-year probability rate was 50%. (Adapted from Fattovich, et al. *Gastroenterology*. 1997;112.)

The general indications for OLT include deterioration in biochemical tests of liver function (coagulopathy, hyperbilirubinemia, and/or hypoalbuminemia), complications of portal hypertension refractory to medical management (ascites, variceal bleeding, portosystemic encephalopathy), development of hepatocellular carcinoma, and deteriorating quality of life for patients as manifested by disabling symptoms

Table 15-1

MEDICAL MANAGEMENT RECOMMENDATIONS FOR THE CIRRHOTIC PATIENT AWAITING LIVER TRANSPLANT

Medical Condition	*Medical Management*
Cirrhosis due to hepatitis B	Antiviral therapy (adefoir dipivoxil or entecavir*) to suppress HBV levels prior to OLT
Esophageal varices	Prophylactic ß-blocker therapy to prevent first bleed
	Band ligation or sclerotherapy for active bleeding
Ascites	2-gram sodium-restricted diet
	Diuretic therapy to induce natriuress
	Oral antibiotics for SBP prophylaxis after GI bleed or in patients with low ascites total protein
Encephalopathy	Aggressive catharsis with lactulose
	Selective bowel decontamination with nonabsorbable antibiotic
	Low-protein diet
	Restrict patient from driving automobile

Use of entecavir should be avoided if lamivudine-resistance is suspected due to the possibility of entecavir cross-resistance.

that disrupt their ability to function at work or perform even basic activities of daily living. In this regard, early referral is paramount, as ideally, OLT should occur before a protracted period of disability in order to minimize the time patients may have to cope with the hardships of unemployment and to increase the chance of rehabilitation to full employment and social functioning post-OLT.

Besides early referral for evaluation, appropriate medical management of the liver failure patient is key to optimize a successful post-OLT outcome (Table 15-1).

DISEASE-SPECIFIC INDICATIONS

The major disease indications for OLT and their prevalence in US adults are shown in Figure 15-3.

Hepatitis C

The principal concern regarding OLT for HCV-related cirrhosis is the burden of recurrence post-OLT. Recurrent HCV viremia occurs universally, but in a subset of HCV-related recipients, severe allograft injury and failure develops. Studies of serial

Figure 15-3. Liver diseases of adult transplant recipients in the United States. Note: n=24,900 patients. (Adapted from the United Network for Organ Sharing Database 1987-1998.)

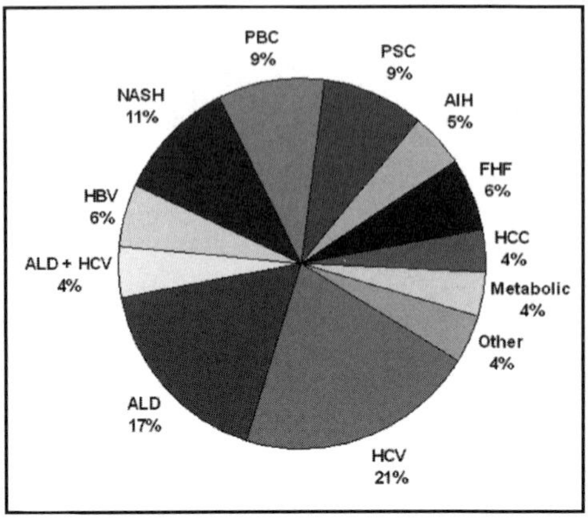

Table 15-2

Factors Associated With More Severe Hepatitis C Recurrence Following Liver Transplantation

Viral	*Other*
High HCV RNA levels pre-OLT and within 2 week post-OLT	High tumor necrosis factor-α production in the graft
Viral genotype Ib (controversial)	Impaired HCV-specific CD4+ T-cell responses
Absence of pretransplant HBV coinfection	Nonwhite recipients
Cytomegalovirus coinfection	Female gender
Immunosuppression	Use of OKT3 for rejection
Severity of illness	Multiple episodes of rejection (indicating a high cumulative prednisone dose)
	Older donor age.
	Older recipient age
	Living donor (controversial)

Adapted from Wiesner et al. Report of the First International Liver Transplantation Society Expert Panel Consensus Conference on Liver Transplantation and Hepatitis C. *Liver Transplantation.* 2003; 9(11), Suppl 3.

liver biopsies from OLT recipients with recurrent HCV have documented accelerated fibrosis progression compared with immunocompetent HCV patients. However, a manifestation of particularly aggressive HCV recurrence characterized by biochemical and histological cholestasis exists, termed "fibrosing cholestatic hepatitis," which is associated with rapid allograft failure. Table 15-2 summarizes several viral and nonviral factors that have been associated with severe recurrence of HCV post-OLT.

In contrast to recurrent HBV infection, there is no effective prophylaxis against recurrent HCV infection. Interferon alpha monotherapy and interferon-alpha in combination with ribavirin given preemptively before histological recurrence of HCV have had limited efficacy in preventing recurrence of HCV. Clinical studies utilizing the long-lasting pegylated interferons preemptively to prevent HCV recurrence are currently ongoing.

Interferon-alpha therapy for the treatment of established recurrent HCV has also been disappointing when compared to treatment in the immunocompetent patient. When interferon is used with ribavirin, the rate of virologic response is increased, but severe side effects often limit the efficacy of antiviral therapy. Leukopenia is a particularly troubling problem in patients undergoing interferon therapy, and adjunctive granulocyte colony-stimulating factor (G-CSF) or erythropoietin (EPO) is often required in order to maintain optimal doses of interferon and ribavirin for continued therapy. However, in individual patients, therapy can result in a sustained virological response with an improvement in graft function. In preliminary studies, pegylated interferon in combination with ribavirin appears to be more effective than standard interferon-alpha in the OLT recipient with recurrent HCV, and larger clinical studies utilizing pegylated interferon are currently ongoing.

Hepatitis B

Allograft reinfection by HBV was shown to result in reduced patient and allograft survival rates by the late 1980s. The importance of active viral replication pre-OLT demonstrated by detectable hepatitis B e antigen (HBeAg) or serum HBV DNA was established as a predictor for recurrence.

The protective effect of passive immunization with long-term, high-dose administration of hepatitis B immune globulin (HBIG) post-OLT led to markedly improved outcomes for patients receiving OLT for HBV-related liver disease. However, the indefinite use of high-dose HBIG administered intravenously is expensive and is associated with adverse side effects such as headache, malaise, nausea, myalgias, and, infrequently, allergic/anaphylactic reactions.

Lamivudine, an oral nucleoside analog that effectively suppresses HBV replication, has also been shown to prevent recurrent HBV infection post-OLT. However, the efficacy of lamivudine monotherapy has been limited by a high incidence (~40%) of lamivudine-resistant mutations in the YMDD sequence of the HBV polymerase gene, leading to allograft reinfection and poor outcomes. Adefovir dipivoxil, a new nucleotide analog, can salvage patients with lamivudine-resistant HBV pre- and post-OLT.

Most recently, the combination of lamivudine and HBIG has been shown to be highly effective in preventing recurrent HBV with an apparently low rate of HBV mutant formation (Table 15-3). The optimal dosing regimen for HBIG remains undefined. Some groups have titrated HBIG doses according to trough serum levels of antibody to hepatitis B surface antigen (anti-HBs). Recent interest has focused on the less expensive intramuscular administration of HBIG, which has equivalent efficacy to intravenous HBIG.

Alcoholic Liver Disease

Alcoholic liver disease (ALD) remains a significant cause of decompensated chronic liver disease. Approximately 20% to 45% of patients undergoing OLT for alcoholic cirrhosis resume alcohol consumption, though only about one third of these exhibit heavy or repetitive drinking.

Table 15-3

Summary of Studies Using the Combination of HBIG + Lamivudine to Prevent Recurrent HBV

Reference	Year	No. of Patients	HBIG Dose	Recurrent HBV (%)	Follow-Up (Mos.)
Markowitz et al	1998	14	10,000 IU IV monthly	0	11.5 (median)
Yao et al	1999	10	1500 IU IM monthly	10	16
Yoshida et al	1999	6	4300 IU to 6800 IU IM monthly	0	18
Angus et al	2000	32	400 IU to 800 IU IM monthly	3	18
Han et al	2000	58	10,000 IU IV monthly	0	15
Marzan et al	2001	26	5000 IU IV monthly	4	30
Rosenau et al	2001	19	2300 IU IV monthly	11	20
Seehofer et al	2001	17	1500 IU to 2000 IU IV monthly	18	25
Han et al	2003	59	750 IU IM monthly	1.7	17

Nonetheless, in well-selected alcoholics, excellent graft and patient survival rates are achieved following OLT for ALD with improvement in health-related quality of life, comparable to outcomes achieved following OLT for nonalcoholic-related cirrhosis. Key factors determining the alcoholic patient's suitability for OLT include 1) acceptance by the patient of the role of alcohol in his or her liver disease; 2) participation in some form of alcohol rehabilitation, such as Alcoholics Anonymous; 3) a stable social support group; and 4) a defined period of abstinence from alcohol, usually 6 months.

Cholestatic Liver Diseases

Although less common than other causes of cirrhosis, primary biliary cirrhosis (PBC) and primary sclerosing cholangitis (PSC) remain important causes for OLT. Patient and graft survival rates after OLT for PBC have been benchmarks for post-

OLT outcomes and generally have been excellent. The Mayo models to predict the course of these disorders, based on the natural history of PBC and PSC, helped in deciding the appropriate timing of referral for OLT before introduction of MELD. The Mayo model for PBC used bilirubin, albumin, age, prothrombin time, and the presence of edema, whereas the model for PSC included bilirubin, age, splenomegaly, and edema to predict survival.

Longer follow-up in patients transplanted for PBC and PSC suggest that these disorders may recur in the allograft. A recent series of more than 700 patients transplanted for these diseases demonstrated the risk of histologic recurrence to increase from 1% to 4% in the first year to 21% to 25% in the tenth year post-OLT. However, allograft loss caused by recurrent PBC and PSC is uncommon. Use of tacrolimus has been implicated in recurrence of PBC. Recurrence of PBC and PSC mimics the histological features of other diseases in the transplanted liver and can be diagnosed only if other causes of graft dysfunction such as chronic rejection or ischemia due to hepatic artery thrombosis have been excluded.

Autoimmune Hepatitis

Failure of immunosuppressive therapy to arrest progression of severe autoimmune hepatitis (AIH) with the development of hepatic decompensation is an indication to consider OLT. Overall, excellent long-term survival is usual after OLT for AIH; however, higher rates of acute cellular rejection occur. Furthermore, recurrence of AIH has been increasingly recognized in recent years, which often requires very aggressive maintenance doses of immunosuppression. Nonetheless, allograft function is generally not diminished by recurrent autoimmune hepatitis. *De novo* autoimmune hepatitis developing in a recipient transplanted for another indication is an increasingly recognized entity with development of autoantibodies and is responsive to steroids.

Nonalcoholic Steatohepatitis

Nonalcoholic steatohepatitis (NASH) is an increasingly recognized cause of hepatic dysfunction that may progress to decompensated cirrhosis or hepatocellular carcinoma in a subset of patients with obesity, diabetes mellitus, or hyperlipidemia. Recurrence of steatosis with progressive fibrosis in the allograft has been observed post-OLT, although graft loss has not been observed to date.

Acute Liver Failure

Acute liver failure (ALF) is an infrequent but important indication for OLT. OLT for ALF can result in excellent patient and graft survival rates if liver failure is recognized promptly and the patient is referred for OLT before irreversible complications have occurred precluding OLT. The clinical syndrome of "fulminant hepatic failure" (FHF) is defined as the onset of hepatic encephalopathy within 8 weeks of the initial symptoms of liver failure and is associated with a particularly poor prognosis without OLT. Aggressive work-up of altered mental status in the setting of FHF, including computer tomographic (CT) scanning of the head and possibly placement of an intracranial pressure monitor to exclude cerebral edema, as it is indistinguishable clinically from portosystemic encephalopathy, which may lead to intracranial hemorrhage and brain stem herniation. Specific criteria to identify patients with FHF who are unlikely to recover spontaneously without OLT include the Kings College criteria (Table 15-4) and the Clichy criteria (Table 15-5), though such criteria remain imperfect. Clinical trials to better clarify and define better prognosticators of FHF are

Table 15-4

KINGS COLLEGE CRITERIA FOR FULMINANT HEPATIC FAILURE

Acetaminophen Patients	*Nonacetaminophen Patients*
Arterial pH <7.3	Prothrombin time INR >6.5
Prothrombin time INR >6.5	*or*
Serum creatinine >3.5 mg/dL	Prothrombin time INR >3.5.
	Age <10 or >40 years
	Disease etiology (cryptogenic or drug-induced)
	Onset of jaundice before encephalopathy (>7 days)
	Serum bilirubin > 18 mg/dL

Table 15-5

CRITERIA OF HOPITAL PAUL-BROUSSE (CLICHY) FOR FULMINANT HEPATIC FAILURE

- Hepatic encephalopathy
- Factor V level <20% in patients with age <30 years
- Factor V level <30% in patients with age >30 years

currently ongoing. Bioartificial liver support as a "bridge to transplant" remains an area of active investigation.

Hepatic Malignancy

Mazzaferro and colleagues, based on a large European experience, developed the currently accepted criteria (Milan criteria) for OLT in patients with HCC: a solitary tumor <5 cm in diameter or, if multiple, three lesions or less with diameters <3 cm without evidence of vascular invasion. With these criteria, overall survival rates in HCC patients (85% 4-year survival) were comparable to patients transplanted without HCC. More recently, some centers have begun transplanting patients with HCC who fall outside of the Milan criteria, so called "expanded criteria." Under this expanded criteria (solitary tumor <6.5 cm, up to three lesions with the largest diameter <4.5 cm, total tumor burden <8 cm), 5-year survival rates of 75% were observed. Metastatic HCC remains an absolute contraindication for OLT.

Pre-OLT local therapy of HCC by transarterial chemoembolization (TACE), radiofrequency ablation (RFA), or alcohol injection has been used to reduce or control tumor growth in patients while awaiting OLT on the list. Such interventions, however, are potentially hazardous in patients with decompensated cirrhosis and are of unproven efficacy.

Cholangiocarcinoma diagnosed pre-OLT has been considered to be a contraindication to OLT based on its typically rapid and aggressive recurrence. However, more recently, a subset of patients with a hilar tumor location and absence of nodal involvement or intrahepatic tumor have been reported to have reasonable tumor-free survival at the Mayo Clinic with pre-OLT irradiation and chemotherapy followed by intraoperative tumor staging.

Metabolic Disorders

Metabolic disorders considered for OLT can be grouped into two broad categories: diseases causing primary hepatocellular injury (eg, Wilson's disease, hemochromatosis) and diseases without clinical or histological hepatic injury (eg, primary hyperoxaluria, familial amyloidosis, familial hypercholesterolemia). In the latter group of disorders, the primary metabolic defect is hepatic; however, systemic manifestations of the metabolic disorder are the usual indications for OLT. Substantial neurologic improvement can occur following OLT for Wilson's disease presenting with decompensated cirrhosis and neurologic involvement. Fulminant Wilson's disease with severe hemolysis is an indication for urgent OLT. Hemochromatosis has been associated with poorer outcomes following OLT than other forms of cirrhosis due to an increased risk of death from cardiac arrhythmias and infections. Furthermore, iron reaccumulation theoretically may occur in the allograft of patients with hemochromatosis.

OLT also has been performed for a variety of systemic disorders, including adult polycystic disease with extensive and symptomatic hepatic cysts. The biliary type of cirrhosis associated with cystic fibrosis can be cured by OLT.

Vascular Disorders

Budd-Chiari syndrome (BCS) is characterized by hepatic venous outflow obstruction of the liver and manifests initially as portal hypertension with eventual progression to hepatic fibrosis and failure. BCS is most often associated with myeloproliferative disorders, hypercoagulable states, and vena caval webs. Medical approaches to management are often disappointing and fail to retard progression to liver failure and death. Decompressive interventions such a transjugular intrahepatic portosystemic shunt (TIPS) or surgical portosystemic shunt may be effective in the early stages of BCS prior to significant hepatic dysfunction. Patients with advanced fibrosis on liver biopsy or clinically significant hepatic dysfunction should undergo OLT, which is associated with good outcomes for BCS. Though BCS is associated with myeloproliferative disorders, the rate of evolution to acute leukemia does not appear to be enhanced following OLT.

Veno-occlusive disease (VOD) is a disorder manifested by necrosis of zone 3 hepatocytes and fibrous obliteration of the central venule lumen, most commonly seen after bone marrow transplantation (BMT). VOD may lead to hepatic failure and death in up to 25% of patients despite an otherwise successful BMT. The experience with OLT for hepatic complications of BMT is limited; however, OLT appears to be the only intervention that may alter the course of advanced VOD.

Table 15-6

ABSOLUTE CONTRAINDICATIONS TO ORTHOTOPIC LIVER TRANSPLANTATION

Acquired immunodeficiency syndrome (AIDS)	Fulminant hepatic failure with ICP >50 mmHg or CPP <40 mmHg*
Extrahepatic malignancy	Advanced cardiac or pulmonary disease
Advanced cholangiocarcinoma	Anatomic abnormality precluding OLT
Hemangiosarcoma	Active alcoholism or substance abuse
Uncontrolled sepsis	Persistent history of noncompliance
Portopulmonary hypertension	

* ICP is intracranial pressure; CPP is cerebral perfusion pressure and equals the mean arterial pressure minus ICP.

ABSOLUTE AND RELATIVE CONTRAINDICATIONS

A clinical condition is considered an absolute contraindication to OLT if it precludes a successful outcome of OLT. Table 15-6 summarizes absolute contraindications to OLT. Conditions considered relative contraindications diminish the prospect of a good outcome, but OLT may still be considered on a patient-by-patient basis.

For the patient with prior extrahepatic malignancy, consideration of OLT is feasible if specific criteria are met: 1) curative therapy (ie, definitive resection) must have been performed; 2) the pathologic specimen must indicate a low likelihood of metastases; and 3) a sufficient tumor-free period must have elapsed since curative therapy, usually 2 years for most nonhepatic malignancies. For certain tumors, such as breast cancer, colon cancer, and malignant melanoma, longer periods of recurrence-free survival are desirable. An oncology opinion should be sought.

Ongoing alcohol or recreational drug use is an absolute contraindication to OLT. Random toxicology screens are appropriate if there is concern about continued abuse. Medicinal marijuana is contraindicated in the setting of OLT because of concerns regarding compliance of users as well as possible pulmonary infections post-OLT, in particular, fungal pulmonary infections. Prescription narcotic abuse is also a cause for concern because it may contribute to difficulties with pain management post-OLT, and non-narcotic alternatives should be explored with a pain management specialist.

Transplant candidates must be rigorously screened for underlying cardiac disease. The frequency of coronary artery disease (CAD) in adult patients presenting for an evaluation for OLT has been estimated to range from 5% to 10%. Clinically significant CAD may be amenable to a revascularization procedure and may render the patient an acceptable OLT candidate.

Severe chronic obstructive pulmonary disease and pulmonary fibrosis are contraindications to OLT, whereas respiratory compromise from ascites, hydrothorax, or diminished respiratory muscle strength is reversible. Specific pulmonary syndromes

Table 15-7

Pulmonary Syndromes Associated With Portal Hypertension

	Hepatopulmonary Syndrome	*Portopulmonary Hypertension*
Incidence	10% to 20% of cirrhotic patients	2% of cirrhotic patients
Clinical Presentation	Dyspnea Cyanosis Digital clubbing Orthodeoxia and Platypnea	Dyspnea Fatigue Chest pain and syncope Elevated pulmonary artery pressures
Diagnosis	Demonstrable pulmonary vascular dilatation by: 1. Technetium 99m-labeled macroaggregated albumin perfusion lung scan 2. Pulmonary angiography 3. Contrast-enhance bubble echocardiography	Mean pulmonary artery pressure >35 mmHg at rest Peripheral vascular resistance >250 dynes/s/cm-5 Pulmonary vascular resistance <300 dynes/s/cm-5 Cardiac output <8 L/min
Management	No proven drug therapy HPS slowly reverses weeks to months following OLT	Intravenous prostacyclin therapy improves functional state, exercise capacity, and survival OLT contraindicated (mortality post-OLT=100% if mean pulmonary artery pressure >50 mmHg and 50% if mean pulmonary artery pressure between 35 mmHg and 50 mmHg)
Prognosis	1-year survival rates of 16% to 38% once PaO_2 50 mmHg	Median survival=57 months

related to portal hypertension exist including the hepatopulmonary syndrome (HPS) and portopulmonary hypertension (Table 15-7). It is critical to make the distinction between HPS and portopulmonary hypertension, as portopulmonary hypertension is associated with high perioperative mortality despite OLT.

Active, uncontrolled extrahepatic bacterial and fungal infections are an absolute contraindication to OLT.

Portal vein thrombosis is no longer considered a technical obstacle to OLT. However, if the thrombus involves the superior mesenteric vein, OLT may not be feasible due to lack of a suitable venous anastomosis for the graft. Prior portosystemic shunt surgery, particularly a nonselective side-to-side or end-to-side portocaval shunt, increases the technical complexity of OLT but is no longer considered a contraindication. The presence of a TIPS stent is now commonly encountered in cirrhotic patients and does not typically impact the operative procedure.

Although older age is not considered an absolute contraindication to OLT, close attention must be paid to comorbid conditions and the likelihood that the candidate will be able to return to an active lifestyle after OLT. Generally, patients beyond their late 60s are not offered OLT.

Renal insufficiency in patients with decompensated cirrhosis, including the hepatorenal syndrome (HRS), is not a contraindication to OLT. However, renal failure severe enough to require dialysis or combined liver-kidney transplantation has been consistently associated with poorer patient and graft outcomes. The inclusion of the serum creatinine level in the new model for end-stage liver disease (MELD) score reflects the prognostic importance of renal insufficiency in advanced liver disease.

One of the major systemic manifestations of decompensated cirrhosis is malnutrition. Substantial malnutrition with cachexia and muscle wasting increases the likelihood of perioperative morbidity, the need for more prolonged ventilator support, and poorer patient survival overall. Obesity is now recognized as a predictor of morbidity and mortality following OLT, although attempts at weight reduction in the cirrhotic population are generally only modestly successful.

Transplant Evaluation

The formal OLT evaluation usually encompasses a number of days and provides the patient and his or her family the opportunity to become acquainted with the details of OLT. The components of the liver transplant evaluation are summarized in Table 15-8.

Upon completion of all the required consultations and ancillary testing, the members of the transplant team in closed committee formally discuss the need and appropriateness of OLT for the individual candidate. Upon acceptance for OLT, the candidate is placed on the transplant list, matched by the ABO blood type and weight of potential cadaveric donors. The patient's priority for OLT is based on his or hers disease severity.

Listing Criteria and Policies of the United Network for Organ Sharing (UNOS)

Organ allocation within the United States is administered by UNOS, which considers only disease severity in determining a patient's priority for OLT. With the critical shortage of cadaveric donor organs, a major challenge for UNOS has been to develop a uniform and equitable system of allocation in an effort to ensure that hepatic allografts are not used for patients whose prognosis without OLT remains good. Under the previous allocation system implemented on July 30, 1997, UNOS defined specific categories or statuses, which were based on disease severity as assessed by the Child-Turcot-Pugh (CTP) score. Under the UNOS statuses, the CTP score and waiting time on the transplant list were used to stratify cirrhotic patients, and

Table 15-8

COMPONENTS OF THE LIVER TRANSPLANT EVALUATION

Consultations	Transplant surgeon
	Hepatologist
	Psychiatrist
	Social worker
	Cardiologist
	Pulmonologist
	Oncologist
Radiology	Duplex ultrasound
	Abdominal computed tomographic scan
	Abdominal magnetic resonance imaging
	Abdominal angiography
	Cholangiography
Laboratory	Biochemical hepatic function tests
	Complete blood count
	Viral hepatitis serologies
	HIV test
	Tumor markers
	Toxicology screens
	ABO blood type
Financial	Private payor
	State payor
	Federal payor

allowances were made for complications such as hepatorenal syndrome, variceal bleeding, portosystemic encephalopathy, refractory ascites, and SBP. However, because the clinical components of the CTP score, specifically ascites and encephalopathy stage, were highly subjective, there was concern that a more objective assessment of disease severity for OLT candidates was needed.

In 1998, the Department of Health and Human Services redefined policies and principles for organ allocation, whereby equitable organ allocation among transplant candidates should be based purely on medical urgency, minimizing the importance of waiting time. With this mandate, in 2002, the Organ Procurement and Transplantation Network (OPTN) along with UNOS endorsed the development of a new system based on the Model for End-Stage Liver Disease (MELD) score for patients who are not status 1 or in fulminant liver failure, effective February 27, 2002.

The MELD system incorporates the serum creatinine level, serum bilirubin level, and International Normalized Ratio (INR) into a mathematical formula that predicts survival accurately in four different groups of cirrhotic patients:

$$\text{MELD score} = 9.57 \times \log_e(\text{creatinine}) + 3.78 \times \log_e(\text{bilirubin}) + 11.2 \times \log_e(\text{INR})$$

The MELD score was originally developed to assess prognosis of cirrhotic patients undergoing TIPS, but has since been validated to provide a reliable estimate of short-term survival in patients with end-stage liver disease awaiting OLT over a wide range of disease severity and etiology. Although introduction of MELD for organ allocation has been a major advance, there are some indications for OLT, which may not give individual patients adequate priority for transplant. Thus, in patients with HCC, hepatic function may be well preserved, resulting in a low MELD score and longer waiting time, allowing tumor progression. Accordingly, additional points are allocated for HCC based on stage of tumor and waiting time beyond the calculated MELD score based on degree of hepatic dysfunction.

Additional methods will need to be devised to accommodate special circumstances not well served by the MELD scoring system, such as persons with metabolic disorders like hyperoxaluria or familial amyloidosis, adult polycystic liver disease with normal hepatic function, and intractable pruritus.

Surgical Techniques

Once a potential deceased donor is identified, the local organ procurement organization (OPO) supplies pertinent donor medical information to centers with suitable potential recipients listed with UNOS and coordinates harvesting the donor liver. Unlike other types of organ transplants, including kidney and bone marrow, donor-recipient matching for OLT is based only on ABO blood compatibility and physical characteristics and not HLA. The typical deceased donor has had a catastrophic head injury or an intracerebral bleed with brain death, but without multisystem failure. With the critical shortage of deceased donors, expansion of the donor pool has included acceptance of livers from older donors (age 70 years and greater), nonheart-beating donors, donors with viral hepatitis, and steatotic livers.

The harvesting team assesses the potential donor liver after making a visual and often histological determination for fibrosis and steatosis. Once the circulation is interrupted, the organ is rapidly infused with cold University of Wisconsin (UW) solution to preserve it before hepatectomy. Donor iliac arteries and veins also are retrieved in case vascular grafting is required. The entire organ is then removed and preserved in UW solution to maintain its viability during transport back to the transplant center, which usually allows safe organ preservation for up to 24 hours. After arrival at the recipient institution, further "back table" vascular dissection and arterial reconstruction, if necessary, is performed before implantation.

If liver volume is adequate, splitting cadaveric donor livers into two functioning grafts, either in vivo during harvesting or ex vivo back at the transplant center, allows two recipients to receive portions of the same hepatic allograft. The left lateral segment (segments 2 and 3) can be used for a pediatric recipient, and the right trisegment (segments 4 to 8) can be used for an adult recipient. Figure 15-4 shows the segmental anatomy and vasculature of the liver, which forms the basis of dissection for both split and live donor liver transplantation (LDLT). Acceptable graft and patient survival rates can be obtained with split grafts, although high-risk recipients may have poorer outcomes with this technique.

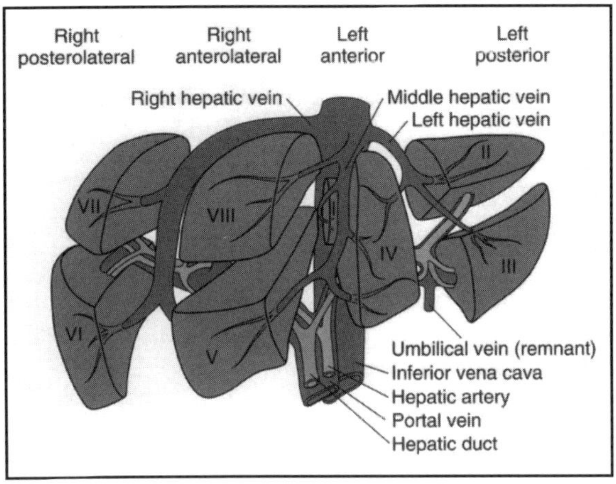

Figure 15-4. Anatomic liver segments with corresponding vascular supply.

Native Hepatectomy and Graft Implantation

Removal of the native liver can be technically challenging due to the presence of severe portal hypertension or prior abdominal surgery, especially portosystemic shunt. In this regard, TIPS has become a favored choice for portal decompression in the OLT candidate.

Hilar dissection is performed first to access the major hepatic vessels and devascularize the liver. During hepatectomy and subsequent graft implantation, venovenous bypass is frequently performed between the femoral and axillary vein to prevent mesenteric congestion, venous stasis in the legs, and renal hypertension when the portal vein and inferior vena cava are clamped. With implantation of the graft, an anastomosis is made between donor and recipient vena cava both above and below the graft. In selected recipients with cardiac instability or a prior portosystemic shunt in whom uninterrupted caval flow during OLT is necessary, graft implantation may be performed using a "piggyback" technique where only a suprahepatic vena caval anastomosis is performed, and the infrahepatic donor vena cava is ligated. Next, the portal venous anastomosis is performed, followed by the hepatic arterial anastomosis. The bile duct anastomosis may be a duct-to-duct anastomosis with or without a T-tube, or a hepaticojejunostomy, which is favored in recipients with primary sclerosing cholangitis or when there is a discrepancy between donor and recipient bile duct diameters. Placement of a T-tube allows easy assessment of bile flow and access for cholangiography post-OLT; however, the risk of bile leakage after T-tube removal has led many transplant centers to abandon routine placement of a T-tube.

After establishment of all vascular anastomoses, the newly implanted graft is reperfused with restoration of normal blood flow. The release of vasoactive agents from pooled blood in the lower half of the body can infrequently result in a "reperfusion syndrome," characterized by potentially lethal cardiovascular instability and tachyarrhythmias. Prompt bile production signals adequate graft function. Hyperacute rejection is a rare, but devastating event and leads to rapid graft necrosis within hours, requiring urgent retransplantation.

Table 15-9

PROTOCOL FOR EVALUATION OF POTENTIAL LIVING-RELATED DONORS

Stage 1	• Complete history and physical examination
	• Laboratory blood tests
	• Hepatic panel, blood chemistry, hematology, coagulation profile, urinalysis, alpha-fetopro-tein, carcinoembryonic antigen, hepatitis serologies, cytomegalovirus, Epstein-Barr virus, and human immunodeficiency virus
	• Abdominal computed tomographic scan
Stage 2	• Complete psychosocial evaluation
	• Pulmonary function tests
	• Echocardiography
Stage 3	• Liver biopsy
	• Celiac and superior mesenteric angiography
Stage 4	• Magnetic resonance cholangiography
	• Informed consent obtained

Live Donor Liver Transplantation

Live donor liver transplantation (LDLT) in adults was introduced in the 1990s as a result of the cadaveric organ supply shortage. The donor (generally a healthy relative of the recipient) undergoes an extensive and thoughtful evaluation by the transplant team to determine suitability for donation. A hepatologist not involved in the care of the recipient usually performs the donor evaluation. Preoperative evaluation of the donor is typically performed in four stages over a period of 1 to 3 months, after which informed consent isS obtained (Table 15-9). After undergoing a complete evaluation, only a relatively small proportion of potential donors are deemed satisfactory candidates. Morbidity and mortality rates in donors undergoing hepatic resection are 10% and 0.5%, respectively. Right lobes (segments 5 to 8), extended right grafts (segments 4 to 8), or left hepatic grafts (segments 2 to 4) have been used successfully in adult-to-adult LDLT. Adult LDLT provides obvious advantages to the recipient, most notably a reduction in the wait list mortality rate. Graft and patient survival rates are equivalent to those reported for recipients receiving deceased donor grafts. Graft rejection rates are not diminished in live donor transplants, and there is concern that the course of recurrent HCV may be accelerated, although this is controversial.

IMMUNOSUPPRESSION

By convention, immunosuppressive regimens have been classified into 1) induction (initial immunosuppression), 2) maintenance immunosuppression, and 3) treatment of acute cellular rejection. The primary goal of immunosuppression is to prevent graft rejection and loss. A secondary goal of immunosuppression is to prevent the adverse effects of the antirejection therapy. Commonly used immununosuppressive agents, modes of action, methods of monitoring, and common adverse effects are summarized in Table 15-10. Common drug interactions involving immunosuppressive agents are summarized in Table 15-11. The calcineurin inhibitors, cyclosporine and tacrolimus, form the basis of the majority of induction and maintenance immunosuppressive regimens. Both agents have substantial toxicity. Tacrolimus has replaced cyclosporine as the primary immunosuppressive agent. Conversion of OLT recipients from cyclosporine to tacrolimus is preferred following glucocorticoid- or OKT3-refractory rejection, late rejection (>6 months post-OLT), histologically diagnosed chronic rejection, severe cholestasis, intestinal malabsorption of cyclosporine, or cyclosporine toxicity (eg, hirsutism, gingivitis, severe hypertension). Use of rapamune in OLT has been restricted, as it has been implicated in a higher frequency of postoperative complications such as hepatic artery thrombosis in some reports.

Post-Transplant Management

Early Postoperative Phase to Discharge from Hospital

The first few postoperative days are spent in the intensive care unit with monitoring by arterial and pulmonary venous lines and ventilatory support. If a T-tube has been placed, production of dark copious bile provides reassuring evidence of good graft function. Neurological recovery with improvement in mental status, good urinary output, and cardiovascular stability also reflect good graft function. Routine antimicrobial prophylaxis includes bowel decontamination with oral nonabsorbable antibiotics, perioperative systemic broad-spectrum antibiotics, antifungal agents, and ganciclovir to prevent cytomegalovirus infection. Markedly abnormal liver biochemical tests are typical during the initial 48 to 72 postoperative hours and reflect a number of insults to the graft including ischemia following harvesting, preservation, and subsequent reperfusion. However, the serum aminotransferase levels should normalize over subsequent days with a corresponding improvement in coagulopathy and fall in serum bilirubin level.

Worrisome clinical features include scanty, pale bile, metabolic acidosis, depressed mentation, continued need for pressor support, and worsening liver biochemistries. Hepatic artery thrombosis (HAT) needs to be excluded promptly by Doppler ultrasound or angiography, as its presence signals the need for urgent re-transplantation. Primary nonfunction (PNF) of the graft is also an indication for urgent retransplantation. Donor characteristics that are associated with an increased likelihood of PNF include marked hepatic macrovesicular steatosis (not microvesicular steatosis), cold temperature in the back table bath during graft preparation for implantation, and livers from nonheart-beating donors. However, with improving graft function, pressor support can be tapered, and weaning from ventilatory support can be initiated. Within the first week post-OLT, liver biochemistries should steadily improve as ischemia and reperfusion injury resolve.

Acute cellular rejection (ACR) becomes an important and frequent cause of graft dysfunction 1 week and beyond post-OLT. ACR is suggested by a rise in serum aminotransferase, alkaline phosphatase, and bilirubin levels. Because the biochemical features are nonspecific, a liver biopsy is often required to evaluate other diagnostic

Table 15-10

Commonly Used Immunosuppressive Agents in Liver Transplantation

Immunosuppressive Agent	*Mode of Action*	*Monitoring*	*Adverse Effects*
Cyclosporine	Calcineurin inhibitor: Suppresses IL-2-dependent T-cell proliferation	Serum drug level	Renal, neurological, hyper-lipidemia, hypertension, hirsutism
Tacrolimus	Calcineurin inhibitor: Suppresses IL-2-dependent T-cell proliferation	Serum drug level	Renal, neurological, diabetes mellitus
Prednisone	Cytokine inhibitor (IL-1, IL-2, IL-6, TNF, and IFN gamma)	None	Hypertension, diabetes mellitus, obesity, osteoporosis, infection
Azathioprine	Inhibits T- and B-cell proliferation by interfering with purine synthesis	White blood cell count	Bone marrow depression, hepto-toxicity
Mycophenolate mofetil	Selective inhibition of T- and B-cell proliferation by interferin with de novo purine synthesis	White blood cell count	Diarrhea, bone marrow toxicity
Sirolimus	Inhibits late T-cell function	Serum drug level	Neutropenia, thrombocytopenia, hyperlipidemia, hemolytic anemia
OKT3	Blocks T-cell CD3 receptor, preventing stimulation by antigen	CD3 count	Cytokine release syndrome, pulmonary edema, increased risk of infections
IL-2 Receptor Blocker (Daclizumab, Basiliximab)	Competitive inhibition of IL-2 receptor on activated lymphocytes	None	Hypersensitivity reactions

Adapted from Everson GT, Karn I. Immediate postoperative care. In: Maddrey WC, Schiff ER, Sorrell MF (eds). *Transplantation of the liver.* 3rd ed. Philadelphia: Lippincott Williams & Wilkins; 131–162.

Table 15-11

Clinically Relevant Drug Interactions With Immunosuppressive Drugs

Drugs that increase blood levels of cyclosporine and tacrolimus	*Antifungals*: fluconazole, ketoconazole, itraconazole *Antibiotics*: erythromycin, clarithromycin *Calcium channel blockers*: diltiazem, verapamil *Others*: bromocriptine, metoclopromide, allopurinol
Drugs that decrease blood levels of cyclosporine and tacrolimus	*Anticonvulsants:* phenytoin, phenobarbitol *Antibiotics*: rifampin, nafcillin
Drugs that increase nephrotoxicity of cyclosporine and tacrolimus	Gentamicin, ketoconazole, nonsteroidal anti-inflammatory drugs
Drugs that interact with mycophenolate mofetil	Acyclovir, ganciclovir, antacids, choleostyramine (inhibitis absorption)
Drugs that interact with azathioprine	Allopurinol, angiotensin-converting enzyme (ACE) inhibitors, warfarin

possibilities including slowly resolving reperfusion injury, biliary tract obstruction, and cholestasis related to sepsis. If ACR is diagnosed, a high-dose glucocorticoid bolus (1000 mg of methylprednisolone or the equivalent) followed by a taper (200 to 20 mg/d) extending over several days is the standard therapy. With successful treatment, resolution of ACR is accompanied by normalization of liver biochemistries. For the occasional patient with ACR who fails to respond to glucocorticoids, additional immunosuppression may be necessary, such as the monoclonal antibody OKT3. Liver biopsy should be repeated to confirm a lack of histologic response before more intensive therapy is initiated and to exclude other important causes of graft dysfunction such as ischemia.

Other important medical issues, which commonly occur in the first weeks following OLT and may require evaluation, are shown in Table 15-12. Neurological dysfunction can present as altered mental status or seizures, and the differential diagnosis includes the lingering effects of hepatic encephalopathy, electrolyte imbalance, poor graft function, sepsis, uremia, and adverse effects of medications, particularly the neurological toxicity caused by the major immunosuppressive agents. Central pontine myelinolysis, often due to overly rapid correction of hyponatremia perioperatively, is another cause of post-OLT altered neurological dysfunction with demyelination demonstrable on magnetic resonance imaging. Overall, management includes correcting the electrolyte imbalance if present, antimicrobial therapy for documented infections, institution of hemodialysis if necessary, and reducing baseline immunosuppression with the calcineurin inhibitors, which has been facilitated in recent years by the availability of mycophenolate mofetil.

Table 15-12

MEDICAL COMPLICATIONS OCCURRING IN THE IMMEDIATE POSTOPERATIVE PERIOD

Infections	Bacterial
	Viral (cytomegalovirus, Epstein-Barr virus)
	Fungal (*Candidiasis*, *Aspergillosis*, mucomycosis)
	Pneumocystis carinii pneumonia
Respiratory complications	Pneumonia
	Pulmonary edema
	Acute respiratory distress syndrome
	Portopulmonary syndrome
	Hepatopulmonary syndrome
Renal failure	Acute tubular necrosis
	Medication-induced
Cardiovascular disease	Hypertension
	Myocardial ischemia
	Arrythmias
	Valvular heart disease
	Cardiomyopathy
	Idiopathic hypertrophic subaortic stenosis
	Hemochromatosis
Neurological complications	Central pontine myelinolysis
	Seizures
	Central nervous system hemorrhage
	Ischemia
	Medication-induced neurotoxicity
Hematological complications	Coagulopathy
	Thrombocytopenia
	Disseminated intravascular coagulation
Metabolic complications	Diabetes mellitus

Adapted from Everson GT, Karn I. Immediate postoperative care. In: Maddrey WC, Schiff ER, Sorrell MF (eds). *Transplantation of the liver.* 3rd ed. Philadelphia: Lippincott Williams & Wilkins; 2001.

Diabetes mellitus can occur in approximately one third of patients for the first time in the post-OLT period and usually requires insulin for control. The pathogenesis is multifactorial and may include immunosuppressive therapy as a major factor because of the hyperglycemic effects of prednisone, cyclosporine, tacrolimus, azathioprine, and mycophenolate mofetil. Recent data suggest that HCV infection further increases the risk of diabetes mellitus in cirrhotic patients.

Renal impairment post-OLT may reflect a number of factors, including pre-OLT hepatorenal syndrome or renal failure of other etiologies, intraoperative hypotension resulting in acute tubular necrosis, and, importantly, the nephrotoxic effects of cyclosporine and tacrolimus. Adjunctive therapy with mycophenolate mofetil allows a reduction in the doses of cyclosporine and tacrolimus while providing adequate immunosuppression. Short-term hemodialysis may be necessary until renal function improves.

In the first 3 to 4 weeks post-OLT, infections are typically bacterial and related to surgical complications such as intra-abdominal bleeding, bile leak, or wound infection.

Following Discharge From Hospital

If the postoperative course is uneventful, discharge may be possible by the second week after OLT. Patients are seen at frequent intervals during the first postoperative month. Any liver test abnormalities or further graft dysfunction is an indication for prompt liver biopsy to distinguish ACR from biliary obstruction, ischemia, or cytomegalovirus (CMV) infection, which becomes an important consideration 3 or more weeks post-OLT. Early recurrence of HCV infection may also become apparent and may mimic ACR histologically.

If the liver biopsy shows features to suggest biliary obstruction or if the patient demonstrates clinical features of cholangitis, such as fever and abdominal pain, a cholangiogram is indicated. Cholangiography may be obtained via the T-tube if present, by endoscopic retrograde cholangiopancreatography (ERCP) if the biliary anastomosis is duct-to-duct, by percutaneous transhepatic cholangiography if a choledochojejunostomy has been performed, or increasingly by magnetic resonance cholangiopancreatography (MRCP). An anastomotic stricture in a choledochocholedochostomy is usually managed by balloon dilation, followed by placement of a temporary internal stent. Surgical intervention is reserved for patients who do not respond to endoscopic or radiological approach, in which case the anastomosis is converted to a Roux-en-Y anastomosis. It is important to distinguish an anastomotic stricture from stricturing caused by ischemia from HAT, as the bile duct in the OLT recipient is prone to ischemia because of its relatively tenuous arterial blood supply. Ischemic stricturing can be hilar, but is generally diffuse and extensive, requiring hepatic retransplantation as endoscopic or radiological intervention is often futile. Biliary stricturing may also herald recurrence of PSC in patients transplanted for PSC. A T-tube, if present, is removed by the sixth postoperative month or when glucocorticoids have been sufficiently tapered to a low dose. Removal is best performed at the transplant center as bile leaks are common and require prompt ERCP with nasobiliary drainage or stenting to allow the tear in the bile duct to heal uneventfully.

Besides graft hepatitis, other important manifestations of de novo CMV infection include pneumonitis and diarrhea. Reactivation of CMV in a previously infected recipient tends to be less clinically severe than de novo infection. The diagnosis of CMV infection is confirmed by culture of tissue or blood. High-dose intravenous ganciclovir is highly effective in the treatment of CMV infection. Other therapies include a CMV hyperimmune globulin and foscarnet.

In the early postoperative months, long-term antibiotics, most frequently trimethoprim-sulfamethoxazole, are prescribed to prevent infection with *Pneumocystis carinii* (PCP). In patients intolerant of sulfa drugs, dapsone or inhaled pentamidine are alternative options. Because PCP infection occurs most commonly in the first postoperative year, prophylaxis needs to be continued for at least this period of time.

Standard antibiotic therapy is appropriate for community-acquired respiratory infections, but a more extensive work-up is indicated for unusually severe symptoms or failure of an infection to resolve rapidly with treatment. Fungal infections pose a major threat to the OLT recipient. When they occur, major sites of infection are mucocutaneous (oral and esophageal), pulmonary, or intracerebral. Despite prolonged therapy with amphotericin or more recently itraconazole or fluconazole, a fatal outcome is usual. Enteric bacteremia may be an initial clue to hepatic artery thrombosis in an otherwise stable recipient. Reactivation of tuberculosis may present in an atypical fashion post-OLT. Bronchoscopy to obtain cultures or lumbar puncture may be necessary for diagnosis if clinically suspected.

LONG-TERM MANAGEMENT

GENERAL PREVENTIVE MEDICINE

Long-term management of the OLT recipient requires continued cooperation and communication between the primary care physician and the transplant center. Many of the disorders related to long-term survival after OLT are common diseases, including systemic hypertension, hyperlipidemia, and diabetes mellitus. Regular determination of a complete blood count, electrolytes, liver biochemical tests, and immunosuppressive drug levels should be arranged and the results forwarded to the transplant center.

Systemic hypertension is a frequent complication post-OLT and may be related to calcineurin inhibitor-induced renal vasoconstriction, as well as other drugs such as glucocorticoids. Other etiologies include mild renal insufficiency, which is frequent post-OLT even when absent preoperatively. Initial antihypertensive therapy usually consists of a calcium channel blocker. Nifedipine is the agent of choice, as verapamil and diltiazem tend to increase cyclosporine and tacrolimus levels. β-blockers are the second-line antihypertensive agents used. Angiotensin-converting enzyme inhibitors and potassium-sparing diuretics are relatively contraindicated because of their propensity to exacerbate hyperkalemia, which is frequent in OLT recipients because of renal tubular acidosis caused by the calcineurin inhibitors. Diuretics are generally avoided due to concern of exacerbating renal insufficiency and electrolyte imbalances in the OLT recipient, but if deemed necessary, furosemide is the diuretic of choice. In the minority of patients in whom hypertension is not controlled, a centrally acting agent such as clonidine may be used. For the occasional patient with intractable hypertension on cyclosporine-based immunosuppression, conversion to tacrolimus may aid blood pressure control.

Osteopenia is a frequent cause of morbidity in OLT recipients. In the initial several months post-OLT, osteopenia is accelerated further by high-dose glucocorticoid therapy, as well as the other major immunosuppressive agents. Atraumatic fractures may occur in trabecular bone such as vertebrae or ribs. Fortunately, patients begin to rebuild bone mass after immunosuppressive doses are reduced and the patient's mobility increases. Supplemental calcium and vitamin D are frequently prescribed for patients with symptomatic osteopenia.

De novo malignancies are increased in frequency following OLT. Post-transplant lymphoproliferative disorder (PTLD) varies from a low-grade indolent process to an aggressive neoplasm. Uncontrolled proliferation of B cells post-OLT, typically in response to primary Epstein-Barr virus infection, can be polyclonal or monoclonal. Intensive immunosuppression with OKT3 for severe rejection increases the risk of PTLD. Clinical features suggestive of the diagnosis of PTLD include lymphadenopathy, unexplained fever, and systemic symptoms such as weight loss. Diagnosis is made histologically after biopsy of suspected lymph nodes or the liver graft. Therapy includes a reduction in the level of immunosuppression and antiviral therapy directed against Epstein-Barr virus with acyclovir or ganciclovir. Systemic chemotherapy may be required in patients who present with a malignant lymphoma.

Hyperlipidemia is observed in up to 50% of OLT recipients and may be related to diabetes mellitus, obesity, renal dysfunction, and immunosuppressive agents—especially cyclosporine. Pharmacologic therapy is indicated if hypercholesterolemia fails to respond to weight reduction and tight diabetic control. Pravastatin, a 3-hydroxy-3-methylglutaryl coenzyme A (HMG-CoA) reductase inhibitor, is well tolerated and efficacious in OLT recipients.

Obesity is frequent in OLT recipients, even in those who were profoundly malnourished preoperatively. Factors responsible for weight gain post-OLT include glucocorticoid use, increased caloric intake, and decreased physical activity during recuperation from surgery. Immunosuppression with tacrolimus has been reported to result in less weight gain than cyclosporine. Management of obesity in this population includes a reduction in the dose of glucocorticoid and complete withdrawal if possible. The advent of mycophenolate mofetil may permit effective immunosuppression without glucocorticoids.

Standard surveillance for other malignancies should be continued. Screening for prostatic carcinoma should be performed by yearly digital rectal examination in male OLT recipients over age 40 years, in conjunction with serum prostate specific antigen (PSA) testing. Screening for colorectal cancer should be performed by colonoscopy every 3 to 5 years after age 50 in asymptomatic recipients and annually in patients with a history of PSC and ulcerative colitis. In the setting of chronic immunosuppression, it seems appropriate to screen female transplant recipients over age 40 years for breast cancer by yearly mammography, although the cost-effectiveness of this approach is undefined.

Immunizations and Bacterial Prophylaxis

Immunization against hepatitis A and B, influenza, pneumoccocus, tetanus, and diphtheria is part of the standard pretransplantation evaluation. However, a substantial proportion of patients may not be able to mount adequate antibody responses. Vaccines based on live or attenuated microorganisms (eg, measles, mumps, rubella, oral polio, bacille Calmette-Guérin [BCG], vaccinia) are contraindicated in post-OLT recipients because of the risk of reactivation. It is recommended that prophylactic antibiotics be taken for any dental procedure, even basic cleaning.

When to Notify the Transplant Center

Any evidence of graft failure needs to be attended to immediately by referral to the transplant center. Certain signs, symptoms, and situations warrant a call by the local

Table 15-13

WHEN TO NOTIFY THE TRANSPLANT CENTER

Signs	Fever
	Jaundice
	Abdominal tenderness
Symptoms	Abdominal pain
	Neurological symptoms
Situations	Medication changes
	Anticipated surgeries (elective or emergent)
Laboratory Abnormalities	Hyperbilirubinemia
	Elevated transaminases
	Leukocytosis or neutropenia
	Anemia

physician to the transplant center (Table 15-13). Although the patient's local physician can obtain a liver biopsy, it is critical that the specimen be reviewed at the transplant center so that appropriate decisions regarding management can be made. Additionally, many transplant centers prefer to perform complex interventional biliary tract studies, because therapeutic intervention often is required, and immediate access to the transplant team permits more rapid decision-making.

BIBLIOGRAPHY

Everson GT, Kam I. Immediate postoperative care. In: Maddrey WC, Schiff E, Sorell M, eds. *Transplantation of the liver.* 3rd ed. Philadelphia: Lippincott Williams & Wilkins; 1999:131-162.

Gane EJ, Portmann BC, Naoumov NV, et al. Long-term outcome of hepatitis C infection after liver transplantation. *N Engl J Med.* 1996;334:815-820.

Ghobrial RM, Amersi F, Busuttil RW. Surgical advances in liver transplantation. Living related and split donors. *Clin Liver Dis.* 2000;4:553-565.

Han SH, Ofman J, Holt C, et al. An efficacy and cost-effectiveness analysis of combination hepatitis B immune globulin and lamivudine to prevent recurrent hepatitis B after orthotopic liver transplantation compared with hepatitis B immune globulin monotherapy. *Liver Transpl.* 2000;6:741-748.

Kamath PS, Wiesner RH, Malinchoc M, et al. A model to predict survival in patients with end-stage liver disease. *Hepatology.* 2001;33:464-470.

Keeffe EB. Liver transplantation: current status and novel approaches to liver replacement. *Gastroenterology.* 2001;120:749-762.

Lim JK, Keeffe EB. Liver transplantation for alcoholic liver disease: current concepts and length of sobriety. *Liver Transpl.* 2004;10:S31-S38.

Mazzaferro V, Regalia E, Doci R, et al. Liver transplantation for the treatment of small hepatocellular carcinomas in patients with cirrhosis. *N Engl J Med.* 1996;334:693-699.

Munoz SJ, Rothstein KD, Reich D, Manzarbeitia C. Long-term care of the liver transplant recipient. *Clin Liver Dis.* 2000;4:691-710.

Neuberger J. Transplantation for autoimmune hepatitis. *Semin Liver Dis.* 2002;22:379-386.

Ostapowicz G, Fontana RJ, Schiodt FV, et al. Results of a prospective study of acute liver failure at 17 tertiary care centers in the United States. *Ann Intern Med.* 2002;137:947-954.

Perrillo RP, Wright T, Rakela J, et al. A multicenter United States-Canadian trial to assess lamivudine monotherapy before and after liver transplantation for chronic hepatitis B. *Hepatology.* 2001;33:424-432.

Rosen HR, Martin P. Hepatitis B and C in the liver transplant recipient. *Semin Liver Dis.* 2000;20:465-480.

Rosen HR. Disease recurrence following liver transplantation. *Clin Liver Dis.* 2000; 4:675-7x.

Samuel D, Muller R, Alexander G, et al. Liver transplantation in European patients with the hepatitis B surface antigen [see comments]. *N Engl J Med.* 1993;329:1842-1847.

Yao FY, Ferrell L, Bass NM, et al. Liver transplantation for hepatocellular carcinoma: expansion of the tumor size limits does not adversely impact survival. *Hepatology.* 2001;33:1394-1403.

chapter 16

Drug Hepatotoxicity

Raúl J. Andrade, MD; Javier Salmerón, MD;
and M. Isabel Lucena, MD

INTRODUCTION

Chemical hepatic injury caused by drugs is an increasing health problem and a major challenge in modern hepatology. This is because hepatotoxicity mimics all forms of acute and chronic liver disease, and in spite of recent advances in the understanding of the mechanisms involved in toxic liver cell injury and cholestasis, reliable tests for the specific diagnosis of hepatotoxicity remain unavailable. In addition, many of the hepatic reactions induced by drugs are severe and life-threatening. A recent survey of the cases of acute liver failure admitted in 17 US hospitals showed that drugs (including acetaminophen) accounted for more than 50% of such cases.[1]

EPIDEMIOLOGY

The true incidence of drug-related liver disease is generally unknown. There are several explanations for this fact. First, it is believed that just a minority of the actual cases—"the tip of the iceberg"—is reported to the regulatory agencies by the spontaneous reporting system (yellow card). These reports often focused on new adverse effects or unusual and more severe (fatal) instances of known hepatotoxic reactions. In fact, in a recent community-based prospective study performed in France over a 3-year period, the annual incidence of hepatic reactions to drugs was 139 cases per million people (16 times as high as the number notified to the French reporting system of adverse drug reactions).[2]

In addition, the lack of an accurate diagnosis is an important limitation. Approximately 50% of the reactions reported to regulatory authorities have been found to be unrelated to the incriminated drug when evaluated carefully later.[3] At best, scattered data for the numerator (total number of affected subjects) are available for some medications, but information on the denominator is derived mainly from prescribing data (as a surrogate for data on number of persons and time of exposure), which inaccurately reflect the population exposed.[4]

Nevertheless, analysis of the hepatic reactions reported to the Danish National Agency of Pharmacovigilance over 2 consecutive decades indicates that the incidence of drug-induced hepatotoxicity is increasing.[5] This is probably due to a combination of factors including greater exposure to drugs, a better knowledge of toxic effects on the liver, and a more rigorous exclusion of alternative causes of liver damage thanks to the availability of new specific tests for diagnosing viral hepatitis.[6]

The diagnosis of drug hepatotoxicity is considerably less common than that of other causes of liver disease. As the whole of jaundiced patients admitted to a general hospital, toxic liver injury accounted for 3% to 5% of instances, and up to 20% among geriatric patients.[4] In a study carried out in England of patients hospitalized with serum transaminase levels greater than 400 IU/L, the prevalence of drug hepatotoxicity was 9%. In a large cohort of patients with severe acute hepatitis, 30% were of unknown cause, and most of them had previous exposure to drugs. In this study, the incidence of serious acute liver disease probably related to drugs was 7.4 per 10^6 inhabitants per year.[7]

Antibacterial agents, nonsteroidal anti-inflammatory drugs (NSAIDs), and analgesics rank in most large case series as the main compounds incriminated,[2,7-8] probably because they are also the most commonly used drugs. Some studies (mainly retrospective) have yielded consistent figures upon the absolute frequency of hepatotoxicity for a few drugs (eg, isoniazid, aspirin, or diclofenac). Although data are lacking, the frequency of unpredictable hepatotoxicity associated with the use of most medications is believed to be between 1 per 10,000 to 1 per 100,000 exposed persons.[4]

Pathogenesis

Some marketed drugs (acetaminophen and acetylsalicylic acid being the most prominent examples) and environmental hepatotoxins may cause dose-related liver damage and are termed intrinsic hepatotoxins. However, the vast majority of hepatic reactions to drugs usually occur in fewer than 1 per 10,000 individuals exposed, and in persons who were receiving therapeutic doses. These types of reactions are considered idiosyncratic and are largely due to genetic (host-dependent) and environmental factors.

The mechanisms involved in drug-related hepatic cell dysfunction and necrosis are poorly understood. Within the hepatocyte, all foreign substances that cross the intestinal barrier (necessarily lipophilic) should render more hydrophilic compounds, before they can be excreted in urine or bile. This process encompasses various metabolic steps, usually starting with oxidative reactions through cytochrome P-450 (CYP) and then inactivation by way of another enzyme system, including glucuronide, sulfate, epoxide hydrolase, or glutathione (GSH). Finally, hydrophilic drug metabolites are exported to the bloodstream and filtrated by the glomerule or to bile by transport proteins located at the hepatocyte apical canalicular membrane.

Although some parent drugs may be directly toxic to the hepatocyte (eg, nucleoside reverse transcriptase inhibitors, which inhibit mitochondrial DNA production), in most idiosyncratic adverse reactions, the damage presumably follows a sequence of rare events that would begin with the generation of reactive metabolites by polymorphic CYP isoenzymes, which cause liver damage either through covalent binding to intracellular proteins or by oxidative stress elicited by GSH depletion (Figure 16-1). This, subsequently, might have various effects on hepatic cells, including an impairment of mitochondrial function (eg, the transition membrane pore), loss of cellular ionic gradients, a fall in ATP levels, and actin disruption, cell swelling, and destruction.[9-10]

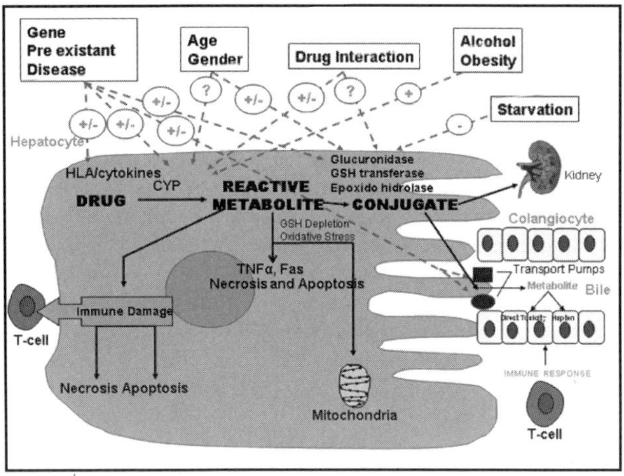

Figure 16-1. Hepatic metabolism of drugs and its interplay with genetic and environmental risk factors for causing hepatotoxicity.

Drug metabolites, which are unlikely to evoke an immune response because of their small size, are able to do so through the covalent binding with hepatic proteins resulting in the formation of adducts. This may result in an alternative pathway for liver damage, because the formed adducts are then exposed on the surface of the hepatocytes, where they can elicit an immune humoral (antibody-mediated cytotoxicity) or direct cytotoxic T-cell response (see Figure 16-1). It appears that the immune response to reactive metabolites forming adducts only occurs if they have previously produced a minor degree of cell death or cell stress (the "danger signal hypothesis"). The human leukocyte antigen (HLA) system is crucial in antigen presentation, and the presence or absence of some alleles, which are genetically defined, may influence immune response and possibly the ultimate predominance of the damaged hepatic cell. Indeed, HLA class I and II molecules may also be responsible for suppression of immune response, once initiated. Secondarily, recruited inflammatory cells and cytokines released by other non-parenchymal cells such as Kupffer's cells may amplify injury.[10]

It has recently been recognized that, in addition to necrosis, an important pathway of toxic liver damage is the activation of apoptotic cascade through intracellular stress (signalling mitochondria to permeabilize, releasing intermembrane proteins). Apoptosis may also occur if a drug or its metabolites sensitize the hepatocyte to the lethal actions of inflammatory mediators and cytokines such as tumor necrosis factor and Fas. Additionally, programmed cell death may be activated by immune-mediated injury (see Figure 16-1).[9-10]

A delicate imbalance exists between proapoptotic and protective survival pathways, as it does between stimuli to up-regulate toxic cytokines and those to up-regulate protective ones, the final result depending on the predominance of one or the other, as has been shown in animal models. Thus, the chemokine receptor 2 and IL-10 (two protective cytokine pathway) null mice develop hepatotoxicity with sub-toxic doses of acetaminophen. This suggests that subjects who have polymorphism or rare genetic defects in the expression of protective cytokines may suffer from uncommon hepatotoxic idiosyncratic reactions to drugs. For instance, a specific IL-10 promoter phenotype, which inhibits IL-10 secretion with subsequent down-regulation of type

2 helper T-cell immune reactions, is associated with diclofenac toxicity.[11] In addition, if suppressor or attenuator pathways are efficient, liver damage may wax and wane, despite continuation of drug exposure.[10]

The role of the canalicular transporting system in drug-induced cholestasis is still being elucidated. Some drugs or their metabolites may alter canalicular transporter proteins, preventing bile flow[12] (see Figure 16-1). Genetic defects in transporters may facilitate the process, as is exemplified by the nonsense mutation in the multidrug resistance-3 transporter,[13] which renders women susceptible to cholestasis during pregnancy and presumably also vulnerable to estrogen-induced cholestasis. Inhibition of the bile salt excretory protein by drugs (metabolites) leads to retention of bile acids and elevated serum bile acids, causing "bland" or pure cholestasis. Other compounds (usually reactive metabolites or labile conjugates of the parent drug) undergo canalicular secretion and damage the bile ductular cells, either directly or through immune response against adducts formed with the duct cell proteins. Such cases are accompanied by inflammation and some degree of hepatocellular injury. Impaired canalicular transport of drugs or reactive metabolites may also produce "retrograde" hepatocellular damage. In addition, retention of a drug due to abnormal canalicular secretion may theoretically induce CYP, mediated by orphan receptors/transcription factors, such as pregnane X receptor and constitutive androstane receptor, leading to enhanced production of toxic metabolite of the same or of another drug.

Clinical and Pathological Features and Classifications

Drug hepatotoxicity may present with clinical and pathological features that evoke virtually any other liver disease, with severity ranging from subclinical elevations in liver enzymes to fulminant hepatic failure. A clinical picture resembling acute viral hepatitis with jaundice, malaise, anorexia, nausea, and abdominal pain is the most common presentation, but because every liver cell may be the target of drug toxicity, many other expressions of hepatotoxicity, such as chronic hepatitis, cirrhosis, veno-occlusive disease, or neoplasm, can be seen.[4,14]

Common Presentations of Drug Hepatotoxicity

Liver histology is the most appropriate tool for defining the pattern of hepatotoxicity. However, because a liver biopsy specimen is often unavailable, from a practical standpoint, the pattern of drug-related liver injury is usually classified according to laboratory data, including the activity of serum alanine aminotransferase (ALT) and alkaline phosphatase (AP) expressed as the fold increase with respect to the upper limit of normal (N) and the ratio (R).[15] This classification is somewhat arbitrary and does not accurately convey all types of drug-induced liver damage (eg, vascular lesions and, in general, chronic damage), yet it has prognostic value.

The acute *hepatocellular* (cytotoxic, cytolytic) type of liver injury is defined by ALT >2N or ALT/AP ≥5. Patients with this particular type of liver damage have nonspecific clinical features, and they may not be jaundiced. Sometimes, there are manifestations of hypersensitivity, such as fever, rash or peripheral eosinophilia, which argue in favor of drug allergy. Serum levels of aminotransferase are markedly increased. Liver histology shows variable grades of cell necrosis and inflammation, yet the predominance of necrosis in zone 3 (centrilobular) and the abundance of eosinophils in the infiltrate are consistent with a toxic etiology. These expressions of hepatotoxicity can be seen with many drugs (Table 16-1).

Centrizonal necrosis is very marked with some intrinsic hepatotoxins such as acetaminophen overdose, carbon tetrachloride, and mushroom poisoning. In these cases, aminotransferase levels are exceedingly high, usually in the range of ischemic hepatitis.

Acute *cholestatic* injury is defined by an increase in serum AP >2N or by an ALT/AP ≤2 and is classified into two subtypes: 1) pure, "bland," or *canalicular* cholestasis and 2) acute cholestatic or hepatocanalicular hepatitis. Patients with acute cholestasis usually present with jaundice and pruritus. The *canalicular* type is characterized by an increase in conjugated bilirubin, AP, and γ-glutamyl transpeptidase with little or no impairment in serum transaminases. Liver histology shows hepatocyte cholestasis and dilated biliary canaliculi with bile plugs, but inflammation and hepatocyte necrosis are absent or negligible. Anabolic and contraceptive steroids typically produce this type of injury.

Patients with the *hepatocanalicular* type of damage may have abdominal pain and fever resembling acute biliary obstruction as well as hypersensitivity features. Liver biopsy reveals variable degrees of portal inflammation and hepatocyte necrosis, in addition to marked cholestasis of centrilobular predominance. Although the prognosis is better than for hepatocellular lesions and prompt recovery is the rule, in some patients who had destructive cholangitis, a picture of chronic cholestasis with progressive ductopenia may ensue. Drugs that typically cause this variety of liver damage are amoxicillin-clavulanate, macrolide antibiotics, and phenothiazine neuroleptics, but many others are able to do so (see Table 16-1).

The term *mixed* hepatic injury is used when the clinical and biological picture is intermediate between the hepatocellular and cholestatic types, although features of either type may predominate. By definition, the ALT/AP ratio is between 2 and 5. Allergic manifestations are often present, as well as a granulomatous reaction in the liver biopsy specimen. In diagnosing a patient with the mixed type of hepatic damage, physicians should keep in mind that this type of injury is far more characteristic of drug-induced hepatotoxicity than of viral hepatitis.[4] Almost all drugs that produce cholestatic injury are also capable of inducing a mixed pattern.

Unusual Patterns of Drug-Hepatotoxicity

Drugs rarely cause *chronic liver disease,* and, in these cases, the definition of the disease pattern requires a histological specimen. *Chronic hepatocellular* injury presumably results, in most instances, from the persistence of drug exposure once low-grade damage is initiated. Several drugs that cause acute hepatocellular hepatitis are also capable of provoking chronic damage. Examples of these include diclofenac, nitrofurantoin, and methyldopa. If jaundice is absent, the severity of liver lesions is often unsuspected from the clinical and laboratory features, because serum transaminase levels are usually only moderately increased. Withdrawal of the drug is typically followed by rapid normalization in the liver test. In some cases, toxic chronic hepatitis is accompanied by detectably circulating serum autoantibodies and hyperglobulinemia, resembling idiopathic autoimmune hepatitis, but differing from it in that recovery is the rule after drug discontinuation.[4,14]

Table 16-1

Medicinal Compounds Predominantly Associated With Hepatocellular or Cholestatic Damage

Hepatocelullar Damage	*Cholestatic Damage*
Acarbose	Amoxicillin clavulanic acid
Valproic acid	Azathioprine
Allopurinol	Captopril, enalapril, fosinopril
Amiodarone	Carbamazepine
Amoxicillin, Ampicillin	Carbimazole
Anti-HIV:	Celecoxib, Rofecoxib
(didanosine, zidovudine, protease	Cloxacillin, dicloxacillin
inhibitors)	Clindamycin
Nonsteroidal anti-inflammatory drugs	Ciprofloxacin, norfloxacin
(ibuprofen, diclofenac, piroxicam,	Contraceptive steroids
indometacin)	Cyproheptadine
Asparaginase	Erythromycins
Bentazepam	Estrogens
Chlormethiazole	Gold compounds, penicillamine
Diphenytoin	Irbesartan
Disulfiram	Macrolide antibiotics
Fluoxetine and paroxetine	Mirtazapine
Flutamide	Penicillin G
Halothane	Phenotiazines (chlorpromazine)
Lipid-lowering drugs:	Raloxifen
(lovastatin, pravastatin, atorvastatin)	Rosiglitazone, pioglitazone
Isoniazid	Sulfamethoxazole-trimethoprim
Ketoconazole	Sulfonylureas
Mebendazole, albendazole, pentamidine	Tamoxifen
Mesalazine	Terbinafine
Methotrexate	Tetracycline
Minocycline	Ticlopidine
Nitrofurantoin	Thiabendazole
Nefazodone	Tricyclic antidepressants
Omeprazole	
Pyrazinamide	
Risperidone	
Ritodrine	
Sulfasalazine	
Terbinafine	
Tetracycline	
Tolcapone	
Topiramate	
Trazodone	
Trovafloxacin	
Venlafaxine	
Verapamil	
Vitamin A	

Indolent *fibrosis* and *cirrhosis* may occur after prolonged therapy with methotrexate, as a result of increased cumulative doses. Rapid evolution to cirrhosis has also been documented in some instances of drug hepatotoxicity that begin as acute hepatitis (eg, ebrotidine hepatotoxicity).

If hepatocyte mitochondrial β-oxidation and respiration are impaired, *steatosis* and *steatohepatitis* may develop. Liver histology shows variable degrees of steatosis, inflammation and fibrosis, and even Mallory bodies. This is the pattern of injury that typically occurs with amiodarone and tamoxifen hepatotoxicity.

Sinusoidal endothelial cells can also be affected by drug toxicity, primarily on the terminal hepatic venules, leading to *veno-occlusive disease*. Liver biopsy shows intimal hyperplasia in vessel walls and collagen deposition, which causes progressive occlusion and venous outflow obstruction, and, secondarily, necrosis of the surrounding parenchyma. Abdominal pain, jaundice, ascites, edema, and evidence of portal hypertension develop either as an acute fulminant variety or as a more insidious presentation leading to cirrhosis. Several drugs (eg, azatioprine, when given for kidney and bone marrow transplantation, and chemotherapeutic agents) and botanical plants containing pyrrolizidine alkaloids can cause this form of hepatotoxicity. A similar clinical presentation is observed in the thrombotic occlusion of supra-hepatic veins (*Budd-Chiari syndrome*) associated with contraceptive steroid use.

Long-term use of contraceptive and anabolic steroids can also be associated with hepatic *adenomas* and, more rarely, with liver *cancer*.

Risk Factors

Several constitutional and/or acquired risk factors may influence individual susceptibility to drug hepatotoxicity, although incomplete recordings of the reactions and the lack of reliable figures on the incidence of injury have hindered their analyses (Table 16-2). It is not known how many of these factors interplay with the potential hepatotoxin in enhancing or protecting from toxic liver injury, but it is probable that most of them act by modifying the hepatic biotransformation of the drug or the detoxification pathways (see Figure 16-1).

Genetic Factors

It is important to stress that genetic studies seeking associations with diseases that do not exhibit a classical inheritance attributable to a single gene locus are subject to a variety of potential pitfalls, especially the risk of type II errors if the sample size is too small, which often limits the significance of the data reported.

Polymorphic microsomal enzymes appear to play a role in hepatotoxicity with various compounds (Table 16-3). Most patients with perhexiline hepatotoxicity (an antianginal drug withdrawn from the market) were deficient in CYP2D6 as were two patients with liver damage from the herbal remedy Kava-Kava. However, the contribution of this particular deficiency to hepatotoxicity is unclear because it is present in 6% to 8% of the White population, and many other drugs are metabolized by this enzyme without evidence of liver damage.[16] Patients with tetrabamate-induced hepatic injury also had a partial or complete deficiency in CYP2C19 in one study.[16]

A deficiency in acetylation capacity leading to increased susceptibility to isoniazid hepatotoxicity has long been suspected but was unconfirmed until recently when, using genomic techniques in a large cohort of Asian patients, a relationship was found

Table 16-2

Clinicopathological Patterns of Drug Hepatotoxicity and Associated Risk Factors

Type of Damage	*Compound*	*Risk Factors*
Hepatocellular hepatitis	Acetaminophen	Alcoholism, fasting, isoniazid
	Isoniazid	Alcoholism, older age, slow NAT-2 genotype, rifampicin, HIV, HBV, HCV
	Diclofenac	Female gender, osteoarthritis
Canalicular cholestasis	Oral contraceptive	Non-sense mutation in MDR-3
Cholestatic hepatitis	Amoxicillin-clavulanate Erythromycin Chlorpromazine	Male, older age, several exposures
Granuloma	Phenytoin	Genetic deficiency in epoxide hydrolase
	Allopurinol	Renal failure
	Sulfonamides	HIV, slow acetylators
Chronic hepatitis	Nitrofurantoin Diclofenac, Methyldopa, Bentazepam	Female, older age
Macrovesicular steatosis	Tetracycline	Intravenous administration, pregnancy
Microvesicular steatosis	Valproic acid NRTIs	Children, other anticonvulsant
Nonalcoholic steatohepatitis	Amiodarone Tamoxifen	Prolonged (more than a year) therapy
Fibrosis/cirrhosis	Methotrexate	Daily dosage, alcoholism, obesity, diabetes, chronic hepatitis
Hepatic adenoma	Oral contraceptive	Total dosage and length of therapy

HBV=hepatitis B virus; HCV=hepatitis C virus; HIV=human immunodeficiency virus; MDR-3=multidrug resistance-3 transporter; NAT-2=N-acetyltransferase-2; NRTIs=nucleoside reverse transcriptase inhibitors

between N-acetyltransferase 2 deficiency and the propensity to develop hepatotoxicity from the combination of isoniazid, rifampicin, and pyrazinamide.[17]

Genetic variations in human leukocyte antigen (HLA) molecules might predispose individuals to immunoallergic drug hepatotoxicity. Recently, in a large case series

Table 16-3

Polymorphic Liver Enzymes and Potential Targets for Specific Diagnosis of Hepatotoxicity

A. Deficiency	*Compound*
CYP2D6	Perhexiline
CYP2C19	Tetrabamate
N-acetyltransferase 2	Sulfonamides, Dihydralazine, Isoniazid
Epoxide hydrolase	Phenytoin, carbamazepine
B. Autoantibody Targets	
Antimitochondrial (anti-M6) autoantibody	Iproniazid
Antiliver kidney microsomal 2 antibody (anti-LKM2)	Tienilic acid
Anti-CYP1A2	Dihydralazine
Anti-CYP2E1	Halothane
Antiliver microsomal autoantibody	Carbamazepine
Antimicrosomal epoxide hydrolase	Germander

CYP=cytochrome P450

of drug-induced idiosyncratic liver disease, we found a direct association between cholestatic/mixed reactions (most of which seem to have an immune basis) and the HLA-DRB1*15 and -DQB1*06 alleles. Conversely, the frequency of occurrence of DRB1*07 and DQB1*02 alleles was reduced in patients with this type of reaction.[18] The complete HLA haplotype DRB1*1501-DRB5*0101-DQB1*0602 has also been linked to cholestatic (but not *hepatocellular*) hepatitis related to amoxicillin-clavulanate in two other studies. All these data support the notion that certain HLA class II alleles are important in explaining why a given drug may cause different patterns of liver damage in different individuals.

Pharmacogenomic testing is a promising approach to preventing drug-induced hepatic injury. However, because most rare idiosyncratic reactions involve multiple unlikely events, much has still to be learned. For instance, identification of mutant CYP alleles would only prove that the patient might have altered plasma levels with drugs that are substrates for that specific enzyme, but would not predict hepatotoxicity.

Age

Older persons appear to be more susceptible to drug-induced hepatotoxicity. When cases of hepatitis at a major hepatology center in France were analyzed according to age, the prevalence of drug-induced injury was more than 40% in patients older than 50 years, compared to just 10% in younger patients.[16] The reasons for this are unclear, but might include reduced metabolic capacity, changes in hepatic blood flow and tissue immune response, diminished renal clearance, and greater exposure to drugs and the more frequent use of several concomitant medications by the elderly.[19] In addition, the cholestatic pattern of damage was more frequent than other patterns of damage in older patients in a recent study.[8] Conversely, children appear to be at greater risk of developing liver damage from certain specific drugs such as aspirin and valproic acid.[4]

Gender

Although it is generally accepted that women are more vulnerable than men to the toxic effects of drugs in the liver, gender differences have not always become apparent when large case series were analyzed. Nevertheless, hepatotoxicity with certain medications such as nitrofurantoin, chlorpromazine, tetracycline, halothane, and diclofenac, to mention just a few examples, has been reported more frequently in women, although men seem more likely than women to develop liver damage from azathioprine and amoxicillin-clavulanate.[4,14] In other instances, female predominance could be biased by the propensity for women to use certain remedies. This is likely to be the case for liver damage seen almost exclusively in women that is related to the herbal remedies Germander (a weight-control agent) or Greater Celandine (a therapy for gallbladder stones and dyspepsia). Regarding the clinicopathological expression of hepatotoxicity, the variety of chronic autoimmune hepatitis that is induced by drugs is seen almost exclusively in women.

Metabolic, Hormonal, and Nutritional Factors

Concern over the use of medication during pregnancy is natural, and it is still not known whether this condition makes women in general more vulnerable to the hepatotoxic effects of drugs. There are data indicating that pregnancy increases the susceptibility to hepatic injury from tetracycline. In addition, obesity has been identified as a risk factor for liver damage with halothane, methotrexate, and possibly other drugs. This is not surprising, because obesity is characterized by increased expression of CYP2E1, the isoform responsible for halothane metabolism.[9] Therefore, obesity might theoretically enhance the hepatotoxicity of drugs metabolized by the CYP2E1 fraction. Poor nutritional status has been identified as an important risk factor for acetaminophen hepatotoxicity. A possible explanation for this is the depletion of glutathione (which inactivates the reactive metabolite NAPQI formed through CYP2E1 metabolism of the drug) in liver cells that presumably accompany starvation.

Alcohol and Other Drugs

Alcohol and many other drugs are capable of modulating the hepatotoxic potential of other medications through CYP induction, inhibition, or substrate competition. Alcohol seems to have a dual effect on CYP2E1. During chronic regular intake, ethanol enhances acetaminophen hepatotoxicity by inducting CYP2E1, as well as susceptibility to liver damage from isoniazid, methotrexate, halothane, and cocaine, and perhaps from other drugs that are substrates for this microsomal isoform.[21] During acute intake, however, substrate competition with acetaminophen occurs, actually decreasing the speed of metabolism of this drug to its toxic intermediate.[22] However, this latter effect is partially counteracted by the ability of alcohol to slow the degradation of the CYP2E1 fraction, thus enhancing again the formation of the harmful metabolite once alcohol intake is interrupted.[10] Alcohol also contributes to acetaminophen hepatotoxicity by the direct inhibition of glutathione synthesis and through the malnutrition that frequently accompanies chronic alcoholism.

Some associations of drugs have been clearly identified as being more harmful to the liver than when each drug is taken separately; the later drug presumably results in the induction of CYP, further enhancing the production of toxic metabolites by the former medication. This is the case of rifampicin, which increases the hepatotoxicity of isoniazid, and for phenobarbital, which enhances the hepatotoxicity of halothane and some antidepressant drugs. Conversely, inhibition of CYP3A4 by trioleandomycin increases the availability of estrogens, increasing the risk of cholestasis with these compounds.

Pre-Existing Liver Disease

A major mechanism involved in idiosyncratic hepatotoxicity encompasses the production of "reactive metabolites" during the hepatic metabolism of xenobiotics, a mechanism that, theoretically, requires a relatively intact liver. Therefore, acute severe or chronic liver disease might be a protective factor against hepatotoxicity by interrupting the metabolite-generating pathway as a result of decreased enzyme activity. However, not all enzyme systems are affected in advanced liver disease.[23] Indeed, conjugation reactions with glucuronic acid remain preserved despite a dramatic reduction in hepatic reserve. The activity of CYP2D6 is also intact in severe liver disease, whereas that of CYP2C19 is deeply diminished.

The use of medications that have been associated with hepatotoxicity in patients with underlying liver disease is, nevertheless, an area of continued controversy. In a recent large cohort retroprospective-based study, patients with baseline-raised transaminases did not have an increased risk of hepatotoxicity from statins in comparison to patients with normal transaminase values.[24] In general, patients with liver disease, regardless of the degree of liver function, do not appear to be uniformly at increased risk for hepatotoxicity, although there are some exceptions to the rule[10] (Table 16-4). The fact that patients with chronic hepatitis B (HBV) and hepatitis C (HCV) and HIV infection are at increased risk for drug hepatotoxicity actually suggests a role for cytokine imbalance in these patients.

Pre-existing liver disease may nevertheless hamper the diagnosis of drug-hepatotoxicity, because impaired liver function in this context may be wrongly attributed to the underlying disease. Physicians should be aware of this possibility when prescribing medications of known hepatotoxic potential for patients with underlying hepatic disease. Adequate monitoring, with baseline liver tests before starting therapy, might help to distinguish between these two situations.

Diagnosis

The diagnosis of hepatotoxicity remains challenging in clinical practice. Because no specific markers for toxic liver damage are generally available, causality assessment relies upon circumstantial evidence of exposure to a potential hepatotoxin, as well as the exclusion of other causes of liver injury. Ultimately, the diagnosis of drug-induced liver disease requires a high degree of suspicion (Figure 16-2). It is important to rec-

Table 16-4

PRE-EXISTENT LIVER DISEASE AND THE SUSCEPTIBILITY FOR DRUG HEPATOTOXICITY

Liver Disease	*Agents/Comments*
Chronic hepatitis C	Myeloablative therapy
	Antituberculous therapy (isoniazide+ rifampicin+pyrazinamide) (higher with HIV co-infection)
	HAART
	Flutamide (also with HBV infection)
	Ibuprofen
	Methotrexate
Alcoholic/postnecrotic cirrhosis	Methotrexate
Primary biliary cirrhosis	Rifampicin

HIV=human immunodeficiency virus; HAART=highly active antiretroviral therapy; HBV=hepatitis B virus

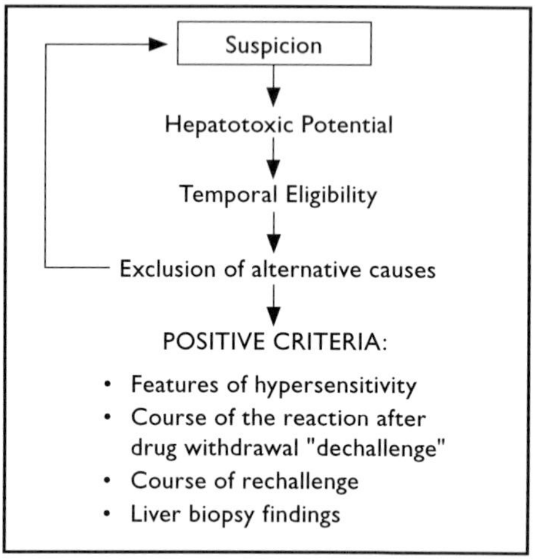

Figure 16-2. Schematic algorithm for a practical approach to the diagnosis of hepatotoxicity. (Adapted from Andrade RJ, Camargo R, Lucena MI, et al. Causality assessment in drug-induced hepatotoxicity. *Expert Opin Drug Saf.* 2004;3(4):329-344.

ognize, if they are present, the risk factors outlined above. Thereafter, several items should be taken into account in the "step-by-step" approach.[6]

DRUG EXPOSURE DATA AND INFORMATION ON HEPATOTOXIC POTENTIAL

A thorough study of drug and chemical history is essential. Prescribed and over-the-counter medications need to be recorded. Consumption of illicit drugs should also be assessed. Although almost all marketed drugs have been incriminated in incidences of hepatotoxicity, their potential for causing liver damage is not the same. For instance, digoxin, streptomycin, and theophylline—which have been used for decades—appear to be relatively free of hepatotoxic potential.[4] Information about the likelihood of liver damage from many other drugs is scanty or vague. In the Summary of Product Characteristics, phrases such as "can produce transient increase in transaminases" or "may cause hepatitis rarely" are common. A search of databases of hepatotoxic drugs, such as HEPATOX (Phytopharmica, Green Bay, Wis),[25] or lists in reference books can be useful. A more up-to-date resource is the Medline-PubMed database of the National Library of Medicine, where searching for the name of the drug together with the terms "hepatotoxicity," "hepatitis," "drug-induced hepatotoxicity," or simply "liver" if the former do not yield details, can be useful.

A special difficulty arises when the patient has been taking a newly marketed drug. In these cases, data regarding the medication's hepatotoxic potential, if known, are only available in pre-approval clinical trials.

Temporal Eligibility

After checking for exposure to a medication or herbal product, the question is whether treatment was begun when the patient was already ill or clearly before presentation. The suspected drug could actually have been prescribed to alleviate early symptoms of hepatotoxicity. If this is not the case, the length of therapy with the suspected drug must be carefully assessed. The time interval between the beginning of treatment and the onset of liver injury varies widely. Intrinsic hepatotoxins (acetaminophen) induce liver damage a few hours after exposure. In most other cases, the latency period is, approximately, between 1 week and 3 months. A shorter period (1 or 2 days) may occur in patients who have been previously treated with the drug and have become sensitized (immunoallergic hepatotoxicity). A delay greater than 3 months may be encountered with compounds that act by metabolic idiosyncrasy.[4,14] Although acute toxic hepatitis very rarely occurs more than 12 months after exposure, it is still possible in unusual forms of chronic liver damage (such as steatohepatitis, fibrosis, and chronic hepatitis) in which the expression of hepatotoxicity is symptom-less, enabling treatment to persist, or simply because the type of lesion requires prolonged exposure to develop (eg, vascular lesions and tumors).

Sometimes, the implication of a drug is difficult to recognize because of a considerable delay between the interruption of therapy and clinical presentation. A classical example is hepatitis associated with halothane and its derivatives, which typically occurs 3 weeks after the first exposure. The phenomenon is extreme with amoxicillin-clavulanate, which may cause hepatitis several weeks after cessation of exposure, but has also been reported recently with other medications such as trovafloxacin and mydecamicin.

Exclusion of Alternative Causes

Exposure to one or more drugs does not in itself prove causality, and due to the nonavailability of biological markers of toxic liver injury, the exclusion of specific causes is mandatory (Table 16-5).

Diagnostic evaluation of any patient with acute liver disease of unknown origin should comprise a careful history, to exclude alcohol abuse, recent episodes of hypotension, epidemiological risk factors of infectious hepatitis, specific serology and molecular biology studies for common viruses involved in viral hepatitis, as well as

Table 16-5

SCREENING FOR ALTERNATIVE CAUSES OF LIVER DISEASE

Test/Clinical Features	*Diseases*
• Viral serology: Always, search for risk factors IgM anti-HAV IgM anti-HBc Anti-HCV, RNA-HCV (RT-PCR) IgM-CMV IgM-EBV	Viral hepatitis
• Bacterial serology: If persistent fever, diarrhea (Salmonella, Campylobacter, Listeria, Coxiella)	Bacterial hepatitis
• Serology for syphilis: Several sexual couples	Secondary syphilis
• Autoimmunity: Women, unspecific (ANA, ANCA, AMA, ASMA, anti-LKM-1)	AIH PBC
• Ceruloplasmine, urine cooper (patients <40 years)	Wilson's disease
• Hypotension, shock, heart failure • Vascular disease, elderly.	Ischemic hepatitis
• Further imaging tests: Cholestasis and negative AU, CT, MRCP, and ERCP	Biliary obstruction

AU=abdominal ultrasonographic examination; AIH=autoinmune hepatitis; Anti-HAV=hepatitis A antibody; Anti-HBc=hepatitis B core antibody; Anti-HCV=hepatitis C antibody; anti-LKM-1=liver-kidney microsomal antibody type 1; AMA=antimitochondrial antibody; ANA=antinuclear antibody; ANCA=perinuclear antineutrophil cytoplasmic antibody; ASMA=antismooth muscle antibody; PBC= primary biliary cirrhosis; CMV=citomegaloviruses; CT=computed tomography; EBV=Epstein-Barr virus; ERCP=endoscopic retrograde cholangiography; MRCP=magnetic resonance cholangiography.

screening for autoimmune hepatitis. All patients should also have an abdominal ultrasound examination to exclude mechanical biliary obstruction. The appropriateness of additional studies depends on the presence of particular symptoms or analytical features (see Table 16-5).

POSITIVE (INCRIMINATING) CRITERIA

Once alternative causes of liver injury have been ruled out, the role of one or more drugs can be highlighted by a careful scrutiny of the presence of hypersensitivity features, the course after drug withdrawal and after a challenge dose, as well as by typical biopsy findings. Direct evidence for hepatotoxicity is rarely available, but can include serum circulating autoantibodies for some drugs (see Table 16-3), most of which have been withdrawn from the market, and blood levels of intrinsic hepatotoxins such as acetaminophen and aspirin. Nevertheless, testing for these autoantibodies is an investigational tool at present. In vitro tests such as the lymphocyte transformation test comprise another tool to search for evidence of drug allergy. Although a positive response has long been considered specific evidence that the drug is responsible for the injury, such a response may merely reflect previous exposure to the drug. Ultimately, in vitro tests are difficult to standardize, are poorly reproducible between laboratories, and have not gained clinical acceptance.[4]

Allergic Features

As clinical symptoms of drug-induced hepatic injury are nonspecific, focusing on unusual manifestations may be helpful in the diagnostic evaluation. Extrahepatic features such as accompanying skin rash, fever, peripheral eosinophilia, cytopenia, and other organ involvement, although present in only a minority of cases of drug-induced liver disease, implicate an adverse drug reaction. Hematologic features including granulocytopenia, thrombopenia, or hemolytic anemia can be seen in drug allergy. Renal and pancreatic involvement may also accompany some instances of drug-induced immunoallergic hepatic injury. However, because these manifestations occur in only a minority of cases of hepatotoxicity,[8] their absence is not a helpful sign. In fact, it is likely that immunologic and metabolic idiosyncrasies operate concurrently in many cases of drug hepatotoxicity.[4,10]

Course After Drug Withdrawal (*Dechallenge*)

Rapid improvement after withdrawal of the drug is strong evidence in favor of a toxic etiology of the liver disease. In cases of hepatocellular injury, the role of a drug is supported by a decrease of at least 50% in the levels of liver enzymes within 30 days after cessation of exposure. The association is even stronger if the 50% decrease occurs in the first 8 days after stopping therapy. However, other atypical outcomes make laboratory scrutiny unhelpful after drug withdrawal; some cholestatic reactions, for instance, subside very slowly, with abnormal enzyme levels persisting for more than 1 year. In other cases, the injury may progress over several days despite drug cessation, or even evolve to fulminant hepatic failure. This outcome makes attempts to determine the toxic etiology particularly difficult. Conversely, a phenomenon of "adaptation or tolerance" to injury occurs with some drugs (eg, statins) and is responsible for the spontaneous improvement in liver tests despite treatment continuation.

The *Rechallenge* Dose

Currently, the only way to confirm causality in drug hepatotoxicity is to demonstrate a recrudescence of liver injury after re-exposure to the suspected agent. A positive response after exposure can be defined as doubling ALT and AP values for hepatocellular and cholestatic reactions, respectively. Rechallenge, however, can be hazardous, especially in drug-induced *hepatocellular* hepatitis with associated hypersensitivity features, because the provoked reaction is often more severe than the initial episode. Besides, the amount of drug required to provoke the reaction is unknown. Arbitrarily, a single dose is usually chosen; arguably, however, more than a few doses would be necessary to reproduce liver damage in hepatotoxicity caused by the progressive accumulation of toxic derivatives. This false-negative response to rechallenge has been demonstrated for isoniazid, but is probably applicable for many other drugs. Ultimately, re-exposure of the patient to the suspected drug should be considered only if the drug seems essential, as in the treatment of tuberculosis with isoniazid and after written informed consent is obtained from the patient. Testing of laboratory abnormalities in preapproval clinical trials might be an additional indication for rechallenge.[6]

More often, a history of inadvertent re-challenge can be elicited by careful inquiry. In these instances, the index episode may not be accompanied by jaundice, and symptoms that incriminate the drug are frequently nonspecific (malaise, fever) and thus easily overlooked.

Histological Findings and the "Signature" of Liver Injury Due to Particular Drugs

There are no histologic findings that can be considered absolutely specific for the diagnosis of drug-induced hepatotoxicity, and consequently liver biopsy should not be routinely performed for this indication. Currently, the reasons for performing a liver biopsy in patients with suspected drug-induced hepatotoxicity are restricted to the following:

1. When a toxic etiology is less likely and other alternative causes should be ruled out.
2. To characterize the pattern of injury with drugs not previously incriminated in hepatotoxicity.
3. To identify more severe or residual lesions (eg, fibrosis) that could have prognostic significance. For instance, in some chronic variants of hepatotoxicity (eg, methotrexate, amiodarone), clinical and laboratory features are poorly predictive of the severity of underlying liver damage. Furthermore, severe bile duct injury during cholestatic hepatitis has been shown to be predictive of evolution to chronic cholestasis,[26] as was also shown in a retrospective study for the presence of fibrosis in the index liver biopsy for the development of chronic liver disease.[27]

Some histological findings are consistent with a toxic etiology (Table 16-6). In fact, undetected drug intake should be suspected from the presence of any of the pathologic features listed in Table 16-6, which should prompt a search for the causal agent.

Because in most cases a liver biopsy is not available, focus on the biochemical expression of hepatic damage may help in incriminating a drug. It has been claimed that each drug has its own pattern of liver injury "signature."10 Although this is true for some drugs (eg, estrogens induce cholestatic injury and seldom any other pattern of damage), for most others, drug consistency is not so straightforward. For instance, amoxicillin-clavulanate tends to produce cholestatic or mixed damage, although hepatocellular damage has also been reported frequently. Hepatocellular and cholestatic or mixed injury have been noted with nimesulide or troglitazone, to mention only a few examples. Therefore, it is important for physicians to view a suspicion of hepatotoxicity with the awareness that a given drug may produce diverse types of injury.

Causality Assessment Methods

Several groups have developed clinical scales for the causality assessment of hepatotoxicity, providing a uniform approach to determining the likelihood of drug involvement in a suspected episode of hepatitis.[28-30] The qualities usually required for a diagnosis scale are reproducibility and validity. Reproducibility ensures an identical

Table 16-6

Liver Biopsy Findings Suggestive of Drug Hepatotoxicity

Histological Feature	*Examples of Drugs*
Centrozonal necrosis/Confluent necrosis	Acetaminophen
	Isoniazid
	Troglitazone
	NSAIDs (bromfenac)
	Nevirapine
	Ritonavir, Indinavir
	Ebrotidine
	Nefazodone
Combined hepatocellular/Cholestatic injury	Propafenone
	Propoxyphene
	Verapamil
Bile duct injury/Periportal cholestasis	Amoxicillin/clavulanate
	Chlorpromazine
	Erythromycins
	Sulindac
Eosinophil-rich infiltrate/Granuloma	Allopurinol
	Quinidine
	Phenylbutazone
	Phenytoin
Microvesicular steatosis	NRTIs (fialuridine, zidovudine)
	Valproic acid
Veno-occlusive disease	Azathioprine
	Busulfan
	Cyclophosphamide

NRTIs=nucleoside reverse transcriptase inhibitors

result regardless of who the user is and when the scale is used. Validity means the method is able to distinguish between cases where the drug is responsible and cases where it is not.

The first method developed for causality assessment in drug-hepatotoxicity was described in 1992—the CIOMS (Council for International Organisations of Medical Sciences) or RUCAM (Roussel Uclaf Causality Assessment Method) scale.[28] This method provides a standardized scoring system in which the limits and contents of most criteria are decided by consensus among experts, on the basis of organ-oriented characteristics. The parameters are outlined in Table 16-7. The time to onset and

Table 16-7

Scores for Individual Axes of the CIOMS and Maria & Victorino Diagnostic Scales

CIOMS

Axis	Score
Chronological criterion	
From drug intake until onset event	+2 to +1
From drug withdrawal until onset event	+1 to 0
Course of the reaction	2 to +3
Risk factors:	
Age	+1 to 0
Alcohol	+1 to 0
Concomitant therapy	-3 to 0
Exclusion nondrug-related causes	-3 to +2
Bibliographical data	0 to +2
Rechallenge	-2 to +3

Maria & Victorino

Axis	Score
Chronological criterion	
From drug intake until onset event	+1 to +3
From drug withdrawal until onset event	-3 to +3
Course of the reaction	0 to +3
Exclusion alternative causes	-3 to +3
Extrahepatic manifestations	0 to +3
Bibliographical data	-3 to +2
Rechallenge	0 to +3

Adapted from Lucena MI, Camargo R, Andrade RJ, et al. Comparison of two clinical scales for causality assessment in hepatotoxicity. *Hepatology*. 2001;33:123-130.

course are evaluated separately for hepatocellular versus cholestatic/mixed reactions, because the latter can occur after a longer post-cessation interval and resolve much more slowly. The CIOMS/RUCAM scale provides a scoring system for six axes in the decision strategy. The answers correspond to weighted numeric values that are summed to give a total score. The scores are translated into categories of suspicion: definite or highly probable (score >8), probable (score 6 to 8), possible (score 3 to 5), unlikely (score 1 to 2), and excluded (score ≤0). This method was originally validated using cases of drug-induced liver disease with known positive rechallenge (the major type of evidence recognized as demonstrating the role of a drug), and the system performed well when these cases were assessed based on data prior to re-challenge or when concomitant drugs were included.[29]

More recently, Maria and Victorino developed a simplified scoring system, called the Clinical Diagnostic Scale (CDS) (also called the M&V scale), which uses several features of the CIOMS/RUCAM scale but omits some and adds others (Table 16-7).[30] The sum of the points for each parameter can vary from -6 to 20. Correspondence with the five classic degrees of probability of adverse drug reactions is established on the basis of the score as follows: definite (score >17), probable (score 14 to 17), possible (score 10 to 13), unlikely (score 6 to 9), and excluded (score <6). The CDS/M&V scale was validated using real and fictitious cases of immunoallergic drug-induced liver injury (high percentages of positive immunological tests in cases classified as definite or probable) and was compared with the external standard or experts' classification. The authors have noted some limitations of the scale: the instrument performs poorly in atypical cases of drugs with unusually long latency periods or chronic evolution after withdrawal. Point II of the scale, concerning the exclusion of alternative causes of liver injury, could be improved by specifying more clearly the clinical conditions to be excluded and including detailed criteria for exclusion. The main advantage of the CDS/M&V scale is its ease of application in clinical practice.

The CIOMS/RUCAM scale and the CDS/ M&V scale were compared in a population of 215 patients with suspected drug hepatotoxicity reported to a registry.[31] Causality in this population was verified by three experts as drug-induced (185) or as nondrug caused (30 cases). Complete agreement between the CDS/M&V scale and the CIOMS/RUCAM scale was obtained in only 42 cases (18%). The CDS/M&V scale classified only about one third of the cases as probable or definite and tended to underestimate the probability of causality. The best correlation between the two scales was found for drug-induced liver injury with a suggested immunoallergic mechanism. The lowest agreement was observed for patients with cholestatic injury. In cases whose outcome was death, no agreement was found. It appears, therefore, that the CIOMS/RUCAM instrument shows better agreement with "common sense" clinical judgment. Aside from its clinical validity, the usefulness of the CIOMS/RUCAM scale is that it provides a framework that emphasizes topics that need to be addressed in cases of suspected hepatic adverse reaction in order to improve the consistency of judgments.

Future refinements of CIOMS/RUCAM scale have been suggested in the weight given to individual parameters, based on statistical evaluations using large databases.[32] A database with up-to-date lists of hepatotoxins is needed, because one of the parameters evaluated in all causality scales is previous information on the hepatotoxicity of the drug in question. Another current limitation of the scales is that follow-up is required to compute a full score. It has been suggested that an abridged or modified version could be developed and validated for the initial evaluation.[32]

Prognosis and Natural History

Immediate prognosis of drug hepatotoxicity depends on the extension of hepatocyte necrosis. Hepatocellular hepatitis, particularly if accompanied by jaundice, bears a worse prognosis than do cholestatic lesions,[8] although the case fatality rates may vary among drugs. Prompt withdrawal of the agent responsible is essential, as is vigilance for the apparition of signs of impending liver failure. It has been determined that continuation of the offending drug once jaundice develops is a major determinant of outcome to acute liver failure.[4] The prognosis of fulminant hepatic failure due to idiosyncratic reaction to drugs is poor without liver transplantation, with a survival rate of less than 10%. Fatalities are very uncommon in cholestatic toxic hepatitis, but when bile ducts become severely damaged, there is a risk of evolution to the so-called vanishing bile duct syndrome, and biliary cirrhosis may ensue.[26]

The issue of the natural history of drug hepatotoxicity remains controversial because it has not been properly assessed in prospective studies involving a large enough cohort of patients. Evidence from isolated cases indicates that most patients with acute hepatocellular lesions, in whom the initial episode is promptly recognized and the responsible drug is withdrawn, are able to resolve the reaction without residual lesions. Concerns have come from a cohort-based retrospective study in 44 patients with pathological diagnosis of drug-hepatotoxicity showing that when brought back for re-evaluation, a quarter had abnormal laboratory or imaging tests and 3 out of the 5 in whom a liver biopsy was performed had residual fibrosis.[27]

Treatment

The treatment of idiosyncratic drug hepatotoxicity is supportive. Jaundiced patients with acute hepatocellular hepatitis probably need close vigilance in an in-hospital setting. Antidotal therapy is restricted to acetaminophen overdose. *N*-acetylcysteine, by repleting glutathione stores, prevents injury if it is administered within 24 hours after intake.[10]

Anecdotal reports suggest that corticosteroids may be useful in drug-hepatotoxicity associated with a general hypersensitivity syndrome. Similarly, there appears to be a rationale for the use of ursodesoxicolic acid in patients with prolonged toxic cholestasis. However, the lack of properly conducted controlled trials hampers a clear recommendation on the use of these two agents. In addition to cholestiramine, the molecular adsorbent recycling system (MARS) has also been advocated for pruritus relief in isolated case reports of drug-induced toxic cholestasis. Parenteral administration of fat-soluble vitamins in prolonged cholestasis may also be needed.[10]

Prevention and Regulatory Perspectives

Patients and doctors should be aware that various drugs in common use can be hepatotoxic and take into account the importance of drug discontinuation and of seeking medical advice if related symptoms such as dark urine, malaise, abdominal pain, or jaundice ensue. Special caution should be applied in the case of new, recently marketed drugs.[33] Each phase of clinical testing before approval includes close monitoring of liver tests. However, to detect significant drug-induced liver disease with 95% confidence, the number of patients studied must be at least three times the incidence of the reaction ("rule of threes").[34] Finding hepatotoxicity with an incidence of

1:10,000 (the approximate incidence of most idiosyncratic reactions) would therefore require 30,000 treated patients. As Phase III clinical trials usually involve 1500 to 2500 patients, overt hepatotoxic reactions are normally only detected after marketing, when several thousand people have been exposed to the drug. Nevertheless, the appearance in preapproval studies of less alarming signals, such as the incidence of asymptomatic ALT and raised levels of bilirubin, should also be carefully investigated. Of particular importance is the magnitude of any increase in transaminases. An ALT ≥8-fold the maximum normal value, especially if accompanied by an increase in direct bilirubin (≥1.5-fold) deserves attention, because this rarely occurs in the control population.[34] The experience with troglitazone illustrates the importance of pre-marketing identification of signals. In 2500 patients participating in phase III studies, ALT >8-fold occurred in 0.6% of the treated patients (vs none of the control patients), and 2 cases of icteric hepatitis were observed. This issue is critical because it has been estimated—"the Hy`s law"—that approximately 10% of jaundiced patients with acute hepatocellular injury will ultimately progress to fulminant hepatic failure.[4] This was the case with troglitazone, which was withdrawn after its implication in several instances of severe hepatitis and acute liver failure leading to death or liver transplantation.[35]

The issue of postmarketing monthly liver test monitoring remains controversial.[34] The rationale is that because drug-induced subclinical elevation in liver enzymes occurs much more frequently than overt clinical injury, early detection at this time might prevent further damage. This strategy, however, involves several practical problems; it applies only to idiosyncratic "metabolic" drug hepatotoxicity, because the latency period for allergic reactions is usually too small. In addition, the ideal monitoring frequency is unknown. Arbitrarily, a monthly time interval is chosen, but rapid progression to severe liver damage has been found after previous negative monitoring; a shorter time interval, however, may be impractical. On the other hand, transient transaminase elevations might not reflect hepatotoxicity, as this condition occurs frequently in untreated subjects.[34] Ultimately, noncompliance of monitoring by patients and doctors is perhaps the main impediment to its implementation. Actually, monthly liver test monitoring has proven its efficacy in some long-established instances (eg, antituberculosis therapy), but recent experiences with troglitazone and bromfenac have been disappointing.[35]

References

1. Ostapowicz G, Fontana RJ, Schiødt FV et al. Results of a prospective study of acute liver failure at 17 tertiary care centers in the United States. *Ann Intern Med.* 2002;137:947-954.
2. Sgro C, Clinard F, Ouazir K, et al. Incidence of drug-induced hepatic injuries: a French population-based study. *Hepatology.* 2002;36:451-455.
3. Aithal GP, Rawlins MD, Day CP. Accuracy of hepatic adverse drug reaction reporting in one English health region. *BMJ.* 1999;319:1541.
4. Zimmerman HJ. *Hepatotoxicity. The Adverse Effects of Drugs and Other Chemicals on the Liver.* 2nd ed. Philadelphia: Lippincott Williams & Wilkins; 1999.
5. Friis H, Andreasen PB. Drug induced hepatic injury: Analysis of 1100 cases reported to The Danish Committee on Adverse Drug Reactions between 1978 and 1987. *J Intern Med.* 1992;232:133-138.

6. Andrade RJ, Camargo R, Lucena MI, González-Grande R. Causality assessment in drug-induced hepatotoxicity. *Expert Opin Drug Saf.* 2004;3(4):329-344.
7. Ibañez L, Pérez E, Vidal X, et al. Prospective surveillance of acute serious liver disease unrelated to infectious, obstructive or metabolic disease: epidemiological and clinical features and exposure to drugs. *J Hepatol.* 2002; 37:592-600.
8. Andrade RJ, Lucena MI, Fernández MC, et al. Drug-induced liver injury: an analysis of 461 incidences submitted to the Spanish Registry over a 10-year period. *Gastroenterology.* 2005; (in press).
9. Bissel DM, Gores GJ, Laskin DL, Hoofnagle JH. Drug-induced liver injury: mechanisms and test systems. *Hepatology.* 2001;33:1009-1013.
10. Lee WM. Drug-induced hepatotoxicity. *N Engl J Med.* 2003;349:474-485.
11. Aithal PG, Ramsey L, Daly AK, et al. Hepatic adducts, circulating antibodies, and cytokine polymorphisms in patients with diclofenac hepatotoxicity. *Hepatology.* 2004; 39(5):1430-1440.
12. Bohan A, Boyer JL. Mechanism of hepatic transporter of drug: implications for cholestatic drug reactions. *Semin Liver Dis.* 2002;22:123-136.
13. Jacquemin E, Cresteil D, Manouvrier S, Bout O, Hadchouel M. Heterozygous non-sense mutation of the MDR3 gene in familial intrahepatic cholestasis of pregnancy. *Lancet.* 1999;353:210-211.
14. Farrell GC. *Drug induced liver disease.* London: Churchill-Livingstone; 1994.
15. Bénichou C. Report of an International Consensus Meeting. Criteria of drug-induced liver disorders. *J Hepatol.* 1990;11:272-6.
16. Larrey D. Epidemiology and individual susceptibility to adverse drug reactions affecting the liver. *Semin Liver Dis.* 2002;22:145-155.
17. Huang YS, Chern HD, Su WJ, et al. Polymorphism of the N-acetyltransferase 2 gene as a susceptibility risk factor for antituberculosis drug-induced hepatitis. *Hepatology.* 2002;35:883-889.
18. Andrade RJ, Lucena MI, Alonso A et al. HLA class II genotype influences the type of liver injury in drug-induced idiosyncratic liver disease. *Hepatology.* 2004;39(6):1603-1612.
19. Reidenberg M. Drugs and the liver. *Br J Clin Pharmacol.* 1998;46:351-359.
20. Stedman C. Herbal hepatotoxicity. *Semin Liver Dis.* 2002;22:195-206.
21. Thummel KE, Slattery JT, Ro H et al. Ethanol and production of the hepatotoxic metabolite of acetaminophen in healthy adults. *Clin Pharmacol Ther.* 2000;67:591-599.
22. Schmidt LE, Dalhoff K, Poulsen HE. Acute versus chronic alcohol consumption in acetaminophen-induced hepatotoxicity. *Hepatology.* 2002;35:876-882.
23. George J, Murray K, Byth K, Farrell GC. Differential alterations of cytochrome P450 proteins in livers of patients with severe chronic liver disease. *Hepatology.* 1995; 21:120-128.
24. Chalasani N, Aljadhey H, Kesterton J, et al. Patients with elevated liver enzymes are not at a higher risk for statin hepatotoxicity. *Gastroenterology.* 2004;126(5):1287-92.
25. Biour M, Poupon R, Grangé J-D, Chazouilleres O. Hépatotoxicité des médicaments. 13e mise á jour du fichier bibliographique des atteintes hépatiques et des médicaments reponsables. *Gastroenterol Clin Biol.* 2000;24:1052-1091. In French
26. Degott C, Feldmann G, Larrey D et al. Drug-induced prolonged cholestasis in adults: a histological semiquantitative study demonstrating progressive ductopenia. *Hepatology.* 1992;15:244-251.

27. Aithal PG, Day CP. The natural history of histologically proved drug induced liver disease. *Gut.* 1999;44:731-735.
28. Danan G, Bénichou C. Causality assessment of adverse reactions to drugs I. A novel method based on the conclusions of international consensus meetings: application to drug-induced liver injuries. *J Clin Epidemiol.* 1993;46:323-1330.
29. Benichou C, Danan G, Flahault A. Causality assessment of adverse reactions to drugs. II. An original model for validation of drug causality assessment methods: case reports with positive rechallenge. *J Clin Epidemiol.* 1993;46:1331-1336.
30. Maria V, Victorino R. Development and validation of a clinical scale for the diagnosis of drug-induced hepatitis. *Hepatology.* 1997;26:664-669.
31. Lucena MI, Camargo R, Andrade RJ, Perez-Sanchez C, Sanchez de la Cuesta F. Comparison of two clinical scales for causality assessment in hepatotoxicity. *Hepatology.* 2001;33:123-130.
32. Kaplowitz N. Causality assessment versus guilt-by-association in drug hepatotoxicity. *Hepatology.* 2001;33:308-310.
33. Bakke OM, Manocchia M, De Abajo F et al. Drug safety discontinuations in the United Kingdom, the United States, and Spain from 1974 through 1993: a regulatory perspective. *Clin Pharmacol Ther.* 1995;58:108-117.
34. Kaplowitz N. Drug-induced liver disorders: implications for drug development and regulation. *Drug Saf.* 2001;24:483-490.
35. Shah RR. Drug-induced hepatotoxicity: Pharmacokinetic perspectives and strategies for risk reduction. *Adverse Drug React Toxicol Rev.* 1999;18:181-233.

Index